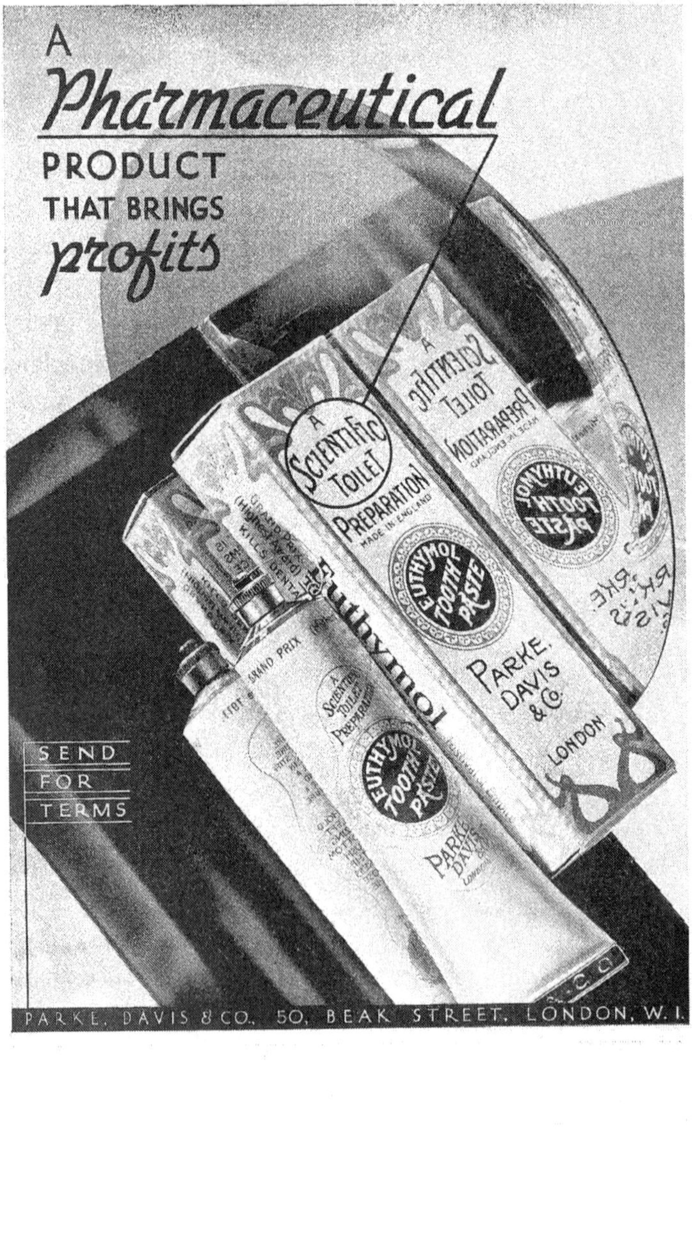
A
Pharmaceutical
PRODUCT
THAT BRINGS
profits
A
SCIENTIFIC
TOILET
PREPARATION
MADE IN ENGLAND
EUTHYMOL
TOOTH
PASTE
PARKE,
DAVIS
& Co.
LONDON
SEND
FOR
TERMS
PARKE, DAVIS & CO., 50, BEAK STREET, LONDON, W. I.

A A

INDEX TO ADVERTISERS

[Continued overleaf.

INDEX—cont.

For Bigger Profits invest in BEECHAM PRODUCTS

BEECHAMS PILLS
BRAND

BEECHAMS POWDERS
BRAND

BEECHAMS
BRAND
LUNG SYRUP

LACTOPEPTINE
BRAND

THE Chemist who is considering the best lines in which to invest his capital is reminded that the Beecham Products are by far the best paying propositions to handle. To begin with the efficacy of Beechams Brand Pills, Beechams Brand Powders, Beechams Brand Lung Syrup and Lactopeptine Brand has placed these products in millions of homes. Secondly, extensive consistent and "telling" advertising is appearing in all the foremost National and Provincial Newspapers. Thirdly, everybody can afford the Beecham Products.

The faith of the Public in Beecham Products is reflected in ever-increasing sales. They are known and bought the world over. A generous margin of profit and no dead stock, make these four lines a particularly attractive proposition.

Keep the Beecham Products before the public and you will reap your reward in bigger profits. A postcard will bring you free display material.

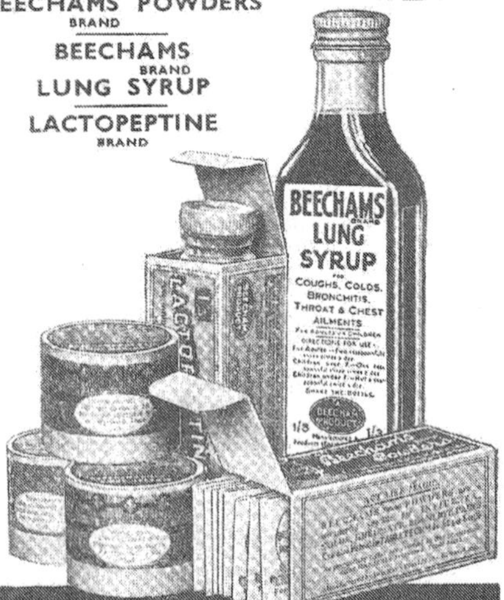

BEECHAMS PILLS LTD.

ST. HELENS. LANCASHIRE.

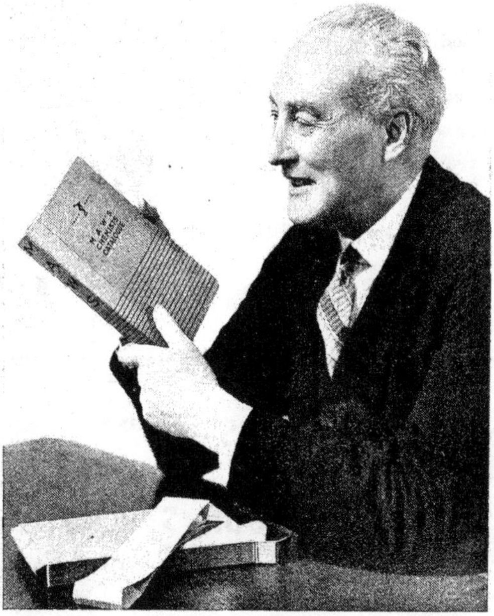

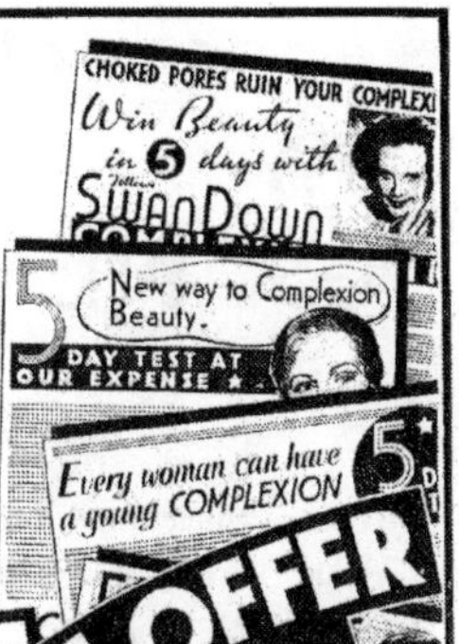
CHOKED PORES RUIN YOUR COMPLEXI
Win Beauty in 5 days with
SwanDown
New way to Complexion Beauty.
5 DAY TEST AT OUR EXPENSE
Every woman can have a young COMPLEXION
BONUS OFFER 13 to doz.

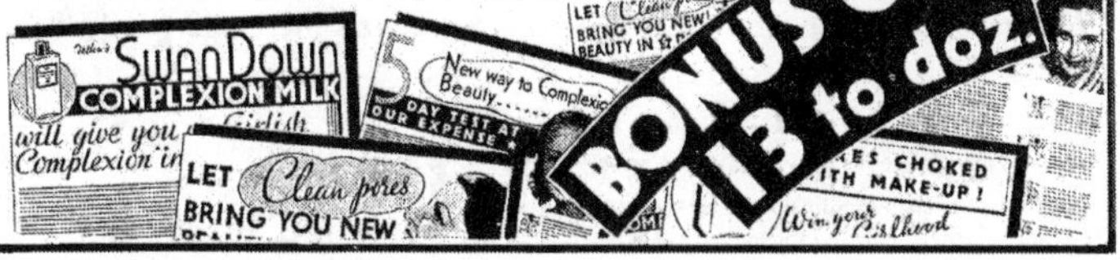
SwanDown COMPLEXION MILK
will give you
Complexion in
New way to Complexion Beauty
DAY TEST AT OUR EXPENSE
LET Clean pores BRING YOU NEW
ES CHOKED
ITH MAKE-UP!

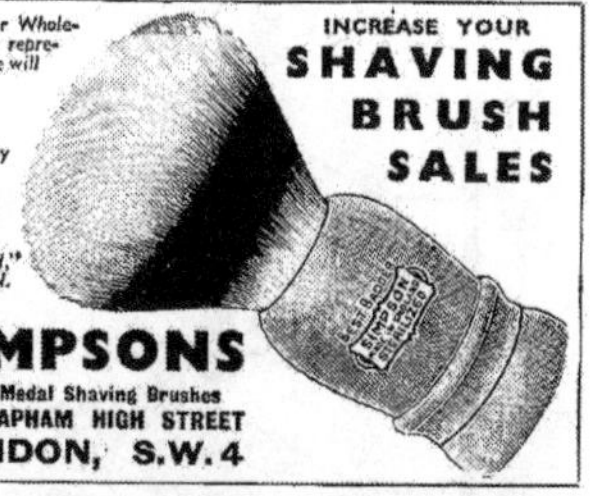

Summer Lines of High Repute

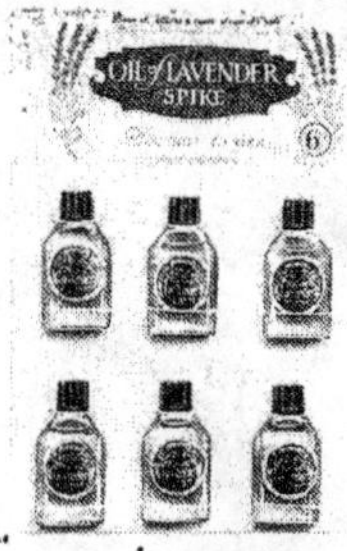

Oil of Lavender Spike
6d. bottles (½ doz. on card) 4/- per doz.
Smartest pack on the market.

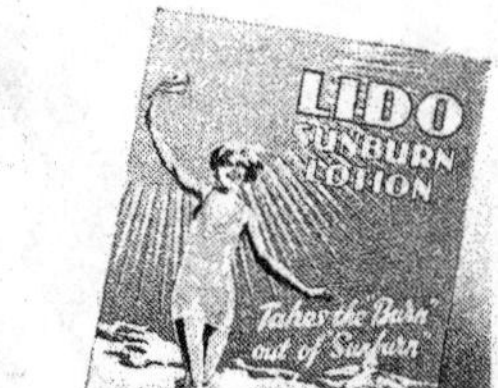

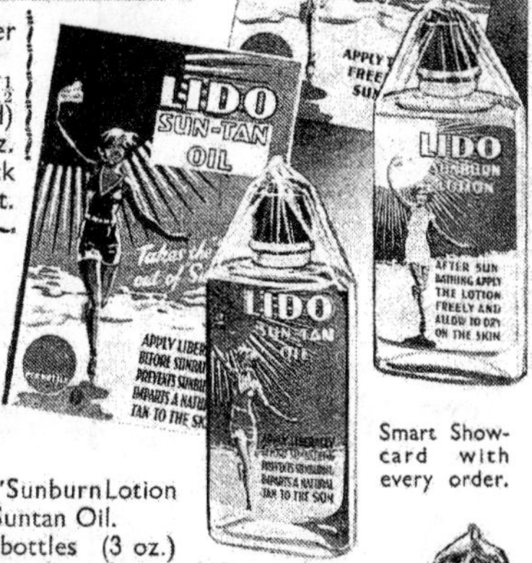

"Lido" Sunburn Lotion and Suntan Oil.
6d. bottles (3 oz.) 3/9 per doz., 3 doz. 3/6 per doz.
10½d. bottles (6 oz.) 6/6 per doz., 3 doz. 7/- per doz.

Smart Show-card with every order.

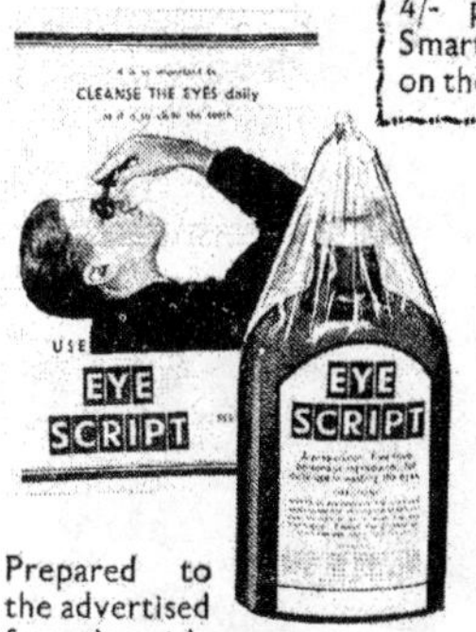

Prepared to the advertised formula, with a very

SPECIAL APPEAL TO MOTORISTS

8d. bottles, 4/6 per doz.
1/- bottles, 8/- per doz.
Showcard as illustrated with every order.

Midge Bite Lotion.
Cures and prevents bites, and stings of Midges, etc.
6d. bottles (3oz.) 3/9 doz.
1/- bottles (6 oz.) 6/6 doz.
Bulk 2/- lb. W.Qt. 1/10 lb.

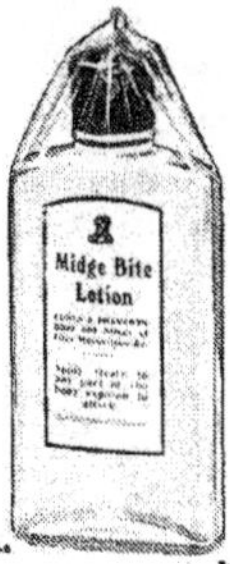

POTTER & CLARKE LTD.

60-64 ARTILLERY LANE, LONDON, E.1
PHONE: BISHOPSGATE 4761 (5 LINES)
GRAMS: "HOREHOUND, PHONE, LONDON"

77 DANTZIC ST., MANCHESTER 4
PHONE: BLACKFRIARS 8734
GRAMS: "HOREHOUND MANCHESTER"

B B

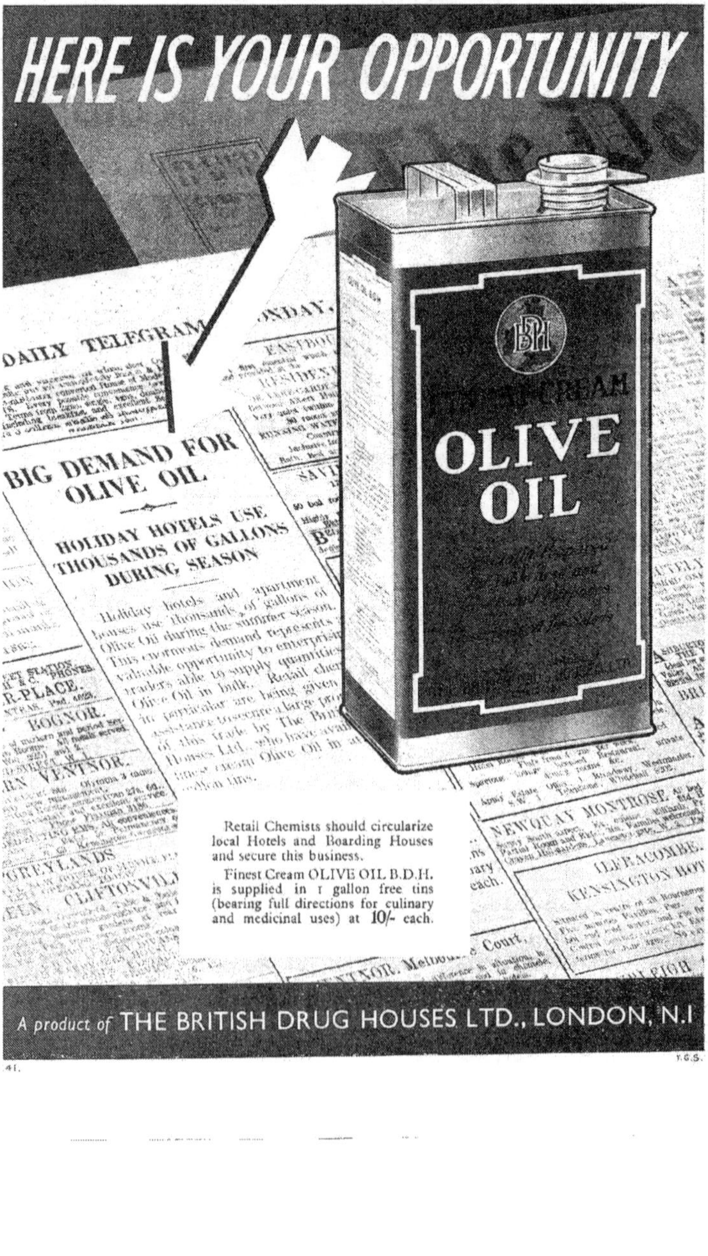
HERE IS YOUR OPPORTUNITY
DAILY TELEGRAM
BIG DEMAND FOR OLIVE OIL
HOLIDAY HOTELS USE THOUSANDS OF GALLONS DURING SEASON

Holiday hotels and apartment houses use thousands of gallons of Olive Oil during the summer season. This enormous demand represents a valuable opportunity to enterprising traders able to supply quantities of Olive Oil in bulk. Retail chemists in particular are being given every assistance to secure a large proportion of this trade by The British Drug Houses Ltd., who have available Finest Cream Olive Oil in attractive tins.

OLIVE OIL
Retail Chemists should circularize local Hotels and Boarding Houses and secure this business.
Finest Cream OLIVE OIL B.D.H. is supplied in 1 gallon free tins (bearing full directions for culinary and medicinal uses) at 10/- each.
A product of THE BRITISH DRUG HOUSES LTD., LONDON, N.1

41. F.G.S.

The
CHEMIST AND DRUGGIST

The Business Newspaper for all Sections of the Drug, Pharmaceutical, Chemical, Cosmetic, Perfumery and Associated Industries

The official organ of The Pharmaceutical Society of Ireland, The Pharmaceutical Society of Northern Ireland, The Chemists' and Druggists' Society of Ireland, and of other Chemists' Societies in Overseas Dominions

Published Weekly at

28 ESSEX STREET, STRAND, LONDON, W.C.2

Telegrams : "Chemicus, Estrand, London" *Telephone : Central 6565 (10 lines)*

BRANCH OFFICES

4 CANNON STREET, MANCHESTER (TEL.: BLACKFRIARS 3052)
54 FOSTER'S BUILDINGS, HIGH STREET, SHEFFIELD (TEL.: 22458)
19 WATERLOO STREET, GLASGOW (TEL.: CENTRAL 2329)
111 NEW STREET, BIRMINGHAM (TEL.: MIDLAND 2921)

372 FLINDERS LANE, MELBOURNE, AUSTRALIA
550 SHORTLAND STREET, AUCKLAND, NEW ZEALAND
155 AVENUE DE WAGRAM, PARIS, XVII[e] (TEL.: ETOILE 19-79)
PLANTAGE FRANSCHELAAN 32 AMSTERDAM-C. HOLLAND

VOL. 125. NO. 2943 JULY 4, 1936

CONTENTS

News of the Week

Key Industry Exemption—Kryofin

The Treasury have made an Order under Section 10 (5) of the Finance Act, 1926, exempting Kryofin from Key Industry Duty from July 3, 1936, until August 19, 1936.

Import Duties Advisory Committee Notice

The Import Duties Advisory Committee give notice of the following applications:—For an increase in the import duties on: (i) Celluloid in sheets, rods or tubes not manufactured beyond the stage of polishing; (ii) endless band knives.

Trade Agreement with Denmark

The Stationery Office has published in the form of a pamphlet particulars of the Trade Agreement between Denmark and this country, supplementary to the Agreement of April 24, 1933, relating to trade and commerce (with Protocol and exchange of Notes), copies of which are now available at the Stationery Office, Kingsway, London, W.C.2, price 2d.

Dangerous Drugs Acts, 1920-32

(From "The London Gazette," June 30, 1936)

(EDWARD INGLEDEW MCGREGOR)

Whereas Edward Ingledew McGregor, M.R.C.V.S., of 3 Cumberland Road, St. Albans, Hertfordshire, has been convicted of offences against the Dangerous Drugs Acts:

And whereas the said Edward Ingledew McGregor cannot, in my opinion, properly be allowed to be in possession of or to supply any of the drugs or preparations to which Part III of the Dangerous Drugs Act, 1920, applies:

Now, therefore, in pursuance of the powers conferred on me by Regulation 6 of the Raw Opium Regulations, 1921, as extended by the Coca Leaves and Indian Hemp Regulations, 1928, and by Regulation 7 of the Dangerous Drugs (Consolidation) Regulations, 1928, I hereby give notice that I withdraw, as from to-day's date, from the said Edward Ingledew McGregor the authority granted by the said Regulations to registered veterinary surgeons to be in possession of and to supply raw opium, coca leaves and Indian hemp and the drugs and preparations to which Part III of the Dangerous Drugs Act, 1920, applies:

And I also direct, as from the same date, that it shall not be lawful for the said Edward Ingledew McGregor to give prescriptions for the purposes of the Dangerous Drugs (Consolidation) Regulations, 1928.

JOHN SIMON,
One of His Majesty's Principal
Secretaries of State.

Whitehall, June 9, 1936.

Grocers and the Chemists' Friends Scheme

At the forty-sixth annual Conference of the National Federation of Grocers' and Provision Dealers' Associations at Southport, on June 23, the president (Councillor A. Cocker) said: "In his presidential address last year Alderman Cobbin made reference to the dictatorial plan of the Retail Trading Standards Association. . . . Now the National Pharmaceutical Union has essayed to dictate to manufacturers of nationally advertised proprietary articles as to what body of traders they may supply. It was a serious attack upon retailers in general, and grocers in particular, who have for many years sold certain articles common to them and to chemists. From the first the Federation boldly met this challenge, which came badly from chemists who live in a glass house of Crystal Palace dimensions in respect of encroachment upon other trades, and the Chemists' Friends scheme is already doomed to failure. We took off our coats to fight this battle, the seriousness of which is shown by the fact that the N.P.U., among other audacious proposals, sought to oblige manufacturers to accept the following limitations upon their relations with traders other than chemists: No window-display material or bonuses for window displays or advertising material; no payment of patent-medicine licences or the equivalent in goods or bonuses of any kind; the words 'Get it at your chemist' to be put at the foot of all advertisements with no reference to other traders. It is pleasing to note that the majority of manufacturers have declined to admit that the N.P.U. Executive are entitled to dictate to them as to how they shall sell their goods, and that the Proprietary Association of Great Britain recommends its members to refrain from joining the Chemists' Friends scheme We thank the manufacturers for their action, and assure them of the full support of this Federation."

A German Tour

On June 7 a party of South-East London pharmacists with their ladies left London for the first organised tour of manufacturing houses in Germany. The party numbered twenty-five. From Cologne the party was collected by a motor coach sent by Bayer Products, Ltd., to convey the visitors to the I.-G. Werk, Leverkusen, where they were received by Dr. Bernhardt (head of the English-speaking departments). In the lecture theatre an outline of the company's organisation, development and activities was given by Dr. Linden, after which the party was taken in appropriate groups to inspect the factory and packing rooms. Everything was laid open for the inspection of the visitors, who were invited to make any inquiry they wished. Points appreciated by the English pharmacists were the scrupulous cleanliness observed and the meticulous care taken to prevent error. Twenty or more girls, each packing ampoules, were singing at their work—a sign of contentment. Luncheon was taken in the Kasino, followed by a brief speech of thanks by Mr. Cecil H. Foster, (president of the S.-E. Metropolitan Branch of the Pharmaceutical Society). Mr. E. Oswald Wells (secretary) also spoke. In the afternoon a cinematograph film entitled "Solar Energy," dealing with departments of the Bayer concern which it had been impossible

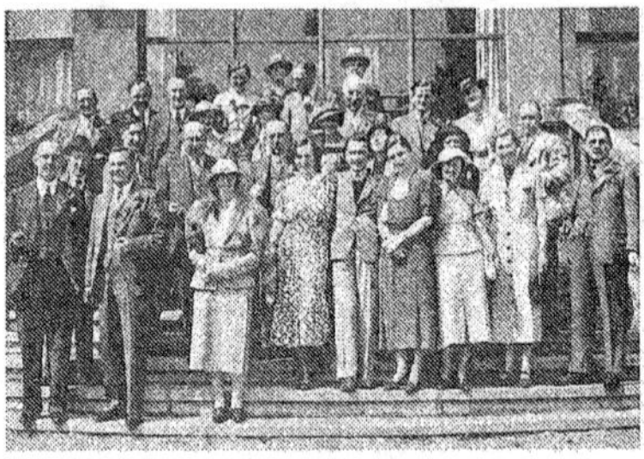

to see, and a humorous film, "The Three Cavaliers," upon the product Cafaspin, were shown, both films being English "talkies." Before leaving, a sheaf of white lilies was laid on the tomb of Carl Duisberg, the "father of the house," by Mrs. Happold. In the evening Dr. Bernhardt, Dr. Linden, Mr. Kratsch and Fräulein Gressler, representing Messrs. Bayer, were guests of the English party to dinner at the Hotel Reichshof, Cologne. The next day the South-Easterners were taken for a conducted tour of Cologne as the guests of "4711" (on arrival at Cologne each lady had been presented with a bottle of 4711 eau de Cologne). In the afternoon a trip by Rhine river steamer was made to Coblenz, and a visit was paid to the Coblenz Wine Garden. On June 12 Zeiss Ikon, Ltd., were hosts of the party at their Dresden factory, Herr Direktor Jurgens officiating. The visitors had the exceptional opportunity of seeing an ordinary working day in a German factory. Everywhere thoroughness and care were the rule. Luncheon was taken at the Hotel Luisenhof, situated high above the Elbe and commanding a wonderful view of the surrounding country. On June 13 the party journeyed to Berlin by the "Berlin Flyer." A conducted tour of Berlin and its environs and an excursion to the Berlin night clubs kept the party occupied until 3 30 on Sunday morning. Later in the day a visit was paid to Potsdam and the Royal Palaces. The party returned to London on June 16.

Inquests

At Battersea, London, S.W., on June 30, an inquiry was held concerning the death of Dr. J. C. Davies, a medical officer at Tooting Bec Hospital, who, the evidence showed, died after taking luminal, 66 gr. of which was found in certain organs of the body. Mr. J. H. Ryffel, Home Office analyst, stated in evidence that a fatal dose of this substance was 20 gr. Sir Bernard Spilsbury's report indicated luminal poisoning as the cause of death. The coroner recorded an open verdict.

At Birmingham, on June 29, an inquest was held on the body of Miss Margaret A. Murphy, Stourbridge. Dr. Denis A. Murphy (brother) said his sister lived with him. For some years she had suffered from a mild form of rheumatism which caused swelling at the finger tips. He had treated her once or twice, and at the beginning of March this year he began to treat her with atoquinol. Sixteen days after beginning the treatment he stopped it, because he heard that there had been two deaths from this type of drug, and he also discovered that a liver-function test should be carried out before it was prescribed. The tablets did his sister good, and after treating her he had administered atoquinol to five patients, including a panel patient. He had given them the same dose as his sister, and had not had trouble with them. On discovering the nature of the drug, he told his sister to stop taking it. He subsequently discovered that while in France she had taken one tablet after lunch and dinner for five days, as she had been instructed when he prescribed them in the first place. Professor K. D. Wilkinson, Professor of Pharmacology at Birmingham University said the drugs in this (cinchophen) group were principally used in gout, but he did not believe it was justifiable to use them except in severe cases. "They relieve pain," added Professor Wilkinson, "and therefore have been used in the past for the treatment of rheumatism, but I do not recommend them. They are very dangerous indeed. This is the twelfth death I have seen from drugs in this group." Professor Wilkinson went on to say that atoquinol was a drug with a cumulative action. He used it only occasionally in very severe cases. The fact that the woman in this case had rather a small dose, and the fact that she was healthy apart from slight rheumatism, showed that the drug was extremely toxic. The Coroner: It is impossible for the public to get this drug except through a medical man?—Yes. The Coroner: This was a healthy woman, and even a hospital test might not have found anything wrong with her liver?—Yes, that is why I say it is a very dangerous drug. These regulations do not convey to the medical man how this drug ought to be used. They do not convey to the doctor the danger which may attend the use of this drug, and this applies to all varieties of the drug. Professor Haswell Wilson, Professor of Pathology at Birmingham University, who conducted the *post-mortem* examination, said his examination showed jaundice of the body. The liver was diminished to half its normal size and it had the appearances of acute yellow atrophy with some attempts at repair. A medical witness called by the representative of Ciba, Ltd., said he specialised in rheumatic diseases. He had been using atoquinol for about twelve years. It had been used in Germany since 1913. He agree with what Sir William Willcox had written about the drug in "The Lancet," that it was undoubtedly of value and could be used, but only following directions as to intermittency of doses and under constant supervision. The first symptom he looked for when using it was loss of appetite. Returning a verdict of "Death by misadventure," the Coroner said he hoped the firm would strengthen or modify their instructions to medical practitioners.

London

A dinner was held at the Restaurant Monico, London, on June 25, to commemorate the 125th anniversary of the foundation of R. Hovenden & Sons, Ltd., Berners Street, W., and City Road, E.C. Presentations were made to Mr. A. J. Carter (joint managing director) and two other members of the staff who had completed fifty years' service.

In Whitechapel County Court, London, on June 25, Mr. Joseph Mayson-Blackburn, manufacturing chemist, Farm Hill, Waltham Abbey, sued Mr. C. A. White, trading as the Jean Bennett Perfumery Co., Princelet Street, Stepney, to recover the sum of £31 3s. as balance due for goods supplied. There was a counterclaim for £40 15s for rent of a room which the plaintiff occupied at the defendant's factory, soap sold to the plaintiff, work done and materials supplied. Judge Lilley, giving judgment, said he believed the plaintiff as to the rent. There had apparently been a system of interchange of goods. He found that the defendant owed the plaintiff £14 19s. 2d, while the plaintiff owed the defendant £11 5s. 5d. in respect of work done, so he would enter judgment for the plaintiff for £3 13s. 9d., with costs, and would dismiss the counterclaim with costs.

Sheffield

Mr. E. Preston, Ph.C., has been elected to represent the Sheffield and District Branch of the Pharmaceutical Society on the court of governors of the Sheffield University.

The local public assistance committee's dispensing service is being taken over by the health committee of the Sheffield Corporation, and will be known as the Medical Service Committee. Chemists wishing to participate in this scheme should make written application to the local medical officer of health, Dr. Rennie.

A set of 300 botanical specimens collected in the Sheffield area and Derbyshire by Mr. Norman Goodyear, Ph.C. (a holder of the Pereria medal), has been presented to the Sheffield and District Branch of the Pharmaceutical Society. Mr. Goodyear, who is now in America, was apprenticed to the late Mr. G. T. W. Newsholme. The collection has been placed under the care of Mr. J. Austen, Ph C, at the local pharmaceutical library's headquarters, 27 High Street, Sheffield.

Miscellaneous

WINDOW ANNOUNCEMENT.—"The Ilkeston Pioneer" of June 26 quotes the following notice seen on the window of a pharmacy.—"This is a CHEMIST'S shop The staff is trained to handle drugs, etc. Grocery from the grocer, nails from the ironmonger, BUT Drugs, Chemicals, POISONS, from the Chemist." We understand that the pharmacy is that of A. A. Williamson, Ltd.

THE combined vacuum still and extraction apparatus illustrated was shown by Bennett, Sons & Shears, Ltd., chemical engineers, 9-13 George Street, London, W.1, at the British Chemical Plant Exhibition. This illustration arrived too late for inclusion with those on pp. 36, 37 of this issue.

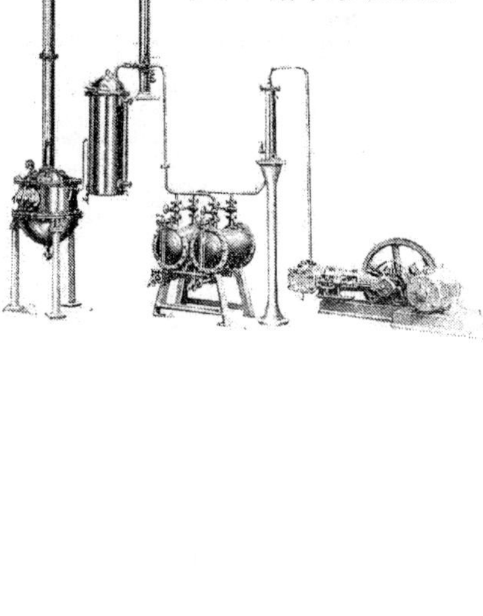

Irish Notes

Pharmaceutical Society of Ireland

The latest dates for making application for entrance to the July examinations of the Pharmaceutical Society of Ireland are Monday, July 6, for the Pharmaceutical Licence examination and Thursday, July 16 for the Pharmaceutical Assistants' examination.

Irish Drug Association

A Committee meeting of the Irish Drug Association was held on June 22, Mr. T. C. Scott (president) in the chair. A date was fixed for the holding of a meeting of the I.D.A. to conclude the agreement with the Chemists' Branch of the Irish Distributive Workers' Union, following which the agreement, which has been accepted by the Union, will become operative. Under this agreement the hours of opening for chemists in the Provinces will be determined by local arrangement. In the Greater Dublin district the hours of business for chemists and druggists will be as follows:—Monday to Friday, 9 a.m to 8 p.m. (instead of 9 a m. to 9 p.m., as at present); Saturdays, 9 a m. to 9 p m. (instead of 9 a.m. to 10 p.m.). On Sundays, shops will open from 11.15 a m. to 1.15 p.m. The new agreement (which applies to all parts of the Free State), while providing for local arrangements regarding hours, offers many concessions to assistants. Only one apprentice is to be allowed to each pharmaceutical chemist in retail trade. Unqualified assistants, after completing their apprenticeship, are to be paid 47s. 6d. per week the first year, rising by yearly increments to 70s. per week in the fourth year. Qualified assistants, if engaged as such, are to be paid 52s. 6d. per week in the first, 57s. 6d. in the second, 70s. in the third, 72s. 6d. in the fourth, and 75s. in the fifth years. Where qualified chemists are employed they are to be paid 67s. 6d. per week the first year, rising by increments to 87s. 6d. the fourth year. Registered druggists, if employed as such, will receive 52s. 6d. per week the first year, 72s. 6d. the fourth year and 82s. 6d. as managers. A bonus at the rate of 2s. 6d. to 7s 6d. per week, according to the turnover, is to be paid to qualified assistants acting as managers. *Locum tenentes* are to be employed for a period of two months or more, and are to be paid rates ranging from four guineas to five guineas per week. All employees are to be allowed 1½ hour for lunch and one hour for tea. Men will have a normal working week of 48 hours, and women of 44 hours. Women are to be paid a sum less by 7s. 6d per week than men in equivalent grades. Workers with twelve months' service will receive twelve working days' leave, with pay. Employees with six months' service will receive one day's leave for each month employed. A conciliation board, consisting of five representatives from each side, is to be set up to deal with all matters affecting each party in the trade; the agreement has been made without prejudice to workers who at present enjoy better conditions in the trade. The Committee have decided to have cards with the new hours printed and distributed to all chemists and druggists—both members and non-members—in the Dublin area. It is stated that the agreement will come into force on July 6. The Committee had complaints before them to the effect that a large number of preparations on the market in the Free State were being changed in pack or price, and sometimes both. In some cases old stocks were being allowed for, where retailers communicated with the agents. The Committee decided that if alterations in prices of preparations were carried out in future without proper adjustment in the interests of the retailers, action would be taken against the manufacturers concerned. A well-known and old-established Dublin firm notified that they had introduced a sheep dip to retail at 1s. 6d., the sales of which would be confined to chemists and druggists. The Committee appreciated the action, and decided to ask their members to support this firm.

Brevities

Mr. Edward Cahill, Ph.C, who is retiring from business, is disposing, by auction, of his Medical Hall at Leeson Street Bridge, Dublin.

The Governor of Northern Ireland has made an Order entitled the Petroleum (Compressed Gases) Order (Northern Ireland), 1936, applying certain provisions of the Petroleum Consolidation Act (1929), to the following gases when compressed in any metal cylinder: air, argon, carbon monoxide, coal gas, hydrogen, methane, neon, nitrogen, oxygen.

Scottish Notes

Brevities

Mr. Allan Morton, chemist and druggist, Rutherglen, who celebrated his silver wedding this week, is well known in the eastern districts of Glasgow and a prominent figure in Scottish Masonic circles.

Mr. William Cumming, chemist and druggist, was a member of a party of bowlers who spoke at the microphone during the broadcast of a midnight bowling match at Thurso. Mr. Cumming led the "Incomers" with a score of eighteen shots.

Twenty-one members of the Edinburgh Chemists' Golf Club took part in a competition played over Dalmahoy East Course on June 17, with the following results: (1) W. J. Rosie 80, (2) R. S. Harvey 82, (3) A. M Edmonds 83. Second class, J. A. Darroch 91.

The Edinburgh Chemists' Assistants' and Apprentices' Association's fourth botanical excursion of the summer session took place to Balerno on June 19, under the leadership of Mr. H. R. Dootson. A large and enthusiastic company attended and many moorland and woodland plants were collected and fully explained by Mr. Dootson.

The general council of St. Andrews University unanimously approved, on June 27, a draft ordinance for the institution of degrees and diplomas in dental surgery. The degrees will be Bachelor of Dental Surgery (B D S.) and Master of Dental Surgery (M.D.S.). It is claimed that St Andrews will now become the leading university in Scotland for dental education.

Mr. James Shields, for sixteen years a member of the Renfrew County Pharmaceutical Committee, was presented, at the Picture House Café, Renfrew, on June 26, with an eight-day boudoir clock, upon the occasion of his taking up a position as an inspector for the Pharmaceutical Society. Mr. MacDonald, Renfrew (chairman), presided. Mr. Trant, in making the presentation, gave a brief *résumé* of Mr. Shield's work for the Committee. Afterwards, toasts of "Pharmaceutical Organisations," "The Checking Bureau" and "The County Pharmaceutical Committee" were proposed.

Mr. James Milne, Broughty Ferry, who recently celebrated his golden wedding, formerly carried on a chemist's business at Comers, Aberdeenshire, for over thirty years. He was a member of both the Comers parish council and the school board, and was for many years representative on the Deeside and district committee of the county council. In Dundee he and his eldest son conducted an aerated water business, and he became president of the Aerated Water Trade Association and a member of the Trade Board for Scotland. He served on the Dundee Parish Council, was latterly chairman of the district board of control, and when these bodies were dissolved was co-opted to the town council.

Glasgow and West of Scotland

A report by the chief constable of Glasgow on the number of shops open on Sundays reveals that on June 7 the total was 5,416, of which 278 were chemists' shops.

An appeal by Dr. John A. McCluskie, Glasgow, against a surcharge of £30 made on him by Glasgow Insurance Committee for excessive prescribing has been dismissed by a tribunal appointed to consider his appeal Dr. McCluskie submitted that his high cost was due to frequency.

At Glasgow, recently, Vita Products, Ltd., London, pleaded "Not guilty" to a summons for breach of warranty arising out of a case previously heard (*C. & D.*, May 2, p. 509). Evidence was given by Mr Thomas Cockburn, F.I.C., city analyst, Mr. A. F. Simpson, managing director of the defendant company, and by other persons. In a reserved judgment the stipendiary magistrate found the charge proved, but in view of the facts of the case decided to admonish the defendants.

Topical Reflections

By Xrayser

The Annual Special Issue

of The Chemist and Druggist is, as you remark on p. 725, a "special among specials." I have rarely, if ever, read a special issue which has been more interesting or which has contained a greater wealth of practical information on subjects of vital interest to pharmacists, be they retail, wholesale or manufacturing. It is not easy to give pride of place to any one contribution, but I have arrived at the conclusion that this should be awarded to the Cosmetic Harmony Chart (p. 729). This will be valuable as a guide for the chemist when advising the customer; that such a chart is needed is proved by the many examples one sees where the colours used for nails, lips and face do not blend harmoniously. Perhaps next in helpfulness to the chemist is the article on opening a surgical department (p. 765). Several British firms selling British-made instruments are prepared to give advice to those pharmacists who decide to go in for this side-line; fitting should be engaged in, however, only when the fitter has expert knowledge of the subject. The subject of colour photography, although a somewhat technical one, is very clearly dealt with, the illustrations making the different processes easy to understand. The historical articles indicate that much research must have been done before such readable contributions could be prepared.

The Article

on the first medicinal patents (p. 758) should appeal to pharmacists, if only to illustrate the ease, to our way of thinking, with which some of the patentees of the medicines in question "got away with it." Under nineteenth-century specifications I note three patents which have had a considerable influence on the progress of pharmacy—pearl coating, capsules and the first aniline dye. I am surprised that in the case of the first such a long time elapsed between the granting of the patent and the general use of the coating on pills As a patent remains in force for fourteen years, presumably anyone could pearl-coat pills in 1868; my recollection is that in the 'eighties very few firms indeed used this method of covering; one of my jobs as an apprentice was to fix up an attachment to the linseed-crushing machine which revolved a pill-coating canister There is a nineteenth-century patent which, in the later developments of the idea, has had a profound effect on the preparation of extracts, etc., *in vacuo*; I allude to J. T. Barry's Patent, No. 4376 (May, 1819), for "distillation, evaporation, and exsiccation." A modification of this was used by the patentee for the preparation of solid extracts, such as henbane, with the claim that they were stronger and more uniform than those made in an open vessel It was not until the early 'eighties that malt extract was made in a vacuum pan, another instance of the length of time which sometimes elapses between the granting of the patent and its general application.

I Was One of Those

who journeyed to Bournemouth to take part in the meeting of the British Pharmaceutical Conference (p. 717). The weather was brilliant throughout, and it was only an hour before the Friday excursion started from Lulworth to return to Bournemouth that rain somewhat marred the enjoyment of the large company who took advantage of the whole-day trip through the Hardy country. I did not hear Mr. Harold Deane's Conference address, although I was not far from the platform This was due to the peculiar acoustics of the building and also to the fact that the microphone provided was not accurately placed. Topics of far-reaching importance were discussed at the meetings of representatives. The Conference will long be remembered for its social amenities and for the delightful setting. The calm summer sea and the illuminated pier seen from the windows of the ball-room, the well-organised functions and the hospitality of the Mayor and Corporation all went to make up a week that will live in the memory. There was ample proof of most efficient organisation on the part of the hard-working secretary and his Committee.

Legal Reports

Claims for Personal Injuries.—In the King's Bench Court, Belfast, on June 23, Mr. W. J. Heatrick, Cliftonville Road, was sued by Mrs. Martha Poots for damages for personal injuries and loss sustained by the plaintiff by reason of the alleged negligence of the defendant or his workmen in the erection and control of premises the property of the defendant. The defendant denied negligence and pleaded that the plaintiff was guilty of contributory negligence. The plaintiff said she slipped and fell across the corner of a platform or concrete area at the defendant's premises and was seven weeks in a nursing home. The jury found for the defendant, and judgment was given accordingly. The judge concurred with the verdict.

In Oldham County Court, on June 25, Taylors (Cash Chemists), London, Ltd., were sued by Mr. and Mrs. Mitchell, Edith Street, for damages for alleged negligence at their pharmacy in King Street, Oldham. Mr. J. G. Rycroft, for the plaintiffs, said that if liability was established the agreed damages amounted to £100 He explained that on December 23 last Mrs. Mitchell visited the shop, and on that day it had been snowing. Mrs. Mitchell fell on the linoleum of the shop floor and fractured her left wrist in two places. Afterwards the manager had papers placed on the floor, and since the accident a mat had been provided at the entrance For the defence, counsel said that the shop floor was no more dangerous than any other floor, and the accident happened without negligence on the part of anyone. The judge said he could not see what the defendants ought to have done. He could not find negligence, and there would be judgment for the defendants.

Pharmacy Acts (Ireland).—In the Dublin District Court, on June 23, Mr. Dominic A. Dolan, Ph.C., 58 Bolton Street, was summoned at the instance of the Pharmaceutical Society of Ireland for breaches of the Pharmacy Act on various dates in February and March. Mr. John J Gaynor appeared on behalf of the Society, and Mr. E. H. Burne defended. On the first summons defendant was charged with having had a prescription compounded by an unqualified assistant. On March 5, it was stated, the defendant sold lysol by an unqualified person. In respect of March 12 a similar offence was alleged. On March 14 a summons was issued in respect of the sale of tablets containing ephedrine, a Part I poison, to a person unknown to the seller. On March 19 there was a further summons for selling lysol and dispensing a prescription, no qualified person being present. Mr. Burne, on behalf of the defendant, pleaded "Guilty" to all the summonses, and in extenuation said his client was a fully qualified chemist, and these sales had taken place in his absence Since the summonses were issued his client had secured a qualified assistant, who would always be in control when Mr. Dolan was absent at meals. Mr. Dolan had been twenty-six years in business, and had never had a prosecution brought against him before. Mr. Gaynor said the defendant had four assistants, none of whom was qualified to act in his absence. The justice said the Court held the case proved, but having regard to the excellent character of the defendant, and his long-standing business, he was not desirous of convicting. On the defendant undertaking to pay the Society £10 10s expenses in connection with the summonses, and £5 5s. costs, he would dismiss all the charges under the Probation Act.

New Companies
and Company News

P.C. means Private Company and R.O. Registered Office

Hughes & Hughes, Ltd. (P.C.).—Capital £5,000. Objects To acquire the business of a chemical and colour merchant formerly carried on by the late Albert Hughes at London House, Crutched Friars, E.C., as "Hughes & Hughes."

Marshalls Malted Milk, Ltd. (P C).—Capital £10,000 Objects: To carry on the business of manufacturers of and dealers in milk powders, malted milk, etc. The first directors are not named. Solicitors: Billinghurst, Wood & Pope, 7 Bucklersbury, E.C.4.

Modern Chemists, Ltd. (P.C.).—Capital £500. Objects: To carry on the business of chemists, druggists, etc. R.O : 231 Westminster Bridge Road, S.E.1.

Davis (Bognor Regis), Ltd. (P.C.).—Capital £2,000. Objects: To carry on the business of chemists and druggists, etc. Charles P. C. Sargent, "Chudleigh," Aldwick Road, Bognor, director.

Oxygenaire, Ltd. (P.C.).—Capital £2,000 Objects: To acquire the business of oxygen therapy equipment sales and rentals now carried on at Chapel Road, Southampton, and at 10A Harrow Road, W.2 John Chilvers, 10A Harrow Road, W.2, managing director

---

Hugh Moore & Alexanders, Ltd.—Report for year ended March 31, 1936, states profit, after charging bad debts, repairs, etc., and income tax, was £1,276 (against £1,897). After adding £2,333, the balance brought forward from previous year, and deducting £1,589 for depreciation and directors' fees, there remains £2,019 to be carried forward. It is not proposed at present to fill the vacancy on the board following the death of the late Mr. J. F. Donagh.

British Glues & Chemicals, Ltd.—As announced recently, this company are resuming ordinary dividend payments after a lapse of five years with a distribution of 7½ per cent., while the preference shares receive a participation of ½ per cent. Accounts show that profits for year to April 30 improved by £15,370, to £86,841, present figure being after writing off cost of goodwill of businesses acquired during year and placing £15,000 to contingencies reserve. Sum of £5,000 allocated to income tax (last year £5,000 taken from tax reserve) and £20,000 (against *nil*) to general reserve, carry-forward being £35,307 (against £36,217), after writing £5,000 off machinery and plant in addition to usual depreciation. A year ago a surplus of £11,044 on sale of investments and £13,716 taken from contingencies reserve were applied in writing down fixed assets and shares in a subsidiary.

Sangers, Ltd.—Net profits showed further expansion in the year ended March 31 last, being £188,723, against £156,370 for 1934-35, the latter figure including a profit on realisation of investments. A provision of £42,683 (against £37,693) is made for income tax, and a final dividend of 16¼ per cent. (against 13¾ per cent.) is proposed on the ordinary shares, making 25 per cent. for the year (against 22½ per cent.), while the balance forward is raised from £80,896 to £100,338. In the balance sheet investments in subsidiaries stand at £961,593, and amounts due from those companies at £181,706, against which there is shown a small amount of £4,412 owing to subsidiaries. Stock, debtors, general investments, and cash total £493,669, against creditors of £320,970. The capital reserve remains at £432,204. In April last 142,000 ordinary 5s. shares were issued at 22s. 6d. each, and the effect of the issue will be shown in the next accounts. It is now proposed to increase the authorised capital by a further 400,000 5s. ordinary shares, the directors considering that this additional reserve capital should be available for issue should any further development arise. Meeting, July 8

Business Changes

Mr. H. M Gardner, chemist and druggist, has opened a pharmacy at 68 High Street, Ramsgate.

Mr W. K. Cooke, chemist and druggist, has taken over the business of Mr. F. Bradbury, chemist and druggist, 273 Lytham Road, Blackpool.

Owing to the expiration of the lease, the business (including prescription-books and private formulas) of the late Mr. Edwin Dawber, chemist and druggist, 15 Hill Road, Wimbledon, has been transferred to Mr. Harry S. Fenton, chemist and druggist, 14 Worple Road, Wimbledon, London, S.W.19.

The partnership subsisting between Mr. J. W. Cox, chemist and druggist, and Mr. B. W. Heaton, chemist and druggist, 1164 Warwick Road, Acocks Green, Birmingham, has been dissolved by mutual consent as from June 8. The business will be continued at the same address by Mr. Heaton

Pharmaceutical Society of Great Britain

Council Meeting

THERE was little discussion at the July meeting of the Council, held at 16 Bloomsbury Square, London, W C 1, on July 1, but among the matters which came up was whether pharmacists should require the payment of a premium from apprentices. It was introduced by Mr. Rowsell, who in moving the adoption of the report of the Education Committee stated that they had considered a letter from the Halifax and District Branch of the Society in which comments were invited upon a resolution under consideration by the branch in the following terms:—"That a minimum premium of £50 in respect of each new apprentice to pharmacy be demanded." The Committee had decided that they could not see their way to recommend that the proposal should be incorporated in the regulations. Mr. Rowsell said that while some pharmacists now insisted on the payment of a premium, there were others who paid their apprentices. He felt that it was a mater, however, to which chemists throughout the country might very well give attention. No further opinion was expressed on the subject, and the Council contented themselves with adopting the Committee's report.

Tuesday's Proceedings

Among the business transacted by the Council at the meeting on June 30 were the following items:—

As Mr. Rutherford Hill would be unable to be present at the Council meeting on Wednesday, the president took that opportunity of expressing to Mr. Hill the congratulations of the Council and of the Society upon the conferment on him of the distinction of Officer of the Order of the British Empire. Mr. Hill, replying, said he had to thank the president and members of Council for their very kind reference and congratulations. He appreciated the honour very highly indeed, and particularly rejoiced in the thought that it was a recognition of the craft of pharmacy. For more than 50 years he had had the honour and privilege of serving as an officer of the Society. During that time he had been able to observe the steady progress of the craft.

The Council considered the statement made by the Chancellor of the Exchequer in the House of Commons on June 25 that he proposed to move for the appointment of a Select Committee to examine the law relating to medicine stamp duty and to recommend what changes appear to be desirable. A committee consisting of the president, the vice-president, Messrs. Rowsell, Melhuish and Neathercoat was appointed to consider what steps the Society might be called upon to take, and if necessary to consult with other pharmaceutical organisations.

Deaths

At the meeting on July 1 THE PRESIDENT (Mr. Thomas Marns) made appropriate reference to the deaths of Mr. Charles William Matthews and Mr. Henry George Mumford.

British Pharmaceutical Conference

THE PRESIDENT and several members of the Council spoke on a resolution expressing appreciation of the hospitality of the Bournemouth Corporation on the occasion of the recent Conference, and of the efforts of the local Committee who organised and carried through the arrangements. Special mention was made of Mr. Bilson, whose long and close association with the Council as well as the Society was recalled with gratification.

Registration Items

Four persons were elected as student-associates and thirteen were restored to the Registers. The registrar reported that several persons had been restored to the Registers on complying with the regulations. The Council approved of the removal from the Registers of the names of nine persons who had failed to pay the retention fee.

Mr. Henry Theodore Smith, Londonderry, residing at Wigan, was registered as a chemist and druggist.

Correspondence

Mr. John Keall wrote thanking the Council for having appointed him a member of the Codex Revision Committee, and said he was always ready to do anything he could for the welfare of pharmacists.

Mr. H. Skinner wrote thanking the Council for allowing the examination for the Fairchild scholarship and prizes to be held at the headquarters in Bloomsbury Square.

Organisation Committee

The Organisation Committee reported that Dr. C. H. Hampshire has accepted an invitation to deliver an address on the British Pharmacopœia Addendum at the next session. The Committee had asked the secretary if he would occupy one of the evenings with a survey of pharmaceutical policy during the immediate future, and he had agreed to do so.

MR. WELLS, in moving the adoption of the Committee's report, referred to the long and distinguished service which Mr. Neathercoat had rendered to the Committee.

Benevolent Fund Committee

The report of this Committee stated that eighteen applications had been considered and grants had been made or were now recommended ranging from £10 to £50. The Committee's report on the last three months' work showed that forty-six grants had been made involving the payment of a total sum of £976.

MR. ANTCLIFFE drew attention to a number of unusual special contributions, including a legacy of £1,000 from the late Mr. P. H. Galloway, £50 from Mr. W. H. Quarrell (the Council's solicitor), and £10 10s. from the Colchester and District Branch.

War Auxiliary Benevolent Fund

The report submitted by the War Auxiliary Benevolent Fund Committee stated that nine applications had been considered and grants made or now recommended ranged from £26 to £240. The Committee's quarterly report showed that fifteen grants had been made amounting to £394.

Establishment Committee

The Committee reported that they had appointed a subcommittee to consider the applications for the Ransom fellowship 1936-38 and Rammell studentship 1936-37, and to make recommendations to the Committee.

The Committee, having considered various matters arising from Mr. Rutherford Hill's retirement, recommended that it should take effect as from October 1, 1936. They also recommended that Dr. J. Tait be appointed resident secretary for Scotland, the appointment to take effect from October 1, 1936.

The president reported that the chairman and he had interviewed five applicants for the post of additional pharmacist to the staff, and recommended the appointment of Dr. Thomas Dewar for the position The recommendation was adopted.

Education Committee

The report of the Education Committee, presented by MR. ROWSELL, compared the expenses to date with the figures included in the estimates for 1936 under the headings "Examinations" and "Miscellaneous." The Committee was satisfied that the expenditure was within those estimates.

The Committee also considered the report of the meeting of the representative body of teachers in schools of pharmacy.

Finance Committee

The financial statement showed that receipts since the last meeting, including a balance of £1 13s. 8d., amounted to £18,855 2s. 8d, comprising the following items:—Retention fees, £211 1s.; premises fees, £159 12s.; subscriptions, £7 17s. 6d; College—Pharmacological Laboratories, £462 5s; registration fees, £54 12s.; restoration fees, £66 13s. 6d.; examination fees, £15,227 2s.; penalties and expenses, £22 11s.; interest, £6 4s. 2d · rentals, £45; "Pharmaceutical Journal," £1,531 12s. 7d.; Pharmaceutical Press, £405 8s. 8d.; Quarterly Journal, £13 8s; F S.S.U. contributions, £18 7s. 4d.; F.S.S.U.

transfer from S.S.S.S., £315 5s. 3d ; loan from premises fund, £300 ; sundries, £6 9s. Payments ordered at the last meeting amounted to £12,102 19s. 5d., and £6,750 had been transferred to deposit account, leaving a balance of £2 3s 3d. The balances on the other accounts were:—Benevolent Fund (current account), £23 13s. 4d.; Benevolent Fund (donation account), £75 14s. 7d.; War Auxiliary Benevolent Fund, £259 12s. 6d.; Hills Orphan Fund, £29 5s. 10d.; Orphan Fund, £27 2s. 8d. Accounts amounting to £10,831 6s. 3d. were passed for payment, and the action of the secretary in making payments amounting to £1,521 12s. 2d. was approved.

Law Committee

The report of this Committee, presented by Mr. Beardsley, showed that in England and Wales 1,124 chemists' shops and 862 drug stores had been visited by the Society's inspectors and agents during the month, and that in Scotland since the last report sixty chemists' shops had been visited.

North British Executive

A meeting of the Executive of the North British Branch was held at 36 York Place, Edinburgh, on June 17, Mr. F. W. M. Bennett in the chair. The chairman referred to the sudden death of Mr. James Nesbit, Portobello. Certain points were raised under the Pharmacy and Poisons Act, 1933, and Poisons Rules. No definite reply had been received from the Home Office in regard to repeat prescriptions for Schedule IV poisons, but chemists had been advised, in the meantime, to treat prescriptions marked "To be repeated" as authorising indefinite repetition. It had been explained that nursing homes could be supplied with such poisons under the provisions of Section 20 (5) (a) on the ground of these substances being required for the trade or business carried on by the nursing home Nursing homes came under the provisions of Rules 27 and 28. It was explained that under Section 19 only prescriptions for Schedule I poisons required to be copied ; in the case of any medicine supplied by a chemist without a medical prescription, all such prescriptions ought to be copied if they contained Schedule I or other Part I poisons.

North British Branch Annual Meeting

The annual general meeting of the members of the Society in Scotland was held in Edinburgh on June 17, Mr. F. W. M. Bennett in the chair.

The chairman, in the course of his address, said that some ten years ago the Departmental Committee on Poisons was appointed, and at last the new legislation was in full operation. Perhaps the matter that had bulked most largely in the work of the Executive had been points relating to the Poisons List and Poisons Rules. A special memorandum had been forwarded to the Council, objecting to the needless increase of facilities for obtaining dangerous poisons through unqualified persons and stressing the principle that the training and qualification of the vendor were the only real means of securing public safety. The memorandum was well received by the Council ; although the defects objected to had not been rectified, a definite promise had been secured from the Home Office that it would insist on local authorities effectually enforcing the regulations applying to listed sellers. Some pharmacists has been removed from the Register owing to failure to pay the retention fee, and had consequently been in danger of being struck off the list of panel chemists. The seriousness of such failure was apparently only slowly being realised. The Executive had in process an inquiry, through the Society's divisional secretaries, as to the position of dispensing throughout Scotland and the arrangements for pharmaceutical service in hospitals and similar institutions. The Executive submitted an important memorandum to the Commission which they had reason to believe was favourably received and in which the advantage of having all public health pharmaceutical work done by duly qualified pharmacists, as provided for under the National Health Insurance scheme, was clearly pointed out. All five branches of the Society in Scotland had been active during the year The idea of holding joint meetings with doctors had again been carried out with very encouraging results. Contributions from Scotland to the Benevolent Fund remained on a rather low level, and members were advised to consider whether they could afford a more generous contribution to the Fund. Scottish demands on the Fund amounted to a larger sum than the Scottish contributions. Membership in Scotland now stood at 2,684, twenty-eight more than last year at the same date and a record number. There had been talk in some quarters of a Consolidation Act, bringing all the Pharmacy Acts into line and placing the whole profession in a clearly defined and worthy position. That was a work to which they might now address themselves with every hope that the original ideal of the Society could be attained, namely, that pharmacy as a distinct profession should have reserved to it the dispensing of medicines.

The resident secretary read the report of the scrutineers. Thirty-seven members had been nominated, of whom twenty signified their willingness to act if elected. Voting papers issued were 2,661 ; returned, 637 ; informal, 10 ; votes recorded, 627. (Names of elected candidates on p. 715 of the *C. & D.* Annual Special Issue.)

Mr. Hossack drew attention to the basis on which the dispensing fee was fixed for public pharmaceutical service, and thought the present system was not satisfactory. He suggested that a dispensing fee based on dosage would be more reasonable. The chairman declared that the present system could not readily be altered. On a motion by himself the matter was remitted to the Pharmaceutical Standing Committee (Scotland), and he thought they might safely leave the point to the Committee. Further discussion took place on this subject

Trade-Mark Applications

The figures in parentheses refer to the classes in which the marks are grouped. A list of classes and particulars as to registration are given in "The Chemist and Druggist Diary and Year-Book," 1936, p. 322.

(From "The Trade Marks Journal," June 10, 1936).

"Dolpholeum" ; for medicinal chemicals (3). By W. G. Kelynack, 83 Thornton Road, Thornton Heath, Surrey. 568,643.

"Rex-o-Lax" ; for laxatives (3). By The United Drug Co., Ltd , 29 Kirkwhite Street, Nottingham. 568,516. (Associated.)

"Pyralvex" ; for all goods (3). By Farmaceuticke Zavody "Norgine," Akc. Spol , Revolucni tr. 1, Prague 1, Czechoslovakia. 568,540.

"Premaline" ; for medicinal chemicals (3) By Société des Usines Chimiques, Rhone-Poulenc, S.A , 21 rue Jean Goujon, Paris (8), France 568,571.

"Dak" ; for photographic apparatus (8). By Kodak, Ltd , Kingsway, London, W.C 2 568,176. (Associated.)

Landscape with letters "XXXX" ("XXXX" disclaimed) ; for surgical goods (11). By J. Schmid, Inc., 423 West 55th Street, New York 563,529.

"Kleford" ; for clinical thermometers (11). By Shamsul Arfeen & Co , 9 Colootolah Street, Calcutta. 564,452.

"Alpha-Latex" ; for india-rubber bandages (11). By Société du Crepe Willot, 196 Boulevard Gambetta, Roubaix (Nord), France, 566,102.

Label design with crown and word "Caron" ("Caron" disclaimed) ; for perfumery, etc. (48) By E. Daltroff & Cie., 10 Rue de la Paix, Paris. 564,801.

"Tattoo" , for cosmetics and toilet articles (48). By Tattoo, Inc., 1 East Austin Street, Chicago, U.S.A. 559,721. (Associated)

"Cetiol" and "Lanedal" ; for cosmetics (48) By Deutsche Hydrierwerke A.-G , Kantstrasse 163, Berlin-Charlottenburg, Germany. 567,667/668.

Monogram in Circle , for perfumery, etc. (48). By J. Lewis & Co , Ltd , 277-288 Oxford Street, London, W.1. 568,107. (Associated.)

"Sanizal" ; for perfumery, etc. (48). By Newton, Chambers & Co , Ltd , Thorncliffe, Sheffield 568,517. (Associated)

(From "The Trade Marks Journal," June 17, 1936)

"Siscomate" ; for photographic chemicals, etc (1) By Sissons Bros & Co , Ltd , Bankside, Sculcoates, Hull 568,632. (Associated)

"Cuprodine" ; for iodine preparations containing copper compounds (3) By A. de St. Dalmas & Co , Ltd , Dalma Works, Junior Street, Leicester. 566,348. (Associated)

Branch Representatives' Meetings
at Bournemouth

A MEETING of representatives from the Pharmaceutical Society's branches was held in the Grand Hall of Bournemouth Town Hall on June 23, the president of the Society (Mr. Thomas Marns) in the chair. The following is an abridgment of the official verbatim report.

In opening the proceedings THE PRESIDENT welcomed the representatives. He called on Mr. F. W. Adams (assistant secretary of the Society) to explain the draft rules of procedure.

MR. ADAMS, after setting forth the origin of the draft rules, said: You will notice in Rule 2 that branches are given until January 23 in order to submit the motions that they wish to have discussed. Assuming that the effective branch year starts somewhere about the end of September, that gives nearly four months for branches to work out their ideas, to discuss them among themselves and to secure the approval of a general meeting of the branch for any motions which it is agreed should be put forward. Then, when the motions have been all received, the Council at their February meeting will review the motions and will exercise a mild form of censorship—one which is defined here fairly clearly, I think, and which everyone will agree is necessary. . . . After this consideration of the list of motions by the Council, they will then be sent to the branches for consideration, and any amendments which the branches wish to put forward must reach headquarters by March 23. These amendments will similarly be reviewed by the Council at their April meeting, and after that they will be sent, together with the original motions, to the branches for final consideration. This procedure has, broadly speaking, been adopted during the past year . . .

After a brief discussion, THE PRESIDENT moved the adoption of the draft rules

THE VICE-PRESIDENT seconded, and the motion was carried.

METHOD OF ELECTION TO COUNCIL

MR. A. H. WARE (Plymouth and District) moved: "That a method of electing members to the Council be instituted embodying a system of territorial representation." The motion, he said, emanated more particularly from members of the Society engaged in retail business. They felt, among other things, that the ordinary retail pharmacist was not satisfactorily represented on the Council. They were not proposing necessarily that the country should be divided up into a number of small territories or that the Council should be composed entirely of representatives of the type of which he was speaking. They might have, for example, seven large territories with three representatives from each.

MR. J. E. CROWE (Sheffield), seconding, said the Council's report was an exceptionally good report on behalf of the Council, but it was definitely defending the present method of election and not bringing forward a new method. Whether territorial representation would be a better method was a matter that wanted proving, and the only way to prove it would be to try it. The suggestion from Sheffield was that the country should be divided into seven separate areas. There would still be twenty-one members. The main point in favour of territorial representation from their point of view was that under the present system they got a definite series of block voting. Then there was the question of expense. It was true West Ham invited candidates to go to London, but not everyone could go to London.

THE PRESIDENT: I should like to hear from the Anglesey, North Carnarvonshire and Colwyn Bay Branch, who have put down an amendment: "That this Conference press for a system of representation on the Pharmaceutical Union which would be more equitable to the needs of Wales."

MR. E. OWEN (Anglesey) said there had been a slight mistake regarding calling this motion an amendment, but he would not quibble about that. He supported Mr. Crowe if he called it, instead of "area," "national representation." They in Wales, as Mr. Crowe pointed out, were not sufficiently strong to exert their will on the Council. (Laughter) They had 1,050 chemists in Wales, 2,500 in Scotland, and all the rest, except those in China and other places, were in England. He wished to withdraw this amendment so that they could get towards the realisation of territorial representation.

THE PRESIDENT: Are you agreeable that this amendment be withdrawn? It is entirely in your hands. (Agreed.) The discussion is now open on the principal resolution.

MR. A. L. TAYLOR (Bristol), in seconding the resolution moved by Mr. Ware, said he did so while fully realising that territorial representation in any one particular form might not necessarily be the best method of remedying certain weaknesses in their constitution. He rather thought that to restrict the choice of a member to one living in the district of his particular branch or branches was a most undesirable limitation. On the other hand, possibly to identify certain members of an already elected Council with certain districts as their particular sphere of interest would have its advantages in bringing together branches and the Council, if only in the annual elections.

MR. W. R. BRACKENBURY (Tees-side) said he always understood that the great argument for territorial representation was that the difficulty of electing new members would thus be overcome. During the last few years they had elected about half a dozen new members to the Council, several at their first attempt, and with regard to the cost of election, one who was elected on this occasion said his total expenses did not exceed £5. Personally he (the speaker) did not approve of territorial representation.

MR. G. R. KNOX-MAWER (Wrexham) suggested that the problem should be looked at from the national point of view. He felt that the Charter should be altered and that Wales should have the power of nominating a certain number of candidates to the Pharmaceutical Council. Some Welshmen felt that they were more than justly entitled to have a resident secretary. What was good for Scotland was good for Wales.

MR. R. E. JACKSON (Newcastle) was all in favour of "this territorial representation." He thought the main thing to be considered was the enormous increase in the size of the electorate. He hoped the resolution would go through.

MR. H. HOCKEN (Redhill) said his association supported this for ten years and was, he thought, the first association to bring it forward. There were thousands of people in the country who were everlastingly running down the Society. If they had territorial representation they would not insult the Society, because each area would be responsible for its members.

MR. E. RATCLIFFE (Harrow) said his branch felt that the report was a very good report from the side of the Council, but they were very dissatisfied with it. It appeared to his branch that unless the state of the voting of the Pharmaceutical Society was improved it did not really matter whether they had territorial representation or any voting at all. They felt that complementary to the change-over to territorial representation should be the reorganisation of branches.

MR. T. B. ROBINSON (Wembley) said his branch was represented there for the first time. They would like to see the Conference do something this year. Had the Council considered calling a commission of the various interests from the various branches to give their opinions and decide on a definite plan and place it before the Council and the branches and then have a vote on it?

MR. F. W. J. HOOPER (North-East Metropolitan) said he was told definitely that his association agreed with the present method of electing the Council. From this point of view they noted a tendency towards a suggestion for territorial representation. It was felt that they had already got that territorial representation. There was the possibility under territorial representation, unless they limited the funds that a particular candidate was going to spend, that they would be worse off than they were now. If they were going to adopt their England, Scotland, Ireland and Wales method, he could see certain branches of pharmacy not represented at all. The North-Eastern felt they could not improve upon their present methods.

A DELEGATE: Hospital pharmacy is already represented on the Council.

MR. J. T. APPLETON (Sheffield), after congratulating the president and the new members of Council, said that, in spite of what his fellow delegate, Mr. Crowe, had said, he would vote territorial representation directly opposite to his own individual opinion. He had had no opportunity of getting a mandate other than the casual mandate to vote for territorial representation. The Sheffield Branch had never had a meeting to discuss territorial representation. He was not a member of the executive. It had been suggested that the Council numbers were quite sufficient for the electorate. If that was so the Council must have been very overcrowded long ago. There were 2,000 members then, and there were approximately 20,000 now. He was going to suggest to the meeting that there might be a mandate from the meeting to the Council, if it received the approval of the meeting, that there shall be no "plump" voting.

MR. T. WILSON (Edinburgh) noted that the name of that meeting was now the representatives' rather than the delegates' meeting. He would like to ask the difference.

THE SECRETARY: I think the distinction Mr. Wilson has drawn is the right one. There was a little feeling in the past that the word "delegate" meant someone delegated to act in a certain way. I think they will prefer to come, possibly with instructions from their branch, but not necessarily so.

MR. E. ROBINSON (Bradford) said he spoke very strongly against territorial representation last year and this year would speak even more strongly. It should be called, not territorial representation, but "localisation, self-centredness and self-importance." This system had been tried by many other organisations and failed miserably.

A SCOTTISH DELEGATE said they all had their "grouse"—he was not satisfied any more than his brothers at the manner of selecting the Council. But he felt they were rushing things. They had now a compulsory membership, and the voting power was a disgrace. (Applause.) He respectfully moved, as an amendment, that they accept the Council's intention to proceed to a new method of selection of the Council at an early date and ask them to proceed with it as speedily as they possibly can.

THE PRESIDENT called upon Mr. Neathercoat, chairman of the Organisation Committee, to say a few words for the Council.

MR. NEATHERCOAT thought they would agree, in fact several speakers had already referred to it, that the subject they had been discussing was by no means a new one. At no time, as far as he had been able to judge, had the members of the Society, or at any rate a majority of the members of the Society, ever given any clear evidence that they were in support of any particular scheme of territorial representation. That afternoon, again, territorial representation had been discussed from many different points of view, but there was not one solid scheme which he thought had been supported whole-heartedly by the majority of the members of the Society throughout the country. In spite of the criticisms that had been made, he did not think anybody would say that that report of the Council did not calmly review the whole situation. It stated the case in favour of territorial representation under four headings and then discussed from all angles both points of view. It was because he felt that this was not the right time to come down on one side or the other that he suggested as an amendment that the report of the Council should be adopted by that meeting. They should overhaul the whole of the Society's activities and deal with the subject as if they were starting afresh but with ninety years' experience behind them. The Council proposed to proceed with this at the earliest opportunity. From his own special point of view he would be sorry to think that he only represented on the Council a section or an area of the members of the Society. The greatest charm and honour of being a member of Council was that they represented all kinds of pharmaceutical interests and were completely untrammelled by any sectional interests. He was speaking also for his colleagues on the Council. He did not believe that in the long history of the Society's development it would be possible to find a serious case of any one section suffering as a result of the Council's legislation or an important occasion when national representation had caused an injury when compared with territorial representation. Finally, there was the legal implication of this question to be considered. The secretary had said that it would be necessary to have a supplementary Charter and to alter Acts of Parliament if they were going to deprive any member of the Society of the right to vote for each candidate at the Council election. After all, there was no other method of election which would give the individual member so much control over the Council or so great an opportunity to secure the right type of councillor that he wanted. It was the most democratic method.

THE VICE-PRESIDENT formally seconded.

The amendment was declared carried, and, being then put as the substantive motion, was passed with only one or two dissentients.

MR. GARSIDE (Oldham and District) moved: "That at the election of Council of the Society the pharmaceutical business qualification (retail, wholesale, company or manufacturing) of the candidate should be stated on the voting paper." He said that his branch considered it necessary to know exactly what relationship the candidate bore to pharmacy.

MR. F. NEWBY (Oldham and District), who seconded the motion, said they desired that candidates for Council should tell more about themselves. Were retailers represented in their right proportion? (Cries of "Yes!") Their calling appeared to have no standing in the eyes of the public, and it was their desire that Council should have 100 per cent. of its interest in pharmacy for the pharmacist and not pharmacy for the financier.

MR. NEATHERCOAT said he did not know whether he was a retailer, a wholesaler, a company director or a manufacturing chemist—he was all of them. He thought there was a large number of other people who would find it very difficult indeed to fill up the form. He thought it was going to be derogatory to the best interests of the Society if they were going to stress these classes. The Society represented all pharmacists, providing they were carrying out the work for which their qualification was given, and the Society had benefited greatly by those engaged in other branches than retail pharmacy.

MR. NEWBY, replying, said the questions that Mr. Neathercoat had put before them were just the reasons that they wanted to know about a candidate and wanted him to answer all those questions. They did recognise how they were helped by the manufacturer, the wholesaler, the hospital pharmacist—and how they had to help themselves. Who got the plums? He could quite understand that the members of Council did not want any alteration in the method of electing them.

The resolution was put to the vote and carried by a small majority.

EDUCATION AND APPRENTICESHIP

MR. D. J. WILLIAMS (Bath and District) moved: "That the Conference discuss the following proposed change in the scheme of training for the C. and D. Qualifying examination:—(1) All college training to precede that of the shop or institution. (2) After matriculation the course to consist of one year's training for the Preliminary Scientific examination, followed by two years' course for the Qualifying examination. (3) At least two years' training in a shop or institution subsequent to passing the Qualifying examination. (4) Certificate of qualification and registration to be given only after completion of the whole course of training at college and shop or institution." He said the problem had for its first object the substitution of a continuous college course in place of the present interrupted one. The difficulty lay in the position to allocate to that portion called the vocational or business training. They in Bath had come to the conclusion that by placing it at the end of the so-called academic course it would produce many more advantages than the losses through removal of apprenticeship. There were many pharmacists who were beginning to say they would not be bothered with apprentices. He had also evidence that the general public had found them out and would not send their sons for three years of very much wasted time, as had been the case in many instances. They must face this. It might account for the extraordinary drop in the number of apprentices. Apprenticeship had been tortuous for many years, and he saw no great hope of its changing. Obviously, in the communal and social life of the college there was that cultural background which was so essential to a pharmacist if he was to regard himself, and get others to believe in him, as a professional man.

MR. T. J. CORNISH (Bath and District) believed that the proposed scheme would mean economy for the student and the parent, and would end the laborious system of cramming which had produced an appalling want of success in the examinations.

Mr. F. Newby (Oldham and District) said this resolution knocks theirs (on restriction of apprentices) "into a cocked hat." How long would it take the Council to consider these questions? There was also the difficulty of controlling apprentices, which would be intensified when they were older. When would the apprentice be expected to register? Their resolution, unnecessary if the Bath motion was carried, was: "That only one apprentice be allowed to any pharmacist during a period of six years." They considered that to be the first step towards improving the standard of the pharmacist. They found in Lancashire generally, which was suffering considerably from ills in the cotton trade, that at the end of their apprenticeship, in the effort to obtain employment when twenty-one or twenty-two, these men offered their services at 30s. or £2 a week; and they had to keep themselves, as their parents could not afford to. From a financial point of view, the more apprentices the more pharmacists and the more the Council would have to spend. At the present rate of increase in the number of pharmacists the number of chemists' shops should double in the next five or six years, and if they all got an apprentice it would happen. Was it not better to limit entrance?

Mr. Garside (Oldham) seconded the motion. The Bath and District resolution, he added, was a very good resolution. The member from Bath said that pharmacists would not bother with apprentices. He would rather say that fair chemists would not take apprentices. If pharmacy once got into the hands of the financial interests it would sink, and above all things they must stop that. They might as well cut down to begin with.

Mr. Taylor (Bristol) said that at present a candidate had to be twenty-one before he sat for his final examination. Under Mr. Williams's system of delayed apprenticeship would he be twenty-one when he passed his final, or at the end of the training?

Mr. F. L. King (Mansfield and District) moved: "That the period be four years instead of six." His branch, he said, suggested four years on the ground that while there should be some limitation it should not be excessive.

The President: Is anyone present to propose the amendment for the West Glamorgan Branch? (No one responded.) Then we wash that out. The amendment of Mansfield Branch is now open for discussion.

Mr. W. J. Tristram (Liverpool) thought it unfortunate that the Bath resolution had been linked up with the other resolutions.

The Secretary: The resolution before the meeting is that moved by Oldham, with the amendment we have had.

Mr. J. E. Crowe (Sheffield) expressed a wish to move an amendment.

Mr. R. Hudson (Burnley) said that in Burnley they did not think very much of the Bath resolution. They felt that it would be too drastic a limitation on the number of apprentices. Whether the shop training preceded or followed the academic it would still remain the most important part. He realised the need for limitation, but it should not be in an arbitrary manner.

Mr. Rowsell said they had covered a pretty wide field in the discussion of apprenticeship. He was deeply indebted to Mr Williams for having brought forward his scheme. It was worthy of the greatest consideration by all the members of the Society in their various branches. On behalf of the Council he could say that this discussion would be very helpful and would be considered in all its bearings. Various things might be said for and against the scheme. There was an amendment from Edinburgh, which he did not think had been put. Would they like him to deal with it?

Mr. T. Wilson (Edinburgh and S.-E. Scottish) moved: "That the Preliminary Scientific examination be recommended to be taken before apprenticeship and further, in all cases, apprenticeship should precede the curriculum of the Qualifying examination." He said it was rather a pity that the Bath proposals had been mixed up with the proposals for apprenticeship. The Bath proposals were very revolutionary proposals. They would mean that the educational system would have to be recast. For a period of years no further burden should be put on a candidate with regard to the number of hours in the curriculum or the scope of the examination. The mover of the Bath resolution spoke as if apprenticeship were to be abolished, and the seconder as if it were to be retained. When was the apprentice to get his training? What kind of examination in practical pharmacy were they going to set to a student who had yet to learn his business? Then the student was to have a period of training under an employer. Was there to be any test at the end of that training? If not, it would be a farce and a delusion. It was not in the institution that the apprentice was going to learn his business. It was in the shop. That should take place in the most plastic age.

Mr. P. Nesbit (Edinburgh) said they could never get rid of the business side of the question. They should be well qualified, but it would never do to have that professional qualification only. He seconded the amendment.

Mr. Rowsell, continuing, said that to his mind the ordinary pupil had quite enough to contend with at present. This year they raised their standard for the Preliminary Scientific to that of Matriculation. Knowing the country fairly well, he thought there would not be the same ease of apprenticeship as in the past. If his friends would accept this very well thought out report of the Council, they would do well to adopt this as their amendment.

The Vice-President formally seconded this proposal.

Mr. Skyrme (Hastings) said that when discussing apprenticeship they must consider the effect of any curriculum on the student as well as on the man who took the apprentice.

The Oldham motion and the Mansfield amendment were withdrawn, and the following motion, submitted by Mr. Crowe (Sheffield) was carried with one dissentient:—"That this meeting of branch representatives accepts the report of the Council and is satisfied with the steps taken by the Council regarding the limitation of apprentices."

Mr. Rutherford Hill's Distinction

On the conclusion of business The President referred to the announcement that morning that his Majesty the King had conferred the honour of O.B.E. on Mr. Rutherford Hill, resident secretary of the Society in Scotland. This reference was greeted with an outburst of loud and prolonged cheering, which did not cease till the president held up his hand for silence.

The President: I can see, ladies and gentlemen, by the spontaneous round of applause that you yourselves appreciate the honour that has been bestowed on Mr. Rutherford Hill, and I will call upon him to speak.

All present rose in a body and sang "For He's a Jolly Good Fellow."

Mr. Hill said: Mr. President, ladies and gentlemen, this must surely be the supreme moment in my career as a pharmacist. It has come upon me very unexpectedly; some of my friends, I think, knew about it before I did—in fact, I read it in the paper this morning, although I had reason to suspect that something was afoot. I would like to regard this not as a personal honour to me, but as some recognition of the profession of pharmacy, because I happen to know that one of the reasons for this most kind and gracious action of his Majesty was that somebody made some mention of some work I had been able to do for the profession of pharmacy. Therefore I would like to regard this as a recognition by his Majesty of the importance and dignity of the profession of pharmacy. Having been now for more than fifty years an officer of the Society, I would like to justify that appreciation by referring to the advances that pharmacy has made. Some say that it has been going to the dogs. I once made the remark that it always had been going to the dogs. I regard pharmacy as in a new position of great responsibility and opportunity. The recent legislation has been far more beneficial to pharmacy than I anticipated it would have been, thanks to the devoted work of my friend Mr. Linstead. (Hear, hear.) We ought not to sit down, but to stand up and go forward and work for the consolidation of the practice of pharmacy that we all hope for, and that was the objective of the Society in 1841. I thank you, Mr. President, for this appreciation of any humble service I may have been able to render to my craft.

The President then declared the meeting adjourned.

(To be continued)

The Chemist a Bureau of Information.—A correspondent (14/4) writes that into his shop came a boy, about ten years old, with a "mangled" message. He was asked to get the message written down, and eventually returned with the following: "Pleas can you tell me whot is Tepid warter."

One Hundred Years of "Smart's Corner," Littlehampton

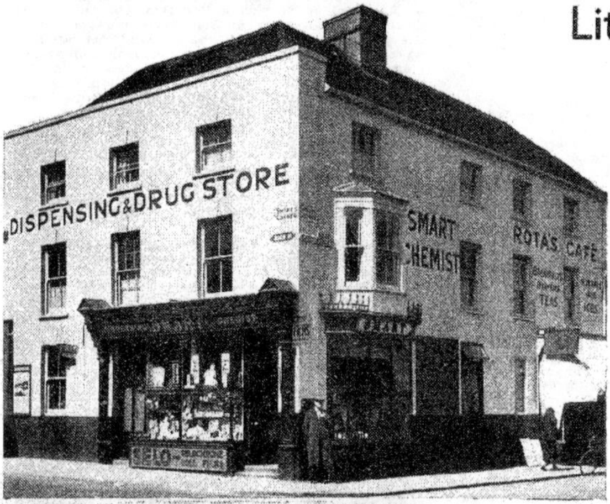

ONE HUNDRED years ago Nevil Smart opened a village shop at what is now officially 62 High Street, Littlehampton, but known popularly as "Smart's Corner." It must have been a veritable department store in miniature, for the stock ranged from chemists' goods to cigars, bibles, fishhooks and wines. It would seem that almost the only commodities missing from advertisements and catalogues of the period were meat and coals! The Pharmaceutical Society's certificate was issued to Nevil Smart in 1853. Prescription-books are preserved in an unbroken line from thirteen years earlier even than that, though the first of the series has apparently been sacrificed at the hand of time. In common with other old relics at the pharmacy, the handwriting in these is of "copperplate" perfection. The enterprising founder was apparently one of the leading public characters of his day and generation. Among other accomplishments must be numbered the conducting of "penny readings" every Saturday evening at the National Schools, for which he was presented with a very handsome silver cup.

Upon his death, in 1881, he was succeeded by his son Charles Frederick, who carried on the business on the old tradition of "good service at a fair remuneration." In spite of increasing competition the chemist's side grew steadily. C. F. Smart retired in 1911 and the business was taken over by his eldest son Harry, the present owner. It is noticeable that each year the business becomes more pharmaceutical, the only present side-line, apart from photography, being wireless apparatus. The owner writes: "There is apparently still bread and cheese in a chemist's business; for notwithstanding that competitors have increased from none to eight chemists (including three multiple shops) and four drug stores, we now employ a manager, two male assistants and a porter."

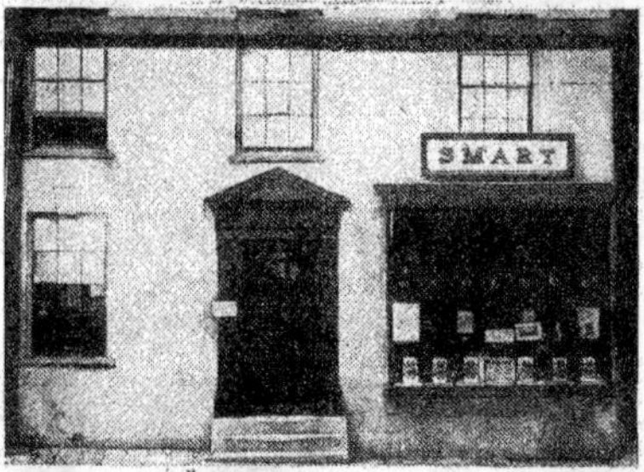

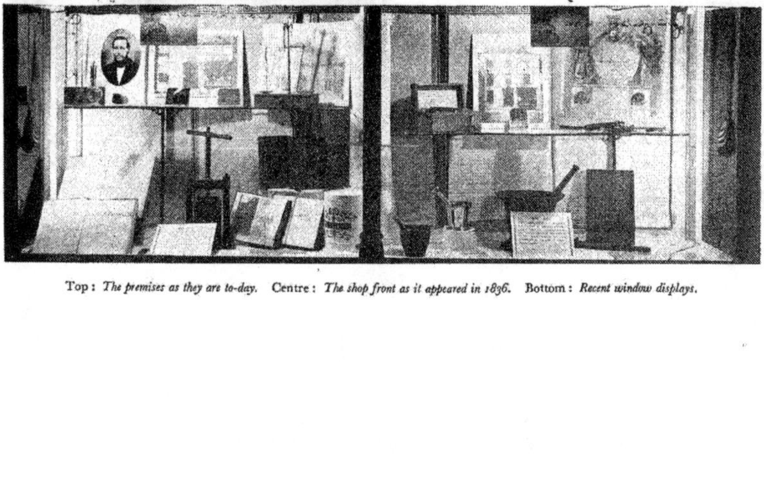

Top: *The premises as they are to-day.* Centre: *The shop front as it appeared in 1836.* Bottom: *Recent window displays.*

Items in Parliament

COMMONWEALTH SCIENTIFIC CONFERENCE

In reply to a question whether it was proposed to summon an Imperial agricultural research conference, the Marquess of Hartington (Under-Secretary for the Dominions) replied: It is hoped to hold a British Commonwealth Scientific Conference in London in September of this year.

PATENT MEDICINES

The Minister of Health was asked whether he proposed to introduce legislation to give effect to the recommendations of the Select Committee on Patent Medicines?

Mr. Shakespeare (Under-Secretary). No, sir. The Government have no present intention of introducing legislation for this purpose. The subject was recently debated on a private member's Bill, which failed to obtain a second reading

"PREPARED" HONEY

The Minister of Health was asked whether he was aware that a mixture of sugar and other ingredients including a small proportion of honey was being sold as honey, and whether he would take steps to protect the public from this deception.

Mr. Shakespeare (Parliamentary Secretary): [The Minister] is aware that a substance which is not pure honey is sold under the name of "prepared honey" with a label indicating that it is a mixture. [He] has no power to take any action in the matter, but if the circumstances of the sale are such as to constitute an offence under the Food and Drugs (Adulteration) Act, the duty of enforcement rests on the local authorities, and it is also open to any person to take proceedings.

EMPLOYMENT OF CHILDREN

The Home Secretary was asked the number of local authorities which had made by-laws permitting children to be employed before school hours and the number of children so employed.

Sir J. Simon: 166 out of 317 local authorities have made by-laws permitting the employment of children for not more than one hour before school commences: similar by-laws made by fifty authorities before the Act remain in force. I have no recent information of the number of children so employed.

AIR RAID PRECAUTIONS

The Home Secretary was asked whether pharmacists were to be employed as gas-detection officers; what qualifications they had for the work; and what steps were to be taken to train them to do the work adequately?

Mr. Geoffrey Lloyd (Under-Secretary): My Department has had under consideration a scheme by which persons with a basic knowledge of chemistry might be recruited as gas-detection officers in populous parts of the country. A scheme of instruction has been devised, and the Civilian Anti-Gas School will be available for the purpose.

Further questioned as to the facilities provided in the London area for doctors wishing to obtain instruction in the treatment of poison-gas cases, Mr. Lloyd replied The General Medical Council and the British Medical Association have been consulted on this matter, and arrangements for giving instruction to medical practitioners in the treatment of poison-gas cases are under consideration.

MEDICINE STAMP DUTY

The Chancellor of the Exchequer was asked whether, in view of the difficulties involved in the administration of the Medicine Stamp Duty Acts, he would undertake a reconstruction of this tax and a revision of the conditions attached to it?

Mr. Chamberlain: The Medicine Stamp Duty is governed by a series of statutes considerably more than a century old. These Acts are in many respects out of date and unsuited to present-day conditions, and they produce a number of anomalies which make the administration of the duty extremely difficult. I have come to the conclusion that the tax needs reconstruction, but a number of conflicting interests are concerned, and in all the circumstances I think the most appropriate course would be for the matter to be considered by a Select Committee of this House. I propose therefore to move for the appointment of a Select Committee to examine the law as it at present stands and to recommend what changes appear to be desirable.

An Artist in Advertising

AN exhibition of commercial art, the first of its kind, has been held in London during the past fortnight. It was opened by Sir William Reid Dick, the sculptor, and about 400 artists—many of them well-known—contributed. One of the organisers said it was estimated that nowadays between 10,000 and 30,000 artists were engaged in advertising.

As a pioneer in the application of art to advertising in trade journalism THE CHEMIST AND DRUGGIST may look back with particular satisfaction to a long line of Special Issues, beginning with the "illuminated covers" of the 'nineties and culminating in the galaxy of photogravure reproductions, colour sections and pictorial insets shown in the advertisement and editorial sections of its latest Special Issue. For forty years there have been artists on the staff of THE CHEMIST AND DRUGGIST. The influence of the pictorial artist on drug-trade advertising has steadily increased, and the results are evident in the highly artistic advertising, now evident not only in the *C. & D.* but also in its many imitators.

In this connexion a thought-provoking article by Mr. Lawrence H. Conrad appears in the current issue of "The Landmark." The question asked by Mr. Conrad is, "Must Realism in Art and Letters Continue?" His ingenious contention is that advertising (particularly in the U.S.A.) has robbed art of all its romanticism, therefore realism must continue "until the business world learns to touch art without leaving crude finger-prints around the edges." In the States, he says, advertising has become in a very genuine sense an art. But the business world, he asserts, has appropriated only certain moods of art—the kind which echoes the theme-song of business.

> "It must have a lift and a leap; it must be an urge and a compulsion; it must suggest high motives, high praise and a high degree of satisfaction to the purchaser. . . . In short, the business world has appropriated all of art's romantic tendencies to its own uses. Romantic art has been 'elevated' to commercial uses; realism has been dropped for the pay roll. The artist, therefore, turns out romantic works for hire. And when he gets a day off for expressing himself he must needs go realistic in order to avoid the appearance of evil."

As corroboration of his theory, Mr. Conrad invites us to study any popular magazine and to compare the snap and sparkle of the world as represented in the advertising pages with the drab and shabby representation of life in the literary pages "where writer and artist work upon their own impulses." To be successful in the arts one must nowadays be of the romantic strain.

> "Yet no one, layman or artist, could stand more glamour and romance than advertising has woven about every commodity that is offered for sale. We have come to a stand; we are on a dead centre."

Advertisers realise that by sponsoring works of art they secure for themselves and their products the highest kind of goodwill; but (Mr. Conrad argues) in associating their products always with one phase of art, they are liable to cause themselves and their goods to be regarded with distaste. The demands which business has hitherto made upon art are, in his idea, extremely short-sighted and ill-advised. He hopes, therefore, for a dawning intelligence among business leaders which will bring to an end the practice of using art solely to bring "a roseate glow to advertising."

"C. & D." Retail Price List

THE drug index of prices for the month of June was 147.0—a slight fall from the preceding month's figure of 147.4. The corresponding figure for June 1935 was 144.7, giving evidence of steadiness in wholesale prices. In surgical dressings the index showed an advance of 0.1 over that of May, being 136.6 against 136.5, and against 136.2 in the corresponding month of last year.

BRITISH PHARMACEUTICAL CONFERENCE

Proceedings

(*Concluded from* THE CHEMIST AND DRUGGIST, *June 27, p.* 721)

Science Session

Tuesday Morning, June 23

The proceedings of the Science Section opened at the Town Hall, Bournemouth, on June 23, in ideal weather. The attendance was so good that the members may be congratulated on resisting—for the time being, at any rate—the other attractions of the town and settling to what, after all, is the primary object of the Conference. The chairman (Mr. Harold Deane) was accompanied on the platform by Mr. T. Edward Lescher (treasurer), Mr. F. W. Gamble, Mr. E. Saville Peck and the general secretaries (Mr. C. E. Corfield and Mr. G. E. Boyes).

THE CHAIRMAN, in opening the proceedings, referred to the distinction conferred on Mr. J. Rutherford Hill, who, as announced in the Press that morning, had been awarded the O.B.E. This mention of a distinguished pharmacist in the Birthday honours would, he was sure, afford gratification to all present, and they desired to offer him their hearty congratulations. (Applause.)

The first paper taken was:—

Effect of Degree of Comminution on Extraction of Belladonna Leaf, Ipecacuanha, and Stramonium

By A. W. BULL

[ABSTRACT]

THE experimental results in this and a previous paper (*C. & D.*, 1935, II, 15) are part of work which is being undertaken in the preparation of a thesis to be submitted for degree. This paper is illustrated by thirteen tables and two graphs.

BELLADONNA LEAF

1. The yield of total extractive increases as the powder size decreases.
2. The alkaloidal yield varies in the same way.
3. The relative proportion of alkaloids to total solids is greatest in the extract from the 22/60 powder and least in that from the 85 powder.
4. The alkaloids are extracted more quickly than are the other soluble constituents of the drug.

IPECACUANHA

1. The yield of total extractive increases as the powder size decreases.
2. A moderately fine powder 44/85 gives a better alkaloidal yield than either a fine powder or a moderately coarse powder.
3. The percentage of alkaloids in the total extractive is greatest in that from the 44/85 powder.
4. The phenolic alkaloids are extracted by alcohol (90 per cent.) more quickly than are the non-phenolic type, and after a time practically all the alkaloids in the marc are non-phenolic.

STRAMONIUM

1. A fine powder, 85, yields more total extractive and total alkaloids than does a moderately coarse powder, 22/60, which in turn gives a greater yield of both than does a moderately fine powder, 44/85.
2. The proportion of alkaloids to total extractive is most in the 22/60 powder and least in the 44/85 powder.
3. The alkaloids are extracted more quickly than is the total extractive of the drug, although in the early stages of the percolation the reverse is the case.

(From the School of Pharmacy, University College, Nottingham.)

DISCUSSION

THE CHAIRMAN said the paper was interesting and important owing to the acknowledged effect of the degree of comminution on the rate of extraction. The paper gave accurate details. In his experience different samples of ipecacuanha behaved very differently in extraction, irrespective of the degree of grinding. Resulting extractives also varied in amount. He (the chairman) had suggested that an alcohol of 80 per cent. should be substituted for that of the Pharmacopœia assay (90 per cent.) as likely to give better results, but in this the Pharmacopœia Commission had not concurred. The difference recorded in the behaviour of belladonna and stramonium was also probably due to differences in menstruum strength.

DR. BULLOCK asked if Mr. Bull would give details of the experimental error met with. The differences of alkaloidal extractive did not appear great. What variation, he asked, might be expected if three experiments were carried out with powder of the same degree of coarseness—say 22/60?

MR. COUTTS asked if Mr. Bull had any comments to make on a paper which was also tabled for the present Conference, that by Mr. Peck on "The Extraction of Vegetable Materials"; as to whether any difference was experienced between results when the powder was percolated dry or previously moistened; and whether a different menstruum would be an advantage in moistening for that used in percolation.

MR. BULL, in reply, agreed with the chairman that different specimens of ipecacuanha yielded different results. The second sample tested had not shown so large a variation in the rate of extraction of the phenolic compared with the non-phenolic alkaloids. The reason for the selection of the particular strength of menstruum used in the extraction of belladonna alkaloids had been for purposes of comparison with belladonna root. The experiments had been performed in duplicate as to the earlier fractions. Although the rates of extraction varied slightly, the total extractive was found to be nearly always equal, later fractions equalising the earlier ones. He had performed no work on the relative merits of dry and moistened powders in percolation. He had found, however, that penetrability of the menstruum varied when extraction was carried out under reduced pressure; in this respect the effect was greater on the coarser powders

The next paper taken was:—

Santonin in English and Welsh *Artemisias*

By JAMES COUTTS

[ABSTRACT]

DESPITE the large amount of work which has been done on many foreign species of *Artemisia*, very little attention seems to have been given by plant analysts to the *A. maritima*, Linn. and *A. gallica*, Willd., growing wild in quite a number of localities in Britain. The few investigations on English plants which have been reported, indicate—inconclusively however—that these plants do not contain santonin, but it has been shown by the present author that these artemisias growing wild in Scotland contain quite an appreciable proportion. It was decided, therefore, to collect *A. maritima* and *A. gallica* from as many localities as possible on the coasts of England and Wales and to examine them for santonin. They were seen to occur in twenty-two of the thirty-one vice-counties visited. In fourteen of these vice-counties sufficient material for the present purpose was found, and batches of plant were collected from twenty-seven localities in them. The author's results are illustrated by six tables and a graph. His conclusions are:—

1. Santonin was found to be present in all of the twenty-seven British populations of *A. maritima* and *A. gallica* examined. One sample yielded 1.24 per cent.
2. *A. maritima* would appear to produce a slightly higher proportion of santonin than does *A. gallica* at the same stage of growth and growing in the same locality.
3. A seasonal variation in santonin content, similar to that reported of the Scottish plant, was found to exist in the two English populations examined for this purpose.

BRITISH PHARMACEUTICAL CONFERENCE 1936

4. Evidence that the soil, alone, or in conjunction with other factors, affects the production of santonin, is incomplete, but it has been suggested that the salinity of the soil may, and it is probable that it does, have a more or less marked effect

Discussion

The Chairman pointed out that the paper showed the wide variation in constitution among wild plants. Santonin was now being largely used in veterinary medicine; the Royal Agricultural Society, for instance, was urging its use for pigs and sheep. This country was largely dependent on Central Asia for supplies, and if santonin were grown commercially in Great Britain competition would no doubt come into play. The chairman inquired whether Dr. Coutts had examined any specimens of artemisia from nurserymen's stocks.

Mr. J. C. Young asked if it was practicable to manufacture santonin in this country.

Mr. Widgery (Weston-super-Mare) remarked that "chromo-santonin" had been recommended for sprue: he wondered whether there was a scientific basis for this.

Mr. Walker inquired what analytical method had been used in the author's determinations.

Dr. Coutts, in reply, said he had examined only two batches of nursery plants: one contained a mere trace of santonin, and the other not more than 0.5 per cent. It might be possible to manufacture santonin commercially in this country after many experiments, but not at present. He had no information about the therapeutic value of so-called "chromo-santonin." The analytical method of determination used was his own, published about three years ago: it gave strictly comparable results.

The next paper was:—

Penetration of Heat into Surgical Dressings

By R. Maxwell Savage

[Abstract]

Certain Government bodies insist to-day on a procedure being applied to their dressings which is not merely unnecessary, but undesirable, and even the British Pharmaceutical Codex, 1934, contains, in the monograph on the sterilisation of surgical dressings, statements which differ in some degree from the facts. The author describes a lengthy series of experiments undertaken with a view to ascertaining the optimal conditions for sterilising dressings. The monograph is illustrated by seven graphs. The summary of conclusions is as follows:—

1. In a vacuum autoclave, steam penetrates packages almost instantly, and it is quite unnecessary to leave the packages open or to arrange them loosely.

2. The size of a package has a small influence on the rate at which it becomes heated at the centre, numerous small packages tightly wedged together, however, do not behave as a large unit, but heat almost as readily as if they were separate.

3. The temperatures and pressures attained within the packages indicate that some superheating of the steam occurs, but reasons are adduced for considering that the material itself remains moist until the end of the sterilising period.

4. When packages of cotton are heated in an oven without added water, heating of the interior portions is partially effected by the condensation of steam generated from the hygroscopic water in the outer layers. Heating is therefore accelerated by wrapping the package and confining the steam, but later retarded by the re-evaporation of the condensed water.

5. The atmosphere of wrapped packages of cotton which are heated in an oven consists not of air, but largely of superheated steam.

6. Dry sterilisation of cotton is a possible procedure.

7. Bacteriological experiments confirm the physical conclusions.

Acknowledgement is made to the author's colleagues, Mr. A. H. Hughes and Mr. S. Whatmough, for co-operation in connexion with the large autoclave, to Mr. G. R. Davenport for assistance in some of the experiments, and to Dr. W. F. Purdy for arranging access to some of the literature. (From the laboratories of S. Maw, Son & Sons, Ltd.)

Discussion

The Chairman commented on the importance of putting such matters to experimental test instead of accepting current views.

Mr. Evers congratulated Mr. Savage on his work and on the interesting conclusions he had come to. At first consideration it would seem that the more tightly dressings were packed the longer the time necessary for penetration. His own experiments confirmed Mr. Savage's that such was not the case.

Mr. Hooper offered one criticism. He suggested that the speaker's conclusion that dry sterilisation methods were worthy of consideration as a possible procedure should be modified by the proviso that no deterioration in tensile strength was suffered by the dressing. He had had experience with the dry sterilisation of a dressing impregnated with vaseline; this had been considerably weakened in the process.

Mr. Peck asked if any work had been done on material in large quantities. He inquired as a matter of interest from a public health rather than a pharmaceutical point of view. Were clothing and bedding taken for disinfection by public authorities thoroughly sterilised? He instanced the experience of a friend who had inserted a clinical thermometer in a mattress before sending to a public authority for disinfection. The thermometer came back unbroken. (Laughter.)

Mr. Gamble hoped the speaker would continue his work. The references to dressings had, he presumed, been to absorbent dressings. He asked if any tests had been made on non-absorbent dressings, and if any difference had been noted Doubts existed as to whether the public and doctors were justified in assuming, as many did, that all dressings sent out were sterile. He thought chemists and purveyors of dressings might consider it advisable to support this point of view. Wood-wool dressings had recently been viewed with suspicion as possible carriers of tetanus bacilli. Had the author any experience? He thought the time was coming when all dressings should be sent out sterile.

Mr. Jackson confirmed that the sterilisation methods of public authorities needed investigation, but thought that ventilating the question was to "put the cat among the pigeons."

Mr. Savage, in reply, was of opinion that the instance given of deterioration of dressing under dry heat sterilisation had been a special case. A point was that great strength was not required by dressings placed in closest proximity to wounds. The method was, he thought, suitable for small dressings. The question of sterilisation of material in quantity had been dealt with many years earlier, and the results had been considered satisfactory. He instanced the case of an operator who, on receipt of complaints of damage to clothing, had turned the valves down and given less than the required amount of heat. In public health work, the authorities deal with non-sporing organisms; while the spores in surgical dressings were not of the sort to cause epidemics. He had done no work on non-absorbent dressings. He had heard of cases of tetanus arising out of the use of wood wool, and believed the cause to be the water used. He agreed in principle that all dressings should be sterile; in a competitive world, manufacturers would be found ready to meet the demand when it arose.

The next paper was:—

Analytical Examination of Commercial Desiccated Hog Stomach Preparations: Relationship of Examination to Clinical Activity

By Kenneth Bullock

[Abstract]

This investigation was undertaken to ascertain to what extent commercial brands of desiccated hog stomach at present on the market differ in the analytical figures which they yield; to see if these differences indicate any great variation in the methods of manufacture employed, and also to ascertain if different samples of the same brand can be produced so as to yield uniform figures. Details of the analytical methods employed are given. The methods were applied to thirteen samples, comprising nine different commercial brands of desiccated hog stomach. The results obtained are given. The Codex requires a defatted powder, yet two preparations included in the

BRITISH PHARMACEUTICAL CONFERENCE 1936

appendix to the book as brands of ventriculus desiccatus contain over 10 per cent. of fat and are clearly not defatted. (Notes on clinical tests, together with certain of the samples analysed, have been supplied to the author by Dr. J. F. Wilkinson, of the Manchester Royal Infirmary.) The manganese content has been estimated.

Among the author's general conclusions are the following:—It would appear desirable to fix upper limits for the moisture-, fat- and ash-contents of commercial hog stomach preparations. Suitable limits would be 5 per cent. for moisture, 5 per cent. for ash, calculated on a fat- and moisture-free basis, and 15 per cent. for fat in the case of a non-fat extracted preparation with a limit of 4 per cent. of fat for the fat extracted preparations. The fact that the activity of a drug can only be determined biologically does not mean that analytical constants are useless in the control of the product. If a standard method of manufacture were laid down, then figures of general application could be worked out which if complied with would to a large extent ensure correct use of the method. Such analytical data would include the peptic activity, the soluble coagulable and non-coagulable nitrogens, together with moisture, fat, ash, insoluble ash, alkalinity of the ash, chloride-content, and acidity of the product.

DISCUSSION

THE CHAIRMAN remarked that this was a very important and useful paper. Several clinically unsatisfactory brands of this type of preparation were on the market.

MR. MANN inquired whether there was any clinical evidence that the manganese present had no biological effect.

DR. CROSSLEY-HOLLAND said the present position appeared to be that manganese was of some definite use. It was a constituent of many of the body tissues, and might play some activating part in the production of blood elements. If it could be given in a form in which it could be utilised, that would be preferable to giving it by injection. The reaction of the body to the injection of manganese could be violent. He congratulated Dr. Bullock on a paper of real constructive value.

MR. FRANKLIN pointed out the differences in flavour between fat-extracted products of hog stomach and others. Was not uniformity in this respect desirable?

MR. BOYES expressed his indebtedness to the author, and hoped that his work would be a step towards the isolation of the active substance.

MR. EVERS inquired why it was considered that hog stomach preparations should have peptic activity. Perhaps the removal of the pepsin could be effected without heat.

DR. BULLOCK, replying, pointed out, with regard to manganese, that only anæmia cases, and particularly pernicious anæmia cases, were under consideration. Though the possibility of manganese having an activating effect was not ruled out, its content in the stomach was less than that in a considerable number of organs of the body. He agreed that the taste of products in which fat remained was objectionable. There was difficulty in devising a standard method of manufacture, as makers would not disclose their processes. Dr. J. F. Wilkinson had never found a product to be free from peptic activity and yet clinically active. It might be possible to remove the pepsin, but the resulting product would no longer be a product of whole hog stomach.

The next paper was:—

Measurement of Proteolytic Activity of Pancreatic Preparations

By NORMAN EVERS and WILFRED SMITH

[ABSTRACT]

THE authors suggest a new method of assaying pancreatin for proteolytic power. They illustrate their findings with two tables and a graph. Their results show that there are wide variations in the proteolytic power of different specimens of pancreatin described as B.P. One of these failed to pass the B.P. test, but two others were more than twice as active as the B.P. requires, in fact, they were equal in proteolytic power to normal specimens of trypsin. The samples examined varied widely in appearance, solubility and price, the price being no criterion of the activity. The authors' summary includes the following points:—

(1) The B.P. method for the determination of the proteolytic power of pancreatin is not entirely satisfactory. It is lengthy and the end-point is not very easy to observe. A further source of error is that the *p*H is not adjusted to a definite point before the addition of the formaldehyde. (2) A method is suggested using purified casein, bringing to *p*H 7 before the addition of formaldehyde and then titrating to *p*H 8.7. (3) It is essential that the quantity of enzyme used should be so regulated as to give a titration varying between narrow limits. (From the analytical laboratories of Allen & Hanburys, Ltd.)

DISCUSSION

THE CHAIRMAN declared that the value of this paper was in the improvements it offered in analytical methods. The commercial position was shown to be far from satisfactory.

MR. POWELL recorded that his experiences with the pharmacopœial methods had been similar. He had found the method of A. R. Smith, referred to by Mr. Evers, superior; the investigations now made into the importance of *p*H would, if put into effect, make it better still.

The last paper taken at this session was:—

Determination of Strychnine in Easton's Syrup

By NORMAN EVERS and WILFRED SMITH

[ABSTRACT]

THE method laid down in the B.P. for the determination of strychnine in Easton's syrup was contained in a paper read before this Conference by Haddock and Evers. While it is fairly satisfactory for the assay of freshly made syrups, difficulties arise when the method is applied to the assay of syrups which have stood for some time. In the authors' view the weakness of the B.P. process is the washing of the alkaloidal residue with the solvent, especially as it was found that the ratio of quinine to strychnine in the residue previous to the washing varied widely. Their investigation (the details of which include two tables) has resulted in the recommendation of the following method:—

Carry out the assay for strychnine exactly as described in the B.P. to the stage when the impure alkaloid is obtained. Dissolve this residue in 10 mils of $N/1$ hydrochloric acid and filter through a 9 cm. filter-paper into a separator. Wash the flask and filter paper with three further quantities of 5 mils $N/1$ hydrochloric acid and then with 25 mils of a saturated solution of sodium chloride. Repeat the extraction of the filtered liquid by shaking with five successive quantities of 25 mils of chloroform, and continue the B.P. process of separation to the same stage as above and weigh the residue, which should be almost white. (From the analytical laboratories of Allen & Hanburys, Ltd.)

There was no discussion on this paper, which THE CHAIRMAN praised as an interesting and useful one. The morning closed with a collective expression of thanks to the authors, and the audience made its way through the Central Gardens to the Pavilion for photography and lunch.

Science Session

Tuesday Afternoon

The audience that assembled in the Science Section on Tuesday afternoon was small, largely on account of the meeting of branch delegates which synchronised with it. A few minutes after the time fixed for opening, THE CHAIRMAN called the members to attention and announced that it would be necessary to take the first paper as read, the author being unavoidably absent. The paper was:—

Extraction of Vegetable Materials

By W. C. PECK

[ABSTRACT]

EXAMINATION of the published work on the extraction of vegetable drugs reveals that little progress has been made for

BRITISH PHARMACEUTICAL CONFERENCE 1936

many years. Reports of various investigators are discussed by the author of this paper, and the need for a more fundamental examination suggested. The nature of vegetable drugs is considered in relation to the processes of maceration and percolation, and the preparation of tinctures and extracts classified into six operations with a view to determining in what ways extraction processes can be improved. Experiments are described in maceration of the drugs of tinct. gent. co., B.P., 1932, at ordinary pressure and *in vacuo*; by the B.P. process and using an electric stirrer; and in maceration of vanilla beans by three alternative methods. The conclusion is put forward that the rate of extraction of these drugs is increased by the application of vacuum and by agitation and circulation of the extracting liquid. The design and operation of several improved types of extraction apparatus are described and diagrams given.

There was no formal discussion, but THE CHAIRMAN made a brief reference to the history of percolation, which, he said, was invented in France about 100 years ago. Mr. Henry Deane was one of the first to advocate its use in this country. The author's suggestions, as a whole, were likely to be very suitable in the case of a long run on one drug, but if frequent changes and smaller quantities were needed another state of things arose. The vacuum extraction principle was good and was already in use—e.g., for creosoting timber. Too rapid extraction was not advisable; the solvent had to penetrate the cells of the drug.

DR. BULLOCK raised a question as to what the author meant by "assay for total solids."

MR. A. J. JONES remarked that the use of vacuum percolation had spread. As to upward percolation, if there was much extractive the percolate might begin to regurgitate. In the case of a coarse powder percolation might take a long time.

MR. BULL suggested that vacuum extraction seemed more applicable to large-scale working.

THE CHAIRMAN expressed thanks to the author.

The next paper was:—

Dry Extract of Stramonium

By A. T. MOORHOUSE

[ABSTRACT]

IT seems reasonable to assume that a dry extract of stramonium, if official, would prove useful. No modern Pharmacopœia, except that of the United States, includes in its formulary a dry extract of stramonium. Extracts have been prepared by the author using various strengths of alcohol as solvents, and the suitability of various diluents has been investigated. It has been found that alcohol (95 per cent.) gives the best results as the solvent, and air-dry starch is most suitable as the diluent. It is suggested the following process be adopted for the production of a dry extract of stramonium:—

Extract 1,000 gm. of stramonium in moderately coarse powder by percolation with alcohol (95 per cent.) until 4,000 mils of percolate have been collected. Determine the total solids present in the percolate. Determine also the proportion of alkaloids in the percolate. Calculate the quantity of air-dry starch that must be added to the percolate to produce a dry extract containing 1 per cent. of the alkaloids of stramonium. Evaporate the percolate to a syrupy consistence at a temperature not exceeding 50° C. and incorporate the whole of the diluent. Dry the product at a temperature not exceeding 70° C. Powder and pass through a No. 22 sieve. The extract should be stored in well-closed containers preferably in the dark. The author wishes to thank Mr. H. Berry for many helpful suggestions. (From the Department of Pharmacy, Technical College, Bradford.) Examples of a number of dry extracts made by the author were passed round for inspection.

DISCUSSION

THE CHAIRMAN congratulated the author on a good paper which showed evidence of much work. It was a pity, he said, that only one sample, and that a particularly good one, had been used. Herbs varied considerably, and it was often impossible to powder a drug extracted with strong alcohol. Coarse powders, though most popular for dispensing, were not equally suitable for tablet-making.

MR. R. R. BENNETT declared that the paper was timely, because it was an open secret that a dry extract of stramonium, probably made with 95 per cent. alcohol, would be included in the next Addendum to the British Pharmacopœia. The difficulty with strong spirit was the greasy or oily nature of the extract; with weak spirit the "snag" was the proportion of sugars contained and the hygroscopic nature of the product. Of the two evils, probably the former was the less.

MR. A. J. JONES detected a superior odour and colour in a sample made with 70 per cent. spirit.

MR. POWELL affirmed that the choice of air-dried starch, if decided upon, would be a wise one, its normal moisture content making for practical uniformity in the varying circumstances in which the extract would be made. He disagreed with the reason of inconvenience as a factor in recommending a diluent other than powdered leaf. Therapeutic use, not convenience, should be the criterion. Keeping power, on the other hand, would be a definite argument. It was a pity, he said, that the B.P. limited the proportion of stem to 20 per cent.

MR. MOORHOUSE, in reply, admitted that all his tests had been made with one sample of crude drug. Similar results had, however, been subsequently obtained with three other samples. He could not hold out any hope, from his experience, that a finer powder than a No. 22 would be practicable. He had found that a homogeneous extract could be made quite satisfactorily and without difficulty using starch as a diluent. His reasons for not using leaf as diluent had not been given in order of importance, and he agreed that therapeutic value should be the chief determining factor.

The next paper was:—

Determination of Cod-Liver Oil in Cod-Liver Oil and Malt Extract

By C. GUNN AND P. F. R. VENABLES

[ABSTRACT]

A METHOD is described for the isolation and quantitative determination of cod-liver oil in extract of malt with cod-liver oil by judicious use of solvents. Precipitation of the dextrin with alcohol of various strengths was tried, and an alcohol of from 70 to 75 per cent. strength was found to give best results. It was not found possible by the authors to standardise the method by the use of solvents alone, but the difficulty was met by precipitating the dextrin in the presence of a small amount of purified kaolin. The results obtained showed a high degree of accuracy. The method has the added advantages that it takes only three hours to complete the assay, and the vitamin content of the oil remains unaffected. The Committee and Principal of Leicester College of Technology are thanked for affording facilities for investigation.

DISCUSSION

THE CHAIRMAN, in inviting discussion, remarked that this was an important paper.

MR. POWELL inquired whether any trials had been made on malt extract alone. About 0.2-0.3 per cent. of an oily extract was obtainable from malt.

MR. EVERS thought the author's method a useful one. With the Rose-Gottlieb method there was sometimes a little trouble.

MR. GUNN, in reply, said that no blanks had been applied. In some cases the results obtained were slightly high. It was found that samples allowed to stand before estimation of blue value yielded none.

The next paper, presented by Mr. R. R. Bennett in the absence of the author through illness, was:—

The Detection of Rhapontic Rhubarb in Galenical Rhubarb Preparations

By SYDNEY K. CREWS

[ABSTRACT]

UPON the knowledge that rhapontic rhubarb contains a fluorescent principle not present in the official varieties and capable of being absorbed on cellulose giving a bright blue fluorescence, the author bases a series of experiments in determining the presence of the unofficial drug in various galenical preparations.

BRITISH PHARMACEUTICAL CONFERENCE 1936

He finds that its presence in galenical rhubarb preparations can be demonstrated with ease, even in very small quantities. The fluorescence test was carried out on a large number of different drugs and galenicals, and of those examined only rhapontic rhubarb gave positive results. Rhapontic rhubarb was found in many galenicals of British and Continental origin, often in amounts suggesting gross adulteration. Attempts to isolate the fluorescent principle are described. Starting in the opposite direction, the author extracted and purified rhaponticin and examined it for physical constants, including ultra-violet absorption. His conclusion was that the absorption fluorescence reaction was due to the presence of rhaponticin. Acknowledgment is made to the directors of The British Drug Houses, Ltd., and to Mr. J. H. Singer.

DISCUSSION

THE CHAIRMAN stated that it was a pity, from the public's point of view, that the sources of the galenicals had not been disclosed.

DR. CROSSLEY-HOLLAND quoted Mr. Bennett's remark that there appeared to be more tannin in the rhapontic than in the official rhubarb, and wondered whether the effect would actually be essentially different. The action of rhubarb was at first aperient, and this was followed by an astringent action not entirely due to tannic acid. He inquired if rhapontic rhubarb had been fully tested clinically; action of some kind was proved by its veterinary applications. It was not always chemical constituents that determined the inclusion of a drug in the Pharmacopœia.

MR. WRAGG asked if Mr Bennett, on behalf of Mr. Crews, could confirm the work of Mr. T. E. Wallis reported at the Conference in 1934. The substance of this was that the fluorescent properties of rhapontic rhubarb underwent modification after exposure.

MR. POWELL asked if any steps had been taken to make the test quantitative. So delicate a reaction as that resulting from one part in three millions did not prove adulteration. The curve given seemed to suggest the possibility of quantitative estimation.

THE CHAIRMAN interpolated a reference to the paper read in 1928 at the International Congress of Pharmacy showing that rhapontic rhubarb had only one-third the activity of the Chinese variety.

MR. BENNETT, in reply, quoted a paragraph in the paper suggesting how tests could be applied showing a very fair approximation to the proportions in which the drug was contained. He admitted that there was much work still to be done. He could not speak, in the absence of Mr. Crews, on the loss of fluorescence.

The next paper, presented by Mr. A. J. Jones in the absence of the author, was:—

Notes on the so-called Magnesium Trisilicate

By NORMAN GLASS

[ABSTRACT]

A GOOD deal has been heard about magnesium trisilicate or "synthetic sepiolite," since the publication of three papers by Mutch at the beginning of this year. It is unusual to employ the term "synthetic" in connection with inorganic salts, but on this occasion such use might be justified as indicating that the laboratory preparation has been made to simulate the composition of sepiolite, while admitting that the actual constitution of the two bodies is not necessarily identical. In the papers already referred to, consideration is primarily given to the properties which magnesium trisilicate exhibits as a mild alkali and absorbent, and how these can be employed for the treatment of peptic ulcer and other gastric complaints. The formula quoted by Mutch is $Mg_2Si_3O_8,xH_2O$, so that the term "tri" merely refers to the number of silicon atoms. This formula may be re-written $2MgO,3SiO_2,xH_2O$. There being at present no recognised standards for magnesium trisilicate, it seems desirable that an indication of the power of the substance, as shown by its analysis, should be given by the manufacturer by whom it is issued. Tests were selected in conformity with two of those employed by Mutch, namely, digestion with acid, and absorption of methylene blue. In addition to these tests, the loss on ignition, and the estimation of silica and magnesium were also performed.

There is no uniformity about the samples in the author's first table, and this points to the absence of a really definite simple compound which can easily be prepared, and to the existence of a material of uncertain constitution. The case is somewhat analogous to that of the magnesium, zinc, and bismuth carbonates of pharmacy. These compounds come out true to type for a given method of preparation so long as the conditions are strictly adhered to, but their chemical composition and their physical properties are determined by the method of preparation. Silica forms many complex alliances of this kind, and the vast array of siliceous minerals is ample testimony to this. The examination of a number of precipitates obtained by the action of magnesium sulphate upon sodium silicate solutions indicated that the primary effect of the addition of a metallic salt was the precipitation of silica; this silica then combined with or absorbed or occluded a certain amount of magnesia, and the extent of this depends upon the opportunity for contact and reaction. Tables show the analyses of twelve different substances prepared in the laboratory. It is considered to be a virtue of magnesium trisilicate that its acid-neutralising properties are gradually manifested, and in the very nature of a water insoluble compound this is only to be expected. If patients were given certain native carbonates of magnesium instead of the usual pharmaceutical preparation, little or no effect would be felt because some of these materials require days of digestion before they are attacked by dilute acid. A comparative test was performed on one of the samples, light and heavy carbonate of magnesia, light oxide of magnesia, and precipitated calcium carbonate, for the rate of neutralisation, by digesting them at 37° C. with excess of decinormal hydrochloric acid. The calcium carbonate, the light magnesium carbonate and the light magnesium oxide dissolved almost instantaneously, but the heavy carbonate of magnesia required about ten minutes for complete solution. At the end of this period the silicate sample was removed from the bath and back titrated. It was found that 88.0 per cent. of the magnesium shown by the standard test outlined above had been neutralised. The conclusion might be formed that there was not a great deal of difference between the rate of neutralisation of magnesium trisilicate and heavy carbonate of magnesia. Such comparisons depend to a large extent on the excess of acid present. There are certain discrepancies in the analyses which call for some explanation. (This work has been carried out in the laboratory of Evans Sons Lescher & Webb, Ltd., Liverpool, by whose permission the paper is published.)

DISCUSSION

THE CHAIRMAN pointed out that obviously a substance of this sort should be uniform.

DR. CROSSLEY-HOLLAND congratulated the author not only on the amount of work done but also on its timeliness. Acidity seemed to be much on the increase, and there was a great tendency to use antacids—salts of magnesium and other alkaloids. The trisilicate was much to be preferred to the carbonate, not only from a chemical standpoint but also on the ground that carbonates could be positively dangerous in certain conditions of the stomach and heart. The paper was a step in the right direction, that of products in forms in which the greatest value was given.

MR. A. J. JONES pointed out that the adsorptive property of magnesium trisilicate with methylene blue might have a different character from that in the stomach. Samples varied much in palatability, some being difficult to swallow. Elegance in pharmacy might be destructive of efficacy, and he hoped this would not happen in the present instance.

MR. POWELL pointed out that there was a considerable difference in the adsorptive properties of different samples mentioned.

MR. R. R. BENNETT said that in his experience it was very difficult to obtain a precipitate which, when dry, was consistently adsorbent.

MR. WRAGG thought that one test was not entirely accurate in the presence of much magnesium.

MR. EVERS suggested that the methylene blue test should preferably be carried out with an excess of methylene blue rather than by the author's method.

MR. JONES, replying on behalf of the author, said he had chosen analytical methods that would be diagnostic at once. He had gone sufficiently far to be able to differentiate samples as suitable and unsuitable. Mr. Evers was very likely correct.

BRITISH PHARMACEUTICAL CONFERENCE 1936

He (Mr. Jones) would like to see other methods of analysis tried. He learned that one manufacturer had added kaolin to magnesium trisilicate in order to increase its adsorptive properties: in doing so he was lessening its antacid value.

The author of the last two papers allotted to this session was absent, and they were taken as read.

Isotonic Solutions for Injection

By F. Wokes

[Abstract]

Tests show that a fairly accurate end-point is discernible in determining the hæmolysing concentration of solutions of sodium chloride and other substances. The author tabulates results found with solutions of sodium chloride, ranging from 0.40 per cent. to 0.50 per cent., on one sample of blood, showing that the hæmolysing concentration corresponds to a figure of 0.475 per cent. Some variation was found with other samples. The hæmolysing concentrations of a number of other substances were determined and compared with their isotonic concentrations. The conclusion is reached that if hæmolysis of normal blood is produced by a solution when diluted with not more than half its volume of distilled water, such a solution is probably not isotonic. Most of the substances recommended by the B.P.C. for the preparation of isotonic solutions are found to have an isotonic hæmolysing ratio equal to, if not greater than, sodium chloride, but it is suggested that boric acid, which produced hæmolysis in every concentration, should be removed from the list. The advice of Dr. G. A. Harrison of St. Bartholomew's Hospital is acknowledged. (From the Pharmacological Laboratory of the College of the Pharmaceutical Society.)

An All-Glass Bacteria-Proof Filter

By F. Wokes

[Abstract]

Advantages such as the avoidance of danger of metallic contamination; ready control of the pressure applied; ease of sterilisation and low cost are claimed for an apparatus described by the author. Essentially, it consists of a glass barrel, flanged at its lower end, separated by Seitz filter-pad, perforated glass disc and rubber washer from a thistle funnel flanged at its upper end, the flanges being clamped together to form a bacteria-proof joint by means of a metal screw-collar. Air under pressure is supplied from a gauge-fitted flask connected, through a tyre valve, to a bicycle pump.

Discussion

Mr. Treves Brown called attention to the fact that certain figures in Table III of the published paper had been based on figures taken from the B.P.C., 1934. These figures had themselves been taken from published researches, but had been incorrectly transferred into the Codex. A figure of 1.12 under potassium sulphate should be 2.11; 1.4 therefore became 2.6. These figures should be taken into account.

The Chairman declared the proceedings of the Section adjourned to Thursday morning, June 25.

Science Session

Thursday Morning, June 25

The Chairman commenced the proceedings on June 25 by asking Mr. G. J. W. Ferrey to present his paper entitled:—

The Determination of Manganese in Iron and Manganese Citrate

By G. J. W. Ferrey

[Abstract]

The B.P.C. method of assay of iron and manganese citrate is defective, owing to the formation of manganese oxides as a heavy brown precipitate. The author investigates the titration of permanganic acid with arsenite under various conditions and determines correct conditions for the complete oxidation of manganese to permanganic acid. Citric acid is shown to interfere with the conversion of manganous salts to permanganic acid. Details of a modification of the Codex method by alternate oxidation and reduction are given.—(From the Analytical Laboratory of James Woolley, Sons & Co., Ltd.).

Discussion

The Chairman remarked that the paper formed a valuable contribution: many experiments must have been needed to clear up the difficulties of the Codex method of assay.

Mr. Powell said that he had noted the low results obtained with certain samples.

The next two papers were presented by Mr. R. R. Bennett:—

Anomalous Viscosity of Tragacanth Mucilage

By G. Middleton

[Abstract]

Although the number of contributions to the study of the viscosity of tragacanth mucilage might appear to suggest that there is little room for further investigation, in reality the subject has not been by any means completely explored; and a general survey of previous work, while revealing much of interest and value, fails to give the complete picture of viscosity relations of the mucilage which is necessary to enable standard methods for determining it to be specified. It has been shown that tragacanth mucilage, like many other lyophilic colloidal solutions such as those of starch, agar, gelatin, nitrocellulose, does not show a true viscosity independent of the rate of flow, but has the property of "anomalous" or "variable" viscosity, i.e., the ratio between applied pressure (rate of shear) and rate of flow is not constant but decreases rapidly as the rate of shear increases. It is therefore impossible to express the viscosity of a tragacanth mucilage by any single figure, but the conditions under which it has been determined must also be specified. The author illustrates his experiments with graphs, diagrams, and five tables. His summary is as follows:—

1. Mucilage of tragacanth does not show thixotropy. Anomalies in viscosity determinations are ascribed to a new phenomenon to which the name of "stream orientation" is given. This is apparently due to orientation of long colloidal particles in the line of flow, and is manifested by an abnormally high reading for the time of all of the first of a series of balls through the mucilage.

2. The effect of accurately defined conditions of heating has been investigated. These conditions cannot be attained by immersing a flask in boiling water.

3. Results showing the effect of dilution and temperature on the apparent viscosity are recorded. The curves relating dilution with the logarithms of the time of fall (falling sphere viscometer) for different grades of gum form approximately a series of parallel straight lines.

The author thanks the directors of The British Drug Houses, Ltd., in whose laboratories the investigation has been carried out, for permission to publish the results.

Standardisation of Tragacanth

By G. Middleton

[Abstract]

The definition of tragacanth in the British Pharmacopœia may be considered to exclude all but first-class samples of the whole gum, but not of powder, for which no definite characters are prescribed. In order to ensure uniformity it is, therefore, necessary to fix a limit for the viscosity of the mucilage. The "viscosity" of tragacanth mucilage is not a definite constant, and it is inaccurate to apply to it the units of viscosity derived from the theory of normal viscous flow. The following is given as a draft specification for a limit test for the strength of powdered tragacanth:—

Add 6 gm. of the gum to 444 gm. of water in a bottle of about 1 litre capacity and allow to stand for two hours or until completely softened. With the aid of suction pass the mixture repeatedly, until uniform, through a strainer of metal gauze, of approximately ⅜ in. diameter and mesh equivalent to the standard sieve No. 36 of the British Pharmacopœia. Allow to stand overnight, adjust the temperature to 20° C. and remove air bubbles by evacuating the air from the bottle,

BRITISH PHARMACEUTICAL CONFERENCE 1936

shaking violently and allowing to stand for five minutes Release the vacuum, and fill the viscometer tube with the mucilage by pouring it down the side of the tube in such a way that no bubbles of air are entrapped. Insert the centralising tube axially, and adjust the apparatus to be exactly vertical. Drop down the centralising tube a steel ball of ⅛ in. diameter and 0.129 to 0.130 gm. in weight. When, or after, the ball has reached the lowest mark allow another ball to fall in a similar manner and time its fall between the highest and lowest marks on the tube, repeating the operation until two successive balls do not show more than 2 per cent. difference in their time of fall. Calculate the mean time of fall per 5 cm. for these two balls. This must not be less than 40 seconds for samples of powdered tragacanth. For whole gum the concentration employed for the limit test should be 1 + 89, the time of 40 seconds being unchanged.

The author thanks the directors of The British Drug Houses, Ltd., in whose laboratories the investigation has been carried out, for permission to publish the results.

Discussion

The Chairman pointed out that a good deal of discussion on this subject had already taken place. Mr. Middleton's paper showed a considerable advance. Tragacanth was not a definite chemical substance but a breakdown of certain tissues; probably some cells from the plant remained in it, and that might be the reason why grinding reduced the viscosity. Pharmacists should realise how much powdering spoils tragacanth. For practical purposes it should be as coarse as possible, not the No. 120 powder usually asked for.

Mr. Brindle agreed with the author as to the effect of heating on viscosity. He suggested that the author was treating the mucilage by a method not in use in the pharmacy. He (Mr. Brindle) had found that he could obtain concordant results by allowing the mucilage to stand for forty-eight hours In one respect he had found a difference of 400 per cent. when using powdered tragacanth. In the author's viscometer the sphere has a diameter of ⅛ in. and the tube of approximately 1 in.; the diameter, however, should be at least ten times that of the falling ball. It was not easy to keep the apparatus (shown in one of the figures) at constant temperature.

Mr. Lescher doubted the relevance of the new expression "stream orientation." As "orientation" literally meant "turning to the east," he hoped that the word would be used in pharmacy only when it meant exactly what its derivation implied.

Mr. Ferrey asked for an exact definition of the factors A, B, C, D in the first equation.

Mr. Frank Browne inquired if there was a possibility of a low viscosity of mucilage being raised by the substance to which it was added.

Mr. Brindle said he was able to throw light on that problem. He had found a difference in the suspending power of tragacanth when certain powders—e.g., calcium carbonate—were added to the mixture in which it was used.

Mr. Bennett, replying on behalf of the author, thanked Mr. Brindle for clearing up one point. He agreed with the chairman on the question of powdered tragacanth: he wished pharmacists could be persuaded to buy this gum in coarse powder. He had never come across a subject which gave rise to so much mild abuse from pharmacists as this question of powdered tragacanth. (Laughter.) He agreed that the author's paper was not the last word, and thanked Mr. Lescher and Mr. Ferrey for their remarks

The next paper was:—

Acriflavine: Solubility and Diaminoacridine Content

By G. F. Hall and A. D. Powell

[Abstract]

The solubility of acriflavine is examined in relation to diaminoacridine content, heat, acidity, and the presence of tarry impurities. The tests described show that solubility is greater with increasing proportions of diaminoacridine dihydrochloride up to 50 per cent. Solutions effected by heat precipitate more slowly, owing to supersaturation. Solutions prepared in the cold show decreasing solubility on standing; the effect is due to hydrolysis. Acidity should not be in excess of a figure equivalent to 1 per cent. of free hydrochloric acid. Acriflavine as usually prepared, which has a diaminoacridine dihydrochloride content of from 30 to 40 per cent., is declared sufficiently soluble for practical requirements. Solubility is affected by the presence of tarry impurities, which render supersaturation more permanent. This, it is stated, is probably the reason why acriflavine, as made to-day, occasionally gives trouble when attempts are made to keep it in concentrated solution. Methods of determining the amount of unmethylated constituent present in acriflavine are discussed; inaccuracies inherent in an electrometric method proposed by one investigator and difficulties in employing a colorimetric method suggested by the same analyst are enumerated. Acknowledgments are made to Boots Pure Drug Co., Ltd., for permission to publish the results, and to Mr. L. R. Ellison for analytical work.

Discussion

The Chairman said that one psychological point arose out of the paper—he referred to the idea that the greater the purity of acriflavine the better. The idea was probably due to subconscious religious associations. (Laughter.) Chemically pure water and chemically pure alcohol were not suitable as beverages. He thought there was a tendency on the part of B.P. compilers to require absence of harmless impurities in an unnecessary degree.

Mr. Treves Brown remarked that there had been complaints in the medical Press of the differing effects of different varieties of acriflavine used intravenously. Had Mr. Powell any information on this point?

Mr. Bull inquired if light had any effect on acriflavine solutions.

Mr. Nutter Smith asked for an explanation of variation in colour.

Mr. Powell, in reply, said that chemical purity was not necessarily a desirable end, but when a chemical could be pure it was as well to have it so. He did not know anything of the differences which caused differing effects. All solutions of acriflavine deposited on standing in light. Variations in colour were probably due to physical differences in composition.

The next paper taken was:—

The Quantitative Determination of Mercury in its Compounds

By H. Brindle and C. E. Waterhouse

[Abstract]

Methods for the determination of mercury in several compounds of mercury are enumerated, examined and discussed. A new volumetric method, to which the title "Reduction Thiocyanate Process" is given, is described. By this process the mercury salt in solution is precipitated as metallic mercury by means of alkaline formaldehyde; the precipitated mercury is collected on a sinter-glass filter, dissolved in nitric acid and titrated with ammonium thiocyanate solution. The process is shown to be applicable in the presence of substances which interfere with most methods for the determination of mercury. It is recommended that calcium chloride be added in the official process for the assay of mercuric chloride to obtain the precipitated mercury in a finely divided form which is readily soluble in the $N/10$ iodine used. The process is a modification of Rupp's method (reduction to metal with alkaline formaldehyde, addition of acetic acid and solution in $N/10$ iodine), and is shown to be applicable to other mercuric compounds. In all cases in which Rupp's method is employed, the addition of calcium chloride is recommended.—(From the Pharmacy Department, Manchester University.)

Discussion

The Chairman pointed out that the determination of mercury was probably one of the earliest operations of the kind, but there was still room for improvement.

Mr. Waterhouse said that since the paper was in type the authors had carried out the quantitative separation of arsenic and mercury in Donovan's solution, and in using their new method of determination the results were only 0.3 per

BRITISH PHARMACEUTICAL CONFERENCE 1936

cent. too low. Precipitation of the sulphide from alkaline solutions in presence of iodides gave results at least 0.5 per cent. high. It appeared that the method was widely applicable.

MR. BERNARD F. HOWARD remarked that all modern methods of determination tended to be volumetric rather than gravimetric. He had attacked thirty-three years ago one of the operations now mentioned in the authors' paper. When dealing with complicated volumetric methods much work had to be done in correcting them.

MR. BATESON said he could confirm the authors' conclusions, as he had made independent experiments.

MR. POWELL congratulated the authors on their work It was very desirable that British Pharmacopœia methods should be co-ordinated if possible. The use of too much reagent gave undesirable results. He had had no difficulty with Rupp's method, but the authors' appeared to be more foolproof. He inquired whether Mr. Brindle had obtained higher results by Rupp's method—a circumstance probably due, he thought, to the formaldehyde used.

DR. BULLOCK pointed out the importance of adding calcium chloride. He had had a series of estimations carried out in duplicate: with the B.P. method the error was anything up to 7 per cent., but with the new method the results were creditably accurate.

MR. A J. JONES remarked that mercury appeared to have derived one attribute from the deity who gave it its name: it appeared in different forms. The personal equation counted for something. Perhaps a committee might be appointed to correlate the results of different workers and to fix a maximum allowance of error. The reduced zinc method for mercuric iodide was rather a nuisance sometimes.

MR. BRINDLE, replying, referred to the factor of speed in choosing volumetric rather than gravimetric methods. Possibly Mr. Howard's attack of thirty-three years ago had not been given sufficient publicity, as the method in question had got into text-books. In the authors' method the mercury was precipitated in the vessel in which the filtration was carried out. He thought the difficulty with Rupp's method was due to acetic acid.

The next paper, which the author humorously described as "a querulous fragment," was:—

Standardisation of Tablets in the Swiss Pharmacopœia

BY BERNARD F. HOWARD

[ABSTRACT]

THE Pharmacopœia Helvetica V, which was published in 1934, is of absorbing interest to the student of pharmacopœias in that it contains certain interesting features which are absent from our own Pharmacopœia and which may to some extent express the trend of pharmaceutical opinion on the Continent. Most interesting of all innovations is perhaps the definite attempt of the new Swiss Pharmacopœia to standardise a number of tablet preparations in separate monographs and also the insertion of a separate monograph on the preparation and character of pharmaceutical products in tablet form under the title "Compressi." It is not perhaps strictly correct to refer to this as an innovation, since the Swedish edition X, published in 1925, and the Danish Pharmacopœia of 1933 both contain some remarks on tablets, but the Swiss have now carried the matter so much further that it becomes worthy of careful consideration in this country.

In the monograph on "Compressi," no specific instructions are given for the preparation of the granule for the tablet machine, but merely a general caveat that no admixture of any substance likely to exert any chemical action on the material must be used. There follows a disintegration test for tablets intended for internal use. In this country such tests have been used for many years, but in the absence of any official edict, each worker has fixed his own arbitrary standard, some ridiculously lax, and some equally ludicrously severe. Such tests have often been distorted to provide stunt experiments for propaganda purposes and a situation has arisen which is, to say the least of it, undignified and also extremely unsatisfactory for both buyer and seller. The author thinks that pharmacists should welcome this departure of our Swiss friends, which should go far to clear the air on the subject in their own fortunate country. This monograph on "Compressi" apparently applies to all tablets of substances mentioned in the Pharmacopœia intended for internal use. Immediately following it appear a number of separate monographs dealing with various substances in tablet form, presumably representing the tablets in commonest use in Switzerland or at any rate those in which special standardisation is considered important. The author deals in detail with that entitled "Compressi Acidi Acetylosalicylici." This Pharmacopœia has taken a definite step towards controlling the dosage of certain tablets in common use. The latest foreign Pharmacopœia, the U.S.P. XI, which only came into force on June 1, 1936, has also made a beginning in this direction and has standardised hyd. perchlor. tablets and trinitrin tablets in separate monographs. In this country no such step has been taken, and the correct standardisation of pharmaceutical preparations in tablet form is left to the manufacturers on the one hand, and the pharmacists on the other, to settle amongst themselves. As analytical control of chemicals becomes each year more thorough and more exacting, the need for a voice of authority becomes even more urgent.

DISCUSSION

THE CHAIRMAN described the introduction of this standardisation into the Swiss Pharmacopœia as important: it was unsatisfactory, he added, that a matter of this kind should be left to the discretion of magistrates.

MR. J. F. SIMON suggested that this subject should have been discussed years ago. A retailer might change his source of supply and receive tablets nominally identical but actually of different size and weight Poisonous tablets should be labelled with skull and crossbones. He thought the allowance of fifteen minutes for disintegration far too liberal.

MR. CORFIELD thought the Americans had made no advance in this respect in the U.S.P. XI. They had standardised nitroglycerin tablets and introduced two others. N.F. VI includes, he added, a large number of monographs of little value from the point of view of tablets. The British Pharmacopœia was in a worse position. He had suggested to the Pharmaceutical Commission some years ago the standardisation of common tablets, but the reception of his suggestion indicated greater interest in the manufacturer than in the retailer. In the B.P. monograph on aspirin the test for free salicylic acid was of little importance. It was impossible to apply any of these B P. tests to aspirin tablets: if they took the B.P. standards they would have to condemn a large proportion of aspirin tablets. The proposed Addendum devoted much attention to things rarely seen in a chemist's shop—vitamins, serums and so forth—and ignored common substances. He could confirm Mr. Simon's experience from his own records. The average weight of 5-gr. aspirin tablets in hundreds of samples tested varied from 5.36 gr. to 6.55 gr.; that of 5-gr. phenacetin tablets from 5.41 gr. to 6.63 gr; that of phenacetin and caffeine tablets similarly; that of 2-gr. quinine sulphate tablets (sugar-coated) from 2.24 gr. to 6.15 gr.—and he was excluding samples in which the medicament was not present in the proper proportion; that of 1-gr. calomel tablets from 1.25 gr. to 2.24 gr.; and that of 2-gr. calomel tablets from 2.21 gr. to 4.56 gr. Another feature was that ½-gr. calomel tablets might weigh 1 gr., while ¾-gr. tablets weighed 1½ gr. and ¼-gr. tablets weighed 2 gr.

MR. R. R. BENNETT said they were greatly indebted to Mr. Howard for introducing an important subject—a subject well worth consideration. He endorsed a good deal of what Mr. Corfield had said.

MR. SIMMONS gave as an example the trouble caused by ephedrine hydrochloride tablets, which were commonly dispensed in ¼-gr., ½-gr. and 1-gr. strengths. It sometimes happened that the ½-gr. tablets of one manufacturer were larger than the 1-gr. tablets of another manufacturer, and patients might be upset. The excuse given was faulty parts of the machinery.

MR. J. C. YOUNG inquired whether the Science Section could take into consideration the varying sizes of capsules, particularly machine-made ones.

MR. NUTTER SMITH pointed out that if a 2-gr. sugar-coated quinine tablet weighed only 2.24 gr., the coating must be extremely thin. Tablets containing medicament weighing less than 1 gr. were usually made up to 1 gr. Punches would

BRITISH PHARMACEUTICAL CONFERENCE 1936

become worn, but with proper analytical control these discrepancies should not arise. In the new Swiss process of extracting with ether, it seemed to him that citric and tartaric acids, if present, might come out to some extent with the aspirin. Tablets for hypodermic injection should dissolve in 15 seconds or less.

MR. F. W. M. BENNETT, speaking as a practising pharmacist, thanked Mr. Howard for bringing forward such a subject. The appearance of a tablet was not a primary object. Calomel tablets were sometimes inactive, owing, he suggested, to undue compression. In the case of Easton's syrup tablets, the amount of sugar coating might determine whether or not they were in the First Schedule.

MR. POWELL pointed out that Mr. Liverseege, in his recent book, had made some reasonable suggestions for variation in accuracy of dosage. Calomel must not be compressed too tightly nor too loosely.

DR BULLOCK inquired as to the exact meaning of the expression "shake the flask gently from time to time." Further, was the addition of hydrochloric acid a question of being realistic?

MR. FRANK BROWNE asked whether Mr. Howard would consent to taking two decimals off the "5.0000 gr." in the paper An analyst should make several examinations of a substance, not one or two only.

MR. HOWARD, replying, said he was delighted to find that his grievance was shared by many fellow-sufferers. He held no brief for the Swiss Pharmacopœia, and in it capsules were not tackled. Perhaps it would be wise to take up the question of tablets first in this country.

The last paper taken at this session was.—

Effect on the Isolated Heart of the Preservative Present in Insulin Solutions, B.P.

By M. M. O. BARRIE

[ABSTRACT]

INSULIN, in amounts equivalent to sixteen times the normal dose, causes a very small increase in the size of the beat of the isolated rabbit heart. In normal dose it has no effect. One mil of solution containing cresol or phenol was found by the author to cause, in the concentration in which these are normally used as preservatives, a marked decrease in the size of the heart beat. The help of Dr. S. W. F. Underhill and the permission of the proprietors of Insulin AB for permission to publish the work are acknowledged —(From the Insulin AB Physiological Laboratories, London)

DISCUSSION

THE CHAIRMAN pointed out that a high degree of purity in these solutions was obviously desirable.

MR. FERGUSON gathered from the author's observations that preservative in such solutions was undesirable.

MISS BARRIE, in reply, said that those who bought and used insulin did not read the label and notice the presence of 3 per cent. of phenols.

THE CHAIRMAN thanked the authors of the papers, and adjourned the proceedings to the afternoon.

Science Session

Thursday Afternoon

At the concluding meeting of the Science Section only two papers were left for presentation; both were read in summarised form by Mr. Morton.

Determination of Official Preparations of Iron by Means of Ceric Sulphate. Assay of Saccharated Iron Carbonate

BY C. G. LYONS AND F. N. APPLEYARD

[ABSTRACT]

THE oxidising action of ceric sulphate and its suitability for use in volumetric reactions are discussed. Its application to the assay of saccharated iron carbonate is considered, ferrous-orthophenanthroline being suggested as indicator. The method recommended is to dissolve about 0 5 gm. of the saccharated iron carbonate by heating it with about 20 mils of dilute sulphuric acid. After cooling, one drop of ferrous-orthophenanthroline sulphate solution is added as indicator, and the solution titrated with standardised approximately decinormal ceric sulphate solution until the orange colour just disappears. The method is convenient and gives a very sharp end-point; methods involving titration with potassium dichromate are described as less accurate. The acid used to dissolve the saccharated iron carbonate causes considerable variation in the proportion of iron retained in the ferrous condition; it is recommended that sulphuric should be used instead of phosphoric acid. Other indicators were tested and found less suitable. The assistance of Hopkin & Williams, Ltd., is acknowledged.—(From the Department of Pharmacy, Bradford Technical College.)

Assay of Saccharated Iron Compounds

By C. MORTON and D. C. HARROD

[ABSTRACT]

IN the determination of ferrous iron by titration with potassium dichromate, both potassium ferricyanide as external and diphenylamine as internal indicators yield high results in the presence of carbohydrates. The authors demonstrate that during the titration with potassium dichromate, oxidation of iron and glucose proceed side by side, and not, as previously believed, in successive stages. It follows that, however the indicator is varied or the procedure modified, no significant improvement can be expected if potassium dichromate is used. It is confirmed that ferrous iron may be accurately determined in saccharated iron compounds by means of sodium iodate, the glucose having no disturbing effect on titrations with this oxidising agent. A grant from the Dixon fund of the University of London is acknowledged.—(From the Chelsea school of Pharmacy.)

Mr. Morton remarked wherever (as was sometimes inevitable) duplication between these two papers had occurred, there had been reasonable agreement. The dichromate method must now be regarded as empirical.

DISCUSSION

THE CHAIRMAN said that when he was working with the late Mr. William Martindale prior to the publication of the 1898 Pharmacopœia, they found that in the assay of pilula ferri their results were too high. This led to the substitution of phosphoric acid for sulphuric acid in the estimation of saccharated iron compounds in that Pharmacopœia.

MR FERREY, after pointing out a textual error in the first equation in the first of the two papers, asked whether the indicator used by Dr. Lyons and Mr. Appleyard kept well and whether it was available. If the ceric sulphate method was accurate, he thought it preferable to the iodate method.

MR. CORFIELD said it was a good thing to have some definite information on ferrous iron. It was difficult to judge a Blaud pill on the ferrous iron itself.

MR. MORTON, in reply, said that the substitution of phosphoric acid for sulphuric acid, referred to by the chairman, had no effect on the oxidation of carbohydrate, but made the end-point clearer. The indicator of Dr. Lyons and Mr. Appleyard was not obtainable in this country, and he did not know its keeping properties. Ceric sulphate, which was coming into rather extensive use, was an interesting oxidant from the physical point of view. The ceric sulphate was more rapid than the iodate titration, but on the other hand the iodate was obtainable in a state of great purity. The authors were concerned only with B.P. standards. It might be suggested that the estimation of total iron should replace that of ferrous iron in the Pharmacopœia.

THE CHAIRMAN, in closing the proceedings, expressed the thanks of the Section to the authors for their contributions, and to the Pharmaceutical Society for the books giving the text of the papers.

BRITISH PHARMACEUTICAL CONFERENCE 1936

Closing Session

The closing session of the Conference was held in the Grand Hall of the Town Hall on the afternoon of June 25, Mr. Harold Deane (chairman) presiding.

THE CHAIRMAN called on the senior general secretary (Mr. C. E. Corfield) to read the annual report of the Executive Committee.

ANNUAL REPORT OF THE EXECUTIVE

The seventy-third annual report of the Executive, read by Mr. C. E. Corfield (senior general secretary), included the following passages:—

Members of the Conference elected by the Executive, known formerly as corresponding members, have in the past paid an annual subscription of 10s. 6d., which has entitled them to the full privileges of Membership and to receive the Quarterly Journal on application without further payment. Your Executive have accepted a proposal by the Council of the Society that such elected members be asked to pay annually a subscription of £1 1s, and at this meeting a proposal to modify Rule 6 will be submitted for your approval.

The Executive regret to report the deaths of several members of Conference, including Mr. Francis Ransom, one of its vice-presidents. Mr. Ransom was president during 1909-1910, in which period the Conference held its annual meeting in Cambridge, and he served the Conference as an honorary general secretary from 1890 to 1903. By his death the British Pharmaceutical Conference has lost one of its most enthusiastic supporters and one who for many years worked with untiring devotion for its advancement, particularly on the scientific side of its activities The generous offer to provide funds for the establishment of the Ransom Fellowship, which is tenable for a period of two years in the Society's laboratories, and the sum of £200 which he left to the Benevolent Fund, illustrate his munificence and his interest in the welfare of pharmacy and pharmacist.

The following subjects require examination or further investigation:

Aconitine.—The composition of commercial aconitine and the methods of standardising aconitine and preparations of aconite.

Alcohol in Galenicals.—Suitable limits for the alcohol content of concentrated infusions and fluid extracts of the B P.C.

Anchusa Root.—The nature of the colouring matters present in anchusa root and Syrian alkanet.

Antiseptics.—The difference in action, if any, between sparingly soluble antiseptics (such as the more complex phenols) in solution and suspension.

Apiol.—Liquid apiol of commerce, with a view to setting up a standard for this article so as to reduce the variation, which appears to be very considerable.

Ash of Crude Drugs.—The value as a standard of the ratio of natural acid-insoluble ash to the total ash of crude drugs.

Barbitone Derivatives.—Qualitative tests for the distinction of barbitone derivatives.

Belladonna and Hyoscyamus—A process for the preparation of dry extracts of belladonna and hyoscyamus without added leaf

Belladonna Plaster—Assay processes for plasters made with a soap basis and for those made with a rubber basis.

Bismuth Salts.—The causes of discoloration of bismuth salts on exposure to light.

Calcium Phosphate.—The composition of calcium phosphate and methods of producing a more uniform product for pharmaceutical purposes.

Cannabis.—The relative activities of extracts and tinctures of cannabis prepared from comparatively fresh cannabis of Indian, African, American and other origin and the effect of storage of the drug upon the activity of the preparations

Cantharidin—The determination of cantharidin in the beetles and in galenicals.

Castor Oil.—The value, or otherwise, of a cooling test for this oil.

Chlorophyll—The composition of commercial chlorophyll.

Colloidal Solutions.—Practical methods or formulas for the preparation of colloidal solutions of elementary substances which are believed to possess valuable therapeutic effects.

Colouring Matters.—(*a*) The colours suitable for pharmaceutical products and their stability on keeping. (*b*) The processes for determining the tinctorial value of cochineal. (*c*) Comparison of the tinctorial values of litmus, cudbear and orchil.

Concentrated Infusions.—The means and substances used in the preservation of concentrated infusions.

Creosote—The composition of medicinal creosote

Crude Drugs—The significance of the official limits for "other organic matter" in unground drugs and methods by which the proportion of "other organic matter" may be determined in the same drugs in the form of powder.

Datura Metel.—The nature and composition of the alkaloids of *Datura Metel.*

Digitalis.—(*a*) A comparison of the results of digitalis assay by physiological and colorimetric methods with clinical effects (*b*) The stability of aqueous solutions containing the glycosides of digitalis.

Disinfectants.—Formulas for disinfectants containing halogen derivatives of phenols.

Drugs in Ultra-Violet Light—The behaviour of drugs and galenicals when exposed to ultra-violet light and the value of such observations for the identification of drugs and their determination in preparations.

Emulsifying Agents—Comparison of the emulsifying powers of different emulsifying agents under different conditions of preparation.

Ephedra.—The determination of ephedrine and pseudo-ephedrine in ephedra herb and the liquid extract prepared from it.

Ergot.—Further examination of ergometrine and the preparation and assay of galenicals containing it.

Extracts.—(*a*) The effect of varying p_H on fungoid growth in aqueous extractives (*b*) The effects produced by various methods (e.g evaporation *in vacuo*, in open air, etc) of concentrating percolates and other solutions of extractive matter, more especially as they affect the composition of their constituents. (*c*) Figures for the relation between the yields of unstandardised extracts and the weights of the drugs from which they are made. (*d*) The extension of the principle of preparing standardised liquid preparations by dissolving standardised solid extract in alcohol, as adopted for the cinchona preparations in the B P. 1932, to other drugs, e g. ipecacuanha, ergot and nux vomica.

Extraction of Crude Drugs.—(*a*) The extraction of crude drugs for the purpose of collecting data as to the relative proportions of active principle and inert material in progressive fractions with a view to determining the economic limits for extractions. (*b*) Data of the amount of extractive yielded by drugs to various menstrua, e.g. alcohol, water, ether, etc.

Extract of Liquorice—The determination of the characters of genuine liquid extract of liquorice.

Extract of Opium.—The processes of manufacture of dry extract of opium so as to reduce the loss of morphine by destruction.

Gland Products—Methods for the identification of animal substances and tissues in desiccated powder form and the possibility of applying pharmacognostic technique for the detection of adulteration, etc.

Glycerin.—The possibilities for increasing the use of glycerin in the preparation of galenicals.

Gums and Mucilages—Methods for the identification of these in mixtures are required.

Injections—Improved formulas for active injections of ergot and digitalis.

Iodised Oil.—Suitable processes for the preparation of products containing a high proportion of iodine in oil.

Limit-test for Sulphates.—The significance of the limit-test for sulphate as applied to various chemicals.

Liver Extract.—The nature of the active principle effective in the treatment of pernicious anæmia and a method of assay

Lobelia—The determination of the total alkaloids of lobelia and its galenical preparations.

Local Anæsthetics.—Qualitative tests for the distinction of local anæsthetics and a differentiation of their relative values in the different types of anæsthesia—spinal, dental, regional, etc.

Magnesium Oxides and Carbonates.—The composition of and impurities in commercial magnesium oxides and carbonates.

Medicinal Dyes.—Suitable qualitative or quantitative tests for controlling the purity of several organic dyestuffs used as colouring agents or for their therapeutic properties, viz. Bordeaux-B, Scarlet Red, Brilliant Green, Methyl Violet, etc.

Mercury with Chalk.—The methods of preparation and of storage of grey powder which will prevent the formation of mercuric compounds.

Mercury Determination.—Methods for the determination of mercury in strong ointment of mercuric nitrate and other mercury ointments, and in certain mercury salts.

Mezereum Bark.—The morphology and histology of various mezereum barks.

Microsublimation.—The value of microsublimation as a means of identifying crude drugs.

Misturæ—The effect of storage upon the stability of dispensed mixtures containing preparations of vegetable drugs, etc., with a view to formulating recommendations on the use of concentrated mixtures and mixtures not freshly or recently prepared.

Mucilaginous Seeds.—The histological characters of certain medicinal mucilaginous seeds of the orders Cruciferæ, Labiatæ, and Plantaginaceæ

Olive Oil—The determination and detection of tea-seed oil in olive oil.

Peptone—The composition of "peptones" suitable for hypodermic injection and other purposes.

Pill Coatings—Formulas for coatings for pills and tablets which will resist wholly the action of gastric secretions and dissolve in the contents of the small intestine, and at the same time have a sufficient degree of expansibility to guard against bursting under normal changes of temperature.

Poppy Capsules.—The re-examination and proximate analysis of poppy capsules.

Potassium Guaiacolsulphonate.—The quantitative determination of potassium guaiacolsulphonate.

BRITISH PHARMACEUTICAL CONFERENCE 1936

Preservatives.—The use of benzoic acid, benzoates and hydroxybenzoates as suitable preservatives for pharmaceutical preparations.

Purgative Drugs.—An examination of the methods of detection of drugs containing oxymethylanthraquinone derivatives in mixtures.

Quinine.—A method for the preparation of ammoniated quinine tablets

Readily Carbonisable Substances.—The sulphuric acid test for "readily carbonisable substances" in organic chemicals with a view to confirming its value as a practical test for purity.

Rhubarb.—Tests for distinguishing East Indian and rhapontic rhubarb and a method for the determination of rhapontic rhubarb in powdered rhubarb.

Senega Preparations.—Means of preventing the formation of deposits in preparations of senega and tests to show that they are of full strength and free from foreign saponin.

Senna Pods and Leaves.—An examination of the active constituents.

Silver Compounds.—The composition of and an investigation of the relative therapeutic actions of colloidal silver compounds and silver salts.

Sodium Morrhuate.—The preparation and standardisation of sodium morrhuate and solutions of sodium morrhuate for injection.

Solubilities.—Figures for the solubilities of a large number of pharmaceutical inorganic and organic chemicals in different solvents.

Solvents.—An investigation of the suitability of ethylene glycol, isopropyl alcohol and similar solvents for use in medicinal products.

Specific Gravities.—Figures for the specific gravity at 25°/25° C. of numerous pharmaceutical substances and preparations.

Sterilisation.—(*a*) An examination of the drugs which are given by injection in order to show (1) how far they are injured by heat sterilisation in aqueous solution, and (2) the stability or otherwise of aqueous solutions on storage. (*b*) The best type of material for apparatus used in the preparation of sterilised water for intravenous injection.

Storage.—(*a*) The effect of light on the physiological activity of quinine salts, apomorphine and other substances which become coloured on exposure or are readily oxidisable, with special reference to the conditions of storage. (*b*) The absorption spectra, visible and invisible, of the various types of glass used as containers.

Syrup of Iron Phosphate with Quinine and Strychnine.—An examination of Easton's syrup with a view to the prevention of colour.

Tin Oxide.—The composition of the compounds of tin suitable for internal administration.

Tragacanth.—The variability of powdered tragacanth and the elaboration of a standard method by which the purity of this drug may be controlled.

Valerian.—(*a*) The active principle of valerian root and an investigation of the difference in constituents of the British root and that from the Continent (*b*) The preparation of a so-called odourless liquid extract of valerian.

Twenty-two papers have been read and discussed at the science meetings, and the Executive desire to express their thanks to the authors of the papers, who have submitted valuable and interesting accounts of their researches to the Conference.

Names of members to form the Executive have, as usual, been recommended by a subcommittee appointed by the Executive, and a proposal will be submitted at this meeting that the following officers be appointed for 1936-37:—

Chairman: T. Edward Lescher *Vice-Presidents:* W. A. H. Naylor, J. F. Tocher, E. H. Farr, E. Saville Peck, David Hooper, W. Kirkby, C. A. Hill *Vice-Chairmen:* F. W. Gamble, D. Lloyd Howard, R. R. Bennett, J. H. Franklin, H. Skinner, C. H. Hampshire, F. W. Crossley-Holland, H. Deane. *Honorary Treasurer:* A. R. Melhuish *Honorary General Secretaries:* C. E. Corfield, G. R. Boyes. *Other Members of the Executive:* H. Berry, H. Brindle, B. A. Bull, H. Davis, N. Evers, E. W. Mann, with W. J. Beardsley, L. Moreton Parry and E. H. Simmons, nominated by the Council of the Pharmaceutical Society. If these recommendations of your Executive are adopted, the above persons will be the officers of the Conference, together with the following, *ex-officio*:—*President:* The president of the Pharmaceutical Society of Great Britain. *Other members of the Executive:* The president of the Pharmaceutical Society of Ireland, the president of the Pharmaceutical Society of Northern Ireland, the chairman of the North British Executive of the Pharmaceutical Society of Great Britain, the chairman of the Local Committee and the honorary local secretary.

In response to the request made by the Executive and reported to the members of Conference at the meeting in Belfast, the Bournemouth Local Committee have arranged a programme of meetings extending to the afternoon of the Thursday of Conference week with a free period on the Wednesday afternoon and an excursion for all members on the Friday. Your Executive feel that this new arrangement has provided that additional time necessary for the scientific and business meetings without damaging the social activities of the Conference. At the same time it has enabled them to make arrangements for the Conference golf and bowls competitions to be held at a time when more members are able to take part in them without losing the enjoyment of the excursion on the Friday. By adopting recommendations made by a subcommittee set up to consider various matters in connection with the sports competitions, your Executive feel that greater interest will now be taken in the competitions and that the new arrangements as a whole will add much to the enjoyment of the week.

The Executive are pleased that the Conference has been given the opportunity of meeting again in Bournemouth and desire to thank the Bournemouth Branch for their hospitality. They wish to place on record their appreciation of the work done by the Local Committee in arranging such exceedingly successful and enjoyable functions and excursions and to congratulate them on the smooth working of their arrangements.

An invitation will be extended at this meeting from the Liverpool and District Branch to visit Liverpool in 1937, and the Executive feel sure that members will receive this invitation with appreciation. As already reported, an invitation has been received from the Bath and District Branch, and an invitation has since been received from the Birmingham and District Branch. The Executive are very grateful to these Branches for having invited the Conference to meet in their cities and they view the future of the Conference with great confidence.

THE PRESIDENT, in moving the adoption of the report, said it needed little comment. He was pleased to find that Mr. Lescher was nominated as chairman of the Conference, and was sure that the members would have a wonderful time at Liverpool. They had great confidence in their old friend (Mr. Melhuish) as custodian of the funds.

THE VICE-PRESIDENT seconded the adoption of the report, which on being put to the meeting by the president was carried unanimously.

TREASURER'S REPORT

THE TREASURER read his annual report, which was in the following terms:—

The accounts for 1935 show that the income from subscriptions paid by elected members was £55 2s 6d. and in addition a composition fee of £25 was received under Rule 2 from the Pharmaceutical Society of Northern Ireland. These amounts have been accredited to the "Quarterly Journal of Pharmacy and Pharmacology" account. On the expenditure side of the account, the general expenses of the Conference were £115 18s. 11d. These figures were included in the Pharmaceutical Society's financial statement presented at the Society's annual meeting in May of this year. The total amount expended is £17 7s. 1d. less than last year. Apart from the figures to which reference has just been made, the Conference account shows a balance in hand of £150 9s. The usual presentation of books in connexion with the Bell and Hills Fund was made to the library of the Pharmaceutical Society of Northern Ireland in 1935. I have finally to report that the financial year of Conference has run its course in uneventful manner, and members will rejoice on learning that the balance at the end of 1935 exceeded that of the previous year by £11 3s. 9d.

THE PRESIDENT moved the adoption of the report.

THE VICE-PRESIDENT seconded the adoption, and the report was carried unanimously.

ALTERATION OF RULE 6

MR. T. EDWARD LESCHER moved an alteration in Rule 6, the effect of which was that 21s. was substituted for 10s. 6d., as the annual contribution of "other members elected."

THE VICE-PRESIDENT, in seconding, remarked that this alteration was an effort to satisfy the wishes of corresponding members to contribute a little more to the funds of the Conference The resolution was carried unanimously.

PLACE OF MEETING FOR 1937

MR. H. HUMPHREYS JONES said it was his pleasant duty to offer the Conference an invitation to visit Liverpool in 1937. Liverpool was the second city in the Empire, "in spite of what our friends from Glasgow say." (Laughter.) History was repeating itself, as it happened that in Bournemouth forty-one years ago a similar invitation was extended. At the Conference of 1920, he (the speaker) was local secretary, and now he was chairman of the Local Executive. It happened that better accommodation for mentally defective persons had lately been discussed in the Liverpool City Council, but he was not associating this fact with the Conference meeting. (Laughter.) In Liverpool they had much that was interesting in science, nature and art, notably the Mersey Tunnel, which with its contents would no doubt have been placed on the First Schedule if it had been ready earlier. (Laughter.) There had been a controversy of late over Liverpool coat of arms; Dr. Crossley-Holland could no doubt settle that matter when he arrived. (Laughter.)

BRITISH PHARMACEUTICAL CONFERENCE 1936

Mr. W. E. Humphreys (secretary of the Liverpool Local Executive), in seconding the invitation, said that Liverpool pharmacists would leave no stone unturned to make the visit a happy one.

Mr. F. W. M. Bennett moved the acceptance of the invitation. Mr. Bennett remarked that, thanks to the present Local Committee, the Scottish ladies were taking away some of the charm of Bournemouth. He was sure that the invitation would be accepted with acclamation.

Mr. W. S. Taylor (president of the Pharmaceutical Society of Northern Ireland), in seconding, said they could rely on having a good time in Liverpool. Thanks were due to members of the Bournemouth Local Committee for their extraordinary efficiency; they had even squared the clerk of the weather.

The resolution to accept the invitation was carried unanimously.

Election of Officers

Mr. D. A. Bryan (chairman of the N.P.U. Executive) proposed the election of the officers nominated in the annual report of the Executive Committee. Mr. Bryan said that the name of Lescher was known in every pharmacy throughout the Empire. Mr. Melhuish was the embodiment of the strictest integrity, and they also welcomed the new members of the Executive.

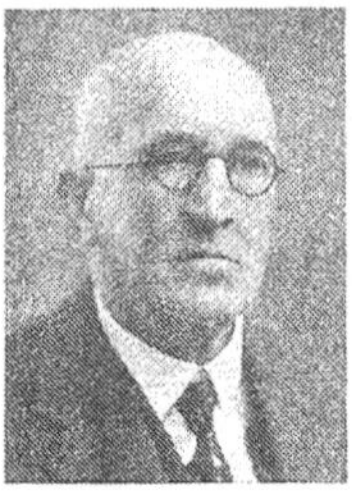

Mr. T. Edward Lescher

Mr. A. D. Powell, in seconding, said that Mr. Lescher would rule in the science session with a firm hand and would keep an eye on the English used. (Laughter.)

The resolution was carried unanimously.

Mr. Lescher returned thanks for the confidence placed in himself and the other new officers. He said he was rather sorry to leave the position of treasurer, which was one entailing light work, for a position of great responsibility and much work. The Conference was recognised in every town as one of the learned societies of the country. In Liverpool they would try to work as a team for the seventy-fourth meeting of the Conference.

Presentation of Books

The chairman made the customary presentation of books from the Bell and Hills Fund to the Bournemouth and District Branch.

Mr. F. E. Bilson, in accepting the gift, said the books would be handed over to the library of the Bournemouth Technical College, where they would be very useful to the students. Years ago he was an assistant with one of the donors, the late Mr. T. H. Hills, at the old shop of John Bell & Co , at 225 Oxford Street, London.

Thanks to the Chairman

Mr. R. R. Bennett moved a vote of thanks to the chairman for his services during the past twelve months, and particularly for his conduct in the chair during the past week. He himself never ceased to be impressed by the good work this Conference did. The chairman bore a name greatly honoured in the history of pharmacy, and they were pleased to have Mrs. Deane, who was also a pharmacist, with them.

Mr. Nutter Smith seconded the vote of thanks briefly in humorous terms, giving reminiscences of his long association with the chairman.

The president put the resolution, which was carried with acclamation.

The Chairman, in acknowledgment, said he had enjoyed this Conference more than any other. He thanked his old friends for their words of appreciation and the audience for their help. He then declared the proceedings of the Conference closed.

Social Side

Passengers travelling from London by train were not as numerous as might have been expected. A few elected to travel by the 10.30 Pullman; we noticed three from West Ham on the platform at Waterloo, where a small Scottish contingent included Mr. J. Rutherford Hill. Mr. H. M. Hirst, of Scarborough, was another member who chose this route. Those who followed by the express two hours later were even less numerous. The Local Committee had thoughtfully provided "B.P.C." slips for members using their own cars to affix to them, in order to facilitate passage through Bournemouth.

* * * *

The reception on Monday evening owed much to its delightful setting. From the windows on one side of the Pavilion ballroom the guests looked over the sea, with the superb sweep of the bay to the west; and on another side the Central Gardens, with their profusion of bloom, formed an attraction of a different kind. The central space was reserved for dancing, and around it those who were not inclined to "foot it featly" sat in groups or "circulated"—the French idiom is useful in this connexion—with the renewal of old friendships and perhaps the formation of new. Everyone was agreed that the Conference had started well.

* * * *

The chairman's address was quite unusual, and was generally approved in spite of its rather pessimistic outlook. It reflected the sociological feeling of thinking people of to-day and put the prospects of pharmacy plainly and without gloss. It likewise indicated the poetic as well as the philosophic bent of the author, who, withal, viewed the situation from the point of view of the agricultural expert. The chairman's influence was reflected, consciously or unconsciously, in the character of the papers produced in the Science Sessions, where Dr. Coutts gave the results of his latest work on the artemisias, Mr. Peck dealt with vegetable extracts, Mr Moorhouse with stramonium extract and Mr. Crews with rhapontic rhubarb.

* * * *

Another unusual paper in the Science Section was that of Mr. Maxwell Savage on the sterilisation of surgical dressings. This was listened to with exceptional interest, and the subsequent discussion was amusing, particularly in the references to public health sterilisation methods. Mr. Savage had the matter entirely at his fingers' ends.

* * * *

The first Conference luncheon (which set the fashion for the others) was a light-hearted function according well with the brilliant sunshine that streamed through the central dome of the Pavilion ballroom. The municipality of Bournemouth, as being well accustomed to such weather, tabled a luncheon that was as discreetly selected as it was faultlessly served; in fine, as creditable an advertisement for the county borough as the "biscuits Pavilion" with which it terminated. Mr. Harold Deane (Conference chairman) presided. A member who moved the microphone to make the announcements of the local secretary (Mr. Scampton) audible at all points was greeted with ironical applause. There seemed some reluctance to disperse at the end, and some at least of the afternoon's activities made a belated start. On the following day at the corresponding meal Dr. Crossley-Holland proposed the health of the women pharmacists present in his well-known and inimitable style amid general hilarity; and Mrs. Skinner, loudly summoned to the microphone, made a felicitous reply.

* * * *

The Conference banquet, held on June 23 in the spacious ballroom of the Pavilion, overlooking the sea, disclosed a sudden increase in the attendance that made the event the principal function of the 1936 meeting. With the chairman and Mrs. Deane at the chief table were the Mayor and Mayoress of Bournemouth, the Mayor and Mayoress of Poole, the Mayor and Mayoress of Christchurch, the president of the Pharmaceutical Society and Mrs. Marns, the president of the Pharmaceutical Society of Ireland, the president and vice-president of the Pharmaceutical Society of Northern Ireland, the chairman of the National Pharmaceutical Union, Dr. S. Watson Smith (past-president, British Medical Association), Councillor W Asten, M.D , Dr. H. Gordon Smith (medical officer of

BRITISH PHARMACEUTICAL CONFERENCE 1936

health for Bournemouth), Mr. T. Edward Lescher, O.B.E. (treasurer of the Conference), and several members of the Council of the Pharmaceutical Society and officers of the Conference.

* * * *

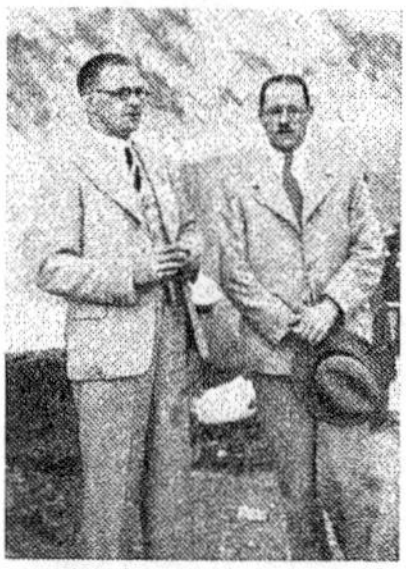

"The Twins"
Left to right: Dr. J. Coutts, Mr. G. R Boyes

* * * *

At an early stage in the evening the chairman announced that a loyal telegram of congratulation had been sent to his Majesty the King on the occasion of his birthday and a gracious reply had been received. With this announcement Mr. Deane combined an expression of gratification that Mr. J. Rutherford Hill had been awarded the O.B.E. At the Science Session in the morning the chairman had made a similar reference, and at the representatives' meeting in the afternoon Mr. Hill had received an ovation on the publication of the same news. After dinner the speeches, eight in all, began, and with a few vocal solos interspersed the proceedings continued till it was time for the more adventurous members to begin dancing.

* * * *

Dr. Crossley-Holland took charge of the first toast, "The County Borough of Bournemouth," in his usual humorous fashion, making fun out of the quarterings of the municipal coat of arms, and suggesting that if the time came for a new device the profiles of "some fine old crusted pharmacists" might be added. He congratulated the borough on the public improvements effected in recent years. The Mayor was full of friendly repartee in responding, chaffing pharmacists on the illegible scripts they handled and on other matters, and promising that if they stayed away from Bournemouth for another forty years they would not know the place.

* * * *

The speech of the evening came from Dr. W. Asten, who submitted in eloquent terms "The Pharmaceutical Society of Great Britain." Dr. Asten reminded his audience of a fact not known, probably, to many of them, that forty-eight years ago he made a contribution to the Conference of that year, and he was pleased to remember that in the record of the subsequent discussion the names of Martindale, Atkins, Greenish and others occurred. He was glad that the Pharmaceutical Society was still in sound and vigorous health; the medical profession was enormously indebted to members of the Society for the manner in which they discharged their duties day and night. He suggested that in the next Pharmacopœia Commission there should be two pharmacists in retail business and two general practitioners in medicine and surgery. The professional and trading aspects of pharmacy would always be in conflict to some extent. As to the Pharmacy and Poisons Act of 1933, he thought that something very much better might have been evolved. The intending poisoner would have trouble in obtaining a small supply from a pharmacist; but if one wanted to poison a town it was quite easy. In Bournemouth they had already registered 164 listed sellers. Mr. Marns, in reply, pointed out that pharmacy had had legislation and plenty of it: the time had come, he suggested, to see what they had and consolidate their position. Better education had been evolved, and they must see that pharmacy kept pace with the general standard.

* * * *

Proposing "The British Pharmaceutical Conference," Dr. S. Watson Smith quoted from Bacon ("Conference maketh a ready man") and Plautus ("It becometh all wise men to confer"). All appreciated the weapons of precision forged by the Conference. He liked to think that the professions of medicine and pharmacy had a common interest and that old scores were forgotten. Men and women of the craft were subject to the work they performed: they became silent, careful, courteous and kindly. Mr. Harold Deane, in reply, said that in his opening address to the Conference he had given examples of the dangers of the handling of poisons by uneducated persons Records of the speech of his grandfather, at the first Conference, also gave many examples of bad adulterations of drugs. To-day most B P. drugs were subject to standards, many of them the result of work contributed to the Conferences. A further extract from the same opening speech was worth quoting: "It is to the united efforts of a few willing heads and hands that all associations must look for their scientific, intellectual and material advancement. These elements of trust we possess to a pre-eminent degree and so long as they exist our success, prosperity and usefulness will exist also."

* * * *

Mr. F. E. Bilson, who proposed "The Guests," singled out a number for special mention. He recalled that Dr. Asten, an earlier speaker, was also a qualified chemist and barrister. The reply was given by Dr. H. Gordon Smith, who declared that, having started with the idea that he should not be a guest since surgeons, physicians, pharmacists and apothecaries were members of one family, he had carried out some researches into old books in which he had discovered a description of the functions of an apothecary. He quoted a few of the twenty-one points from Bullein's "Bulwarke of Defence" (printed in the *C. & D.* of June 30, 1934). After a certain period of friction, physicians and apothecaries had become associated, the latter being given space on the same premises. Later, the assistants of physicians became chemists. It had occurred to him that he could not recall one undesirable member of the profession. This must be taken as a sign, either that they were really exemplary citizens, or that they were exceptionally adept at concealing their misdeeds. (Laughter.) He failed to see that the Pharmacy and Poisons Act, 1933, was going to be very useful.

* * * *

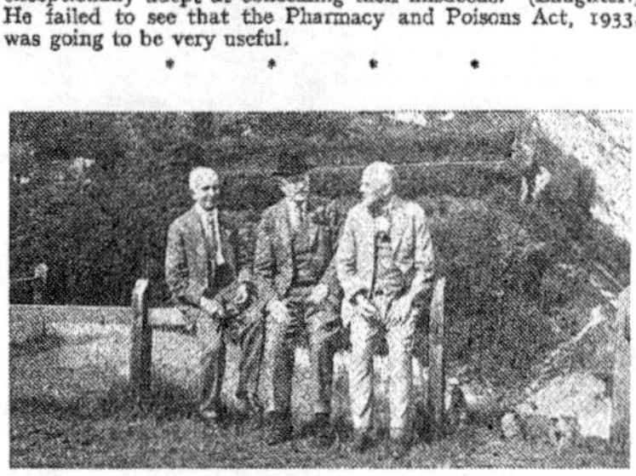

Three Past-Presidents at Lulworth
Left to right: Mr. F. E. Bilson, Mr. A. R. Melhuish, Mr. H. Skinner

* * * *

The honours for speechmaking at the banquet were accorded without question to Dr. Asten. He had the advantage of being able to speak from the point of view of the pharmacist as well as that of the physician. Some amusement was caused

BRITISH PHARMACEUTICAL CONFERENCE 1936

by the innocent introduction by the singer, in his first song, of "Boots! Boots! Boots!" Some folks appeared to be rather intrigued.

* * * *

When the speeches were finished, some 250 of those present adjourned to the Popular Restaurant for dancing until 1 a.m. Paul Jones, veletas, barn dances and "Excuse me" variations were popular items. The atmosphere was one of quiet gaiety, and, though the floor was full, many took advantage of an excellent opportunity to make up informal "round-table conferences" in the wings.

* * * *

The ladies' excursions were all well organised, and the beautiful weather made things comparatively easy for the Local Committee. On the Tuesday afternoon many besides ladies found the cooling breezes of the Channel grateful and comforting on the steamer which voyaged to Swanage and back. Others preferred the shade of the New Forest and tea at the Kettle Inn. The new arrangement regarding Sports Day (Wednesday) left many free to acquire a natural sun tan on the beach or to bathe. The stern, unbending golfers toiled over the Meyrick Links, and at Meyrick likewise a few, but not many, ladies took a detached and dispassionate interest in the bowls tournament.

* * * *

On the Thursday morning Poole pottery attracted connoisseurs in the art of the potters' wheel, whose interest had been whetted by the elegant vase of pottery presented to each lady at the banquet. Ecclesiastically inclined ladies were attracted instead to Wimborne, whose minster had been so learnedly described beforehand by that enthusiastic ecclesiastic, Dr. Crossley-Holland. A third alternative was the visit to Corfe Castle, and this appeared to be the most popular of all. It was certainly well worth inspection, and in spite of the heat many climbed the heights and revelled in the tales—authentic or imaginative—with which the ancient keep is invested. Everyone was interested in the fact that Corfe Castle was being used as a background for "A Midsummer Night's Dream" to be produced by the Balliol Players, who are also about to give the "Alcestis" of Euripides in Professor Gilbert Murray's translation.

* * * *

Quite early in the week it became evident that a very efficient Local Committee had long been at work behind the scenes: only so could the smoothness of the general arrangements be accounted for. Public recognition of their success came at Thursday evening's function, recorded in another paragraph; but we must add our own tribute to the sustained efforts that kept everything going in spite of the brevity of the rest that many of them must have had to be content with. The responsible duties of the chairman and the president were, as usual, carried out with entire appreciation of their relative functions, Mr. Deane's quiet sense of humour forming an excellent foil to Mr. Marns's debonair urbanity.

* * * *

The first dance, held in the Pavilion half way through the week, was a cheery affair, differing from other such functions mainly in the widely varying interests of the pharmacists and their friends who were present. This factor lent attraction to the conversation of the various groups that formed—conversation sometimes with a pharmaceutical undertone, but not always.

* * * *

Sun bathing was very prevalent on the beach, and quite a number of pharmaceutical visitors were enjoying the sunshine, so much so that two lights of the Science Section were caught trying to get an ice cream tricycle and equip it with sunburn oddments. The powder was to be the favourite application, the dusting to be charged at 6d. per two square feet and 3d for every additional square foot.

* * * *

The antithesis to the serene atmosphere of the Science Section was the branch representatives' meetings. The platform was filled from end to end, the president being supported by no fewer than fifteen members of the Council, the secretary, assistant secretary and resident secretary in Scotland. In spite of this formidable array the rank and file had a good run for their money, and many home truths were put bluntly. The hero of the first day's proceedings was Mr. Newby, of Oldham, who succeeded in carrying a resolution which will no doubt be duly recorded when the official report appears. Many subjects, including that hardy annual, "territorial representation," led to animated discussions, but not much else. The ovation given to Mr. Rutherford Hill when the president publicly congratulated him on the honour conferred by the King is mentioned in another paragraph. Mr. Hill made a modest and able reply, describing the honour as being done not to him but to pharmacy.

* * * *

During the Conference it was noticed that an enthusiast (whose name we have so far not been able to ascertain) had mounted and placed on view in the main lounge of the headquarters hotel the *C. & D.* cartoon "Dropping the Pilot" from our issue of June 13.

* * * *

The old term "Sports Day" at the Conference was a misnomer this year, as the experiment was made of a transfer from the Friday (all day) to Wednesday (half day) in order to provide more time for the science papers and the day excursion on Friday. The variety of sports in which competitors joined was, however, not greater than previous years. Tennis was dropped owing to lack of support, while putting, apart from golfers, received no serious entries, and the time for this game was not available to the golfers. There was a good entry for golf, which was played over the Meyrick Park golf course. It was felt that competition for the Edmund White trophy would be keener if played off in the middle of a hectic week; but the results showed the wear and tear of other Conference engagements. Meyrick Park course has more narrow fairways than most links, and the amount of trouble facing the golfer at twelve holes out of eighteen meant many lost balls. Indeed, one golfer at the end of the competition lost a ball at number eleven in the midst of a miniature forest, and in searching therein found seven others; but whether they were all from his pharmaceutical brethren will remain unknown.

* * * *

Many reputations crashed, but a Leeds representative triumphed with a 70 net, excellent for such tantalising links. N. H. Burn, of Leeds, was the winner, 84−14=70 net; W. Gray, of London, 84−11=73 net, the runner-up, was a former winner. T. Miller, of Manchester, had a 75 net, while over some of the others in the list it is kinder to draw a veil. In bowls, the competition was international, England v. Scotland for the London challenge cup, England being the holder. The teams were Messrs. Anderson, Ratcliffe, Hocken and J. Reed (skip) representing England, with Messrs. Hendry, Duff, Nisbet and Culbert (skip) representing Scotland. The game was keen throughout, and finally the Scots ran out winners by 20 points to 15, thereby champions for 1936, the first time for five years. In the open competition in bowls, two teams competed: Messrs. Robinson, Taylor, Alexander and G. A. Tocher, 27 points to 15 by Mr. Kelly, Mr. Barron, Mrs. Glover, and Mr. T. O. Barlow. The prize went to Mr. W. S. Taylor. The trophies and tokens were handed over at the smoking concert on Friday night at the Grand Hotel by Mrs. Harold Deane.

* * * *

On Thursday evening, another exhilarating function was the occasion of well-merited tributes to the Local Committee. To Mr. Herbert Skinner fell the pleasant duty of moving a vote of thanks to these enthusiasts for their triumphant accomplishment of a laborious task. Mr. Skinner remarked that the excellence of the weather that week had only been matched by the kindness and hospitality provided by the Committee, and mentioned by name Mr. Bilson, Mr. Scampton, Mr. Worth and Miss Hardwick, the last-named of whom had presided over the ladies' committee. Mr. Fred Storey said that he was sure the Committee must have had an anxious time, but the Conference had been a magnificent success. The lady visitors especially appreciated the gift of pottery from

BRITISH PHARMACEUTICAL CONFERENCE 1936

the ladies' committee. After the vote of thanks had been carried with enthusiastic applause, souvenirs were presented to Mr. Bilson, Mr. Scampton, Mr. Worth and Miss Hardwick.

* * * *

In each case the gathering called for a speech at the microphone; it is hardly necessary to add that these speeches were brief, sincere and heartily received. Mr. Bilson said that he was greatly touched by the friendship shown on all sides, and the Committee were more than repaid if the visitors had enjoyed the Conference. Mr. Scampton said he had enjoyed every minute of the week and had met many men whose friendship he valued. Mr. Worth managed to escape a speech, but Miss Hardwick was insistently summoned to the microphone, and justified the insistence by remarking that no tact was required to run a ladies' committee and that in any case she had not much—a remark which formed the culmination of a very amusing evening. The chairman of the Conference added an expression of thanks to everyone concerned, including the management of the Pavilion, who had catered to the general satisfaction.

* * * *

The all-day excursion, held for the first time on a Friday, was attended by the Conferencers in more than full strength. It took fifteen touring cars to convey all the sightseers, and many were seen following—or leading—in their own cars. The route chosen was picturesque, showing in turn rhododendron hedgerows, pine forests, cordite factories, Roman earthworks and china clay quarries. Quaint old English villages—comparatively unspoiled—such as Canford Magna and Milton Abbas—were looked upon with longing by jaded city pharmacists, while the literary were interested in the Dorchester district, immortalised by Thomas Hardy. The earthworks at Wareham (visited on the previous day) were eclipsed by Mar-Dun Castle ("The Hill of Strength") outside Dorchester, and then modernity was suddenly reached at Weymouth. There the foreshore and sands were littered with holiday-makers, over whom, it appeared, a battleship and two cruisers were keeping guard just outside the harbour. At Weymouth luncheon was served, and after about an hour's freedom the party proceeded to Lulworth Cove. This romantic beauty spot was seen at its best—and at its second best. On arrival the sun was shining brilliantly, and many took the opportunity of an hour's wait before tea to bathe or to explore the bay in skiff, canoe or motor boat. The most daring appeared to be the president of the Pharmaceutical Society, who canoed with his partner almost out into the open sea. Suddenly a few spots of rain followed by a ten-minute deluge sent everyone rushing for shelter and tea; but even leaking roofs in the tea pavilion did not damp the spirits of the Conferencers, and the homeward journey was accomplished in good time.

* * * *

The lady forming the group with Mr. Rutherford Hill and Mr. H. M. Hirst on p. 718 of our Special Issue of June 27 is Miss H. C. M. Winch, A.I.C., Ph.C., of Sunderland. We are glad to make this tardy recognition of a well-known pharmacist: the fact is that at even the best-regulated Conferences we have to reject numerous snapshots on the ground that the camera has failed to do justice to its victims or even, as in this case, to make them easily identifiable.

* * * *

There was no apparent sadness at the Grand Hotel on Friday evening, although the "Smoker" was the recognised Swan Song of the Bournemouth Conference. The affair was even more informal than usual—and that is saying much. It was difficult to ascertain, through the smoke, who was presiding, but officially it was Mr. Harold Deane. The local secretary, Mr. Scampton, confessed from the platform early in the evening that they had been rather overwhelmed by the attendance, but no one seemed to mind very much. An unofficial interlude increasing the hilarity of the occasion was introduced by Mr. Fred Storey, of Belfast, who insisted on inducing Mrs. Bennett, Mrs. Deane and Mr. Lescher to go on the platform and make a "presentation" to Dr. Crossley-Holland. This was followed by the official presentation by Mrs. Deane of the sports prizes to Mr. N. H. Burns for golf, and to Mr. Culbert (of Airdrie) and Provost Taylor (of Inverurie) for bowls. Speeches were demanded from Mr. Culbert and Provost Taylor, and Mrs. Deane was thanked for presenting the prizes. Thereafter, in a haphazard sort of way, the professional entertainers—all of them good—did a "turn"; at the behest of the President, Mr. Peter Irvine gave two of his clever character sketches, and these appeared to be the best appreciated of all. Presently "Auld Lang Syne" intimated the end of another British Pharmaceutical Conference.

* * * *

Mr. Lescher's apparent reluctance to accept the phrase "stream orientation" during a discussion in the Science Section (p. 19) was probably in the nature of a subtle "leg pull." So great a master of lucid English is, no doubt, well acquainted with the Shorter Oxford English Dictionary, which under "Orientation" has a definition (1.b) apparently suiting the case fairly well: "Position or arrangement (of a natural object or formation) relatively to the points of the compass or to other parts of the same structure." On the face of it Mr. Middleton's "thixotropy" seems more alarming.

* * * *

The local newspaper, "The Bournemouth Daily Echo," gave interesting reports of the principal items of the Conference. On June 24 there appeared an account of the banquet, a photograph of the municipal reception, an interview with Mr. F. E. Bilson extending to nearly a column, and three personal paragraphs on the veteran chairman of the Local Committee. During his interview with the representative of the paper, Mr. Bilson recalled the fact that the old local association, according to the minutes of a meeting it held in May 1894, discussed "the Poisons Act."

* * * *

Copies of the official Conference photograph, price 4s. each, may be obtained from the Panoramic Photograph Co., 50 Osborne Road, Levenshulme, Manchester.

* * * *

The Conference Snapshots

Details of pictures reproduced on other pages of this issue are given below:—

1. *After the closing session, Town Hall.*
2. *At the Conference luncheon.*
3. *Two excursionists at Poole pottery.*
4. *Mr. N. H. Burns, Leeds, winner of the golf trophy.*
5. *Members of the Liverpool executive committee.*
6. *Mr. J. H. Gough, Leeds, with a friend.*
7. *Mr. J. F. Simon, Leeds, relaxes.*
8. *Bowls: the winning team.*
9. *The president and Mr. Herbert Skinner at golf.*
10. *Mr. J. T. Appleton, Sheffield, explains a point.*

At No. 1 Tee:—

11. *Mr. F. W. Gamble, London, and Mr. Davies, Wales.*
12. *Mr. J. G. Twigg, Withernsea, and Mr. J. Judge, Wakefield.*
13. *Mr. C. W. Hobson, Sheffield, and Mr. W. E. Phillipson, Manchester.*
14. *Mr. W. R. Brackenbury and Mr. R. MacDonald Murray, chairman and secretary of the Tees-side branch of the Pharmaceutical Society.*
15. *A party of Welsh visitors.*
16. *Mr. Harold Deane, Chairman of the Conference (right) with Mr. R. R. Bennett and others.*
17. *Mr. Fred Storey (past-president) and Mr. W. S. Taylor (president of the Pharmaceutical Society of Northern Ireland).*
18. *Mr. F. E. Bilson (chairman of the local branch)*
19. *Mr. H. M. Hirst, Scarborough, in good company.*
20. *Mr. S. H. Forrest, Bangor, Northern Ireland.*
21. *A seaside group.*
22. *The New Forest excursion: boarding the coaches.*
23. *Mesdames Melhuish, Noble, Young and Bennett.*
24. *A group of New Forest excursionists.*
25. *Some members of the local committee.*

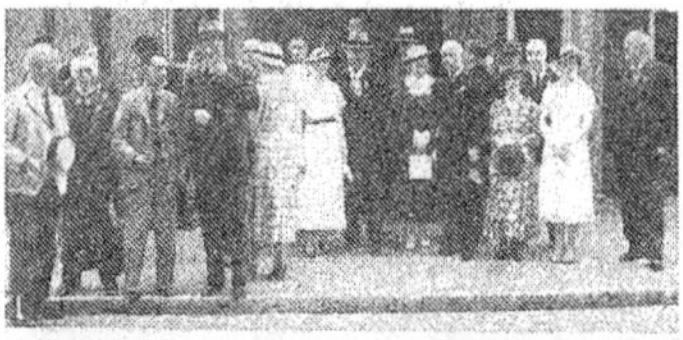
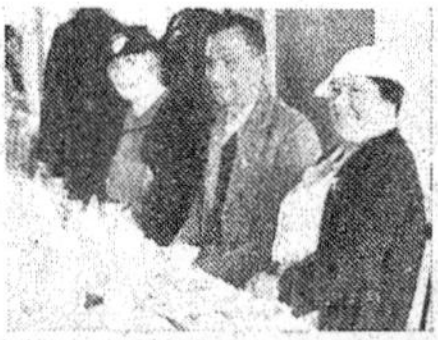
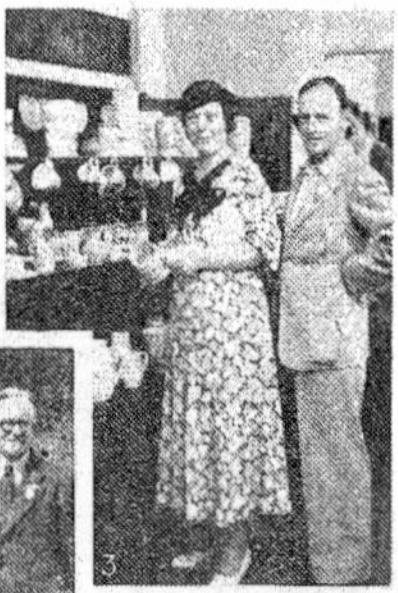
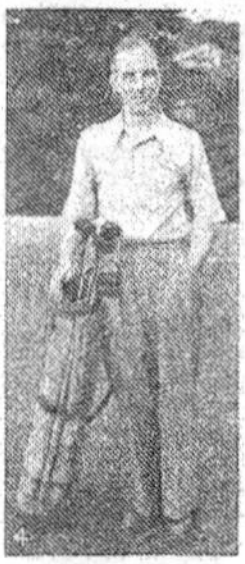
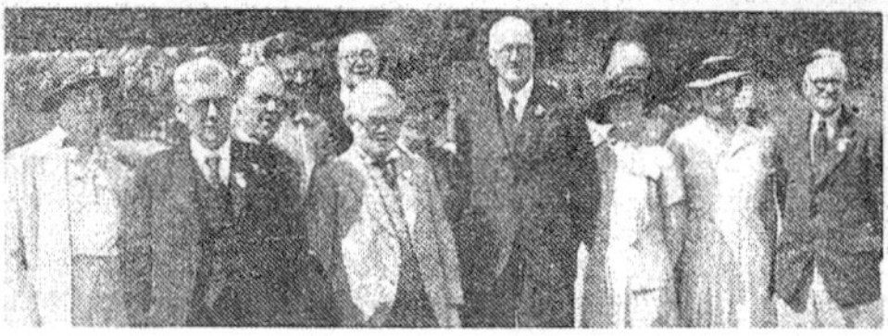

Seen at the BOURNEMOUTH CONFERENCE

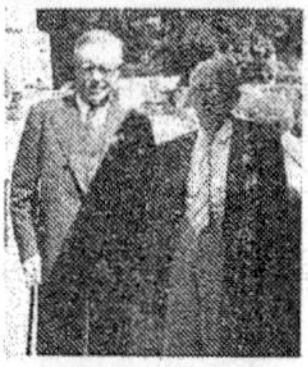
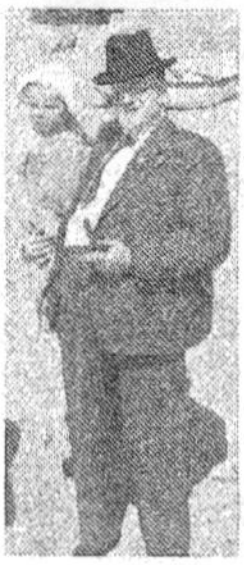
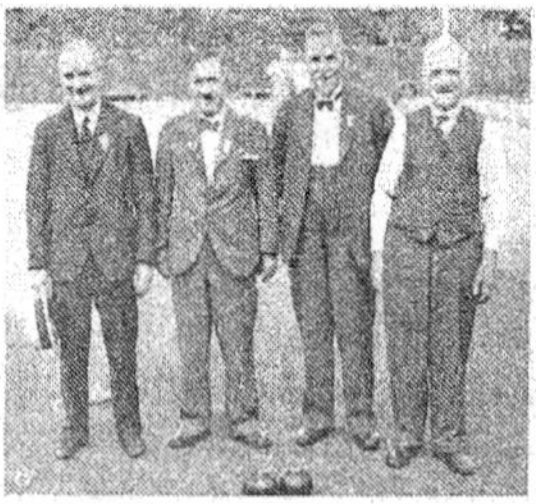
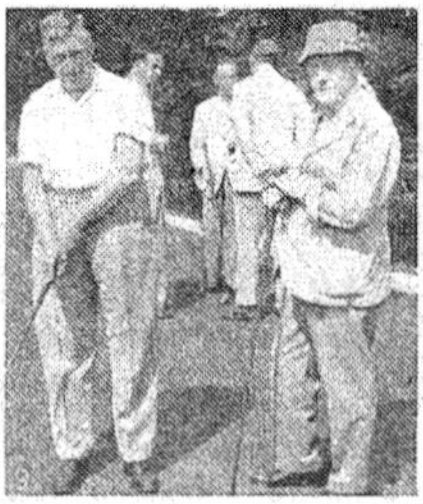
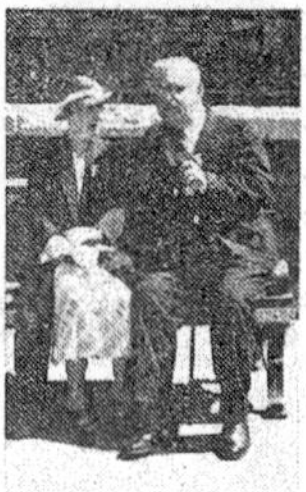
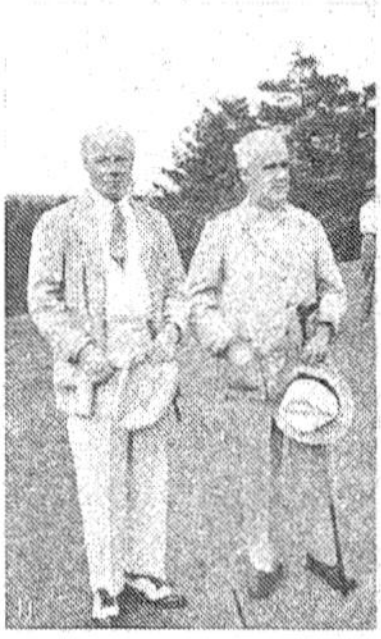
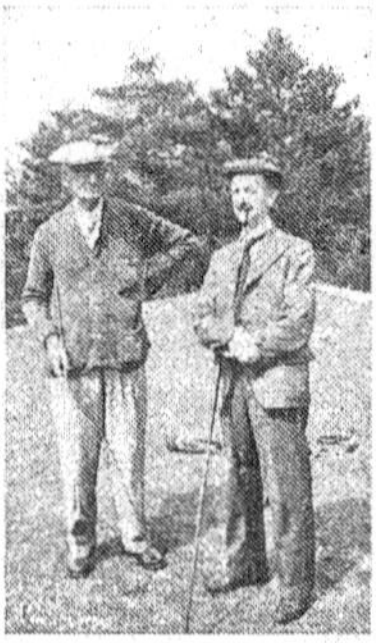
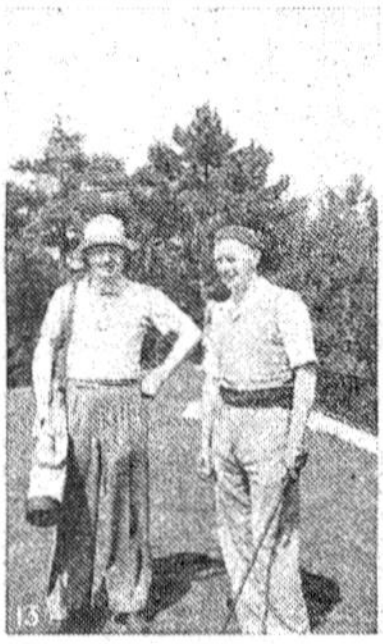
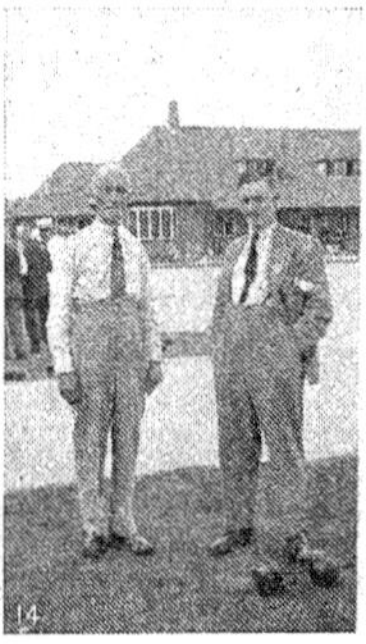

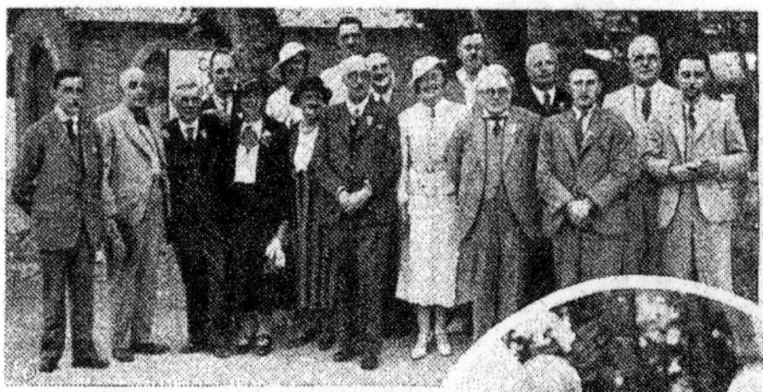

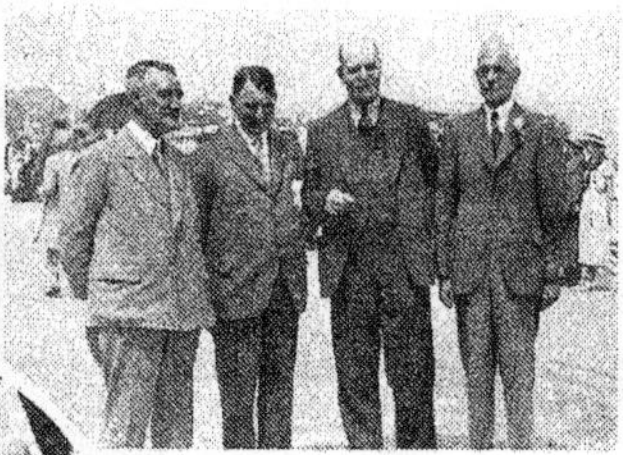

Seen at the BOURNEMOUTH CONFERENCE

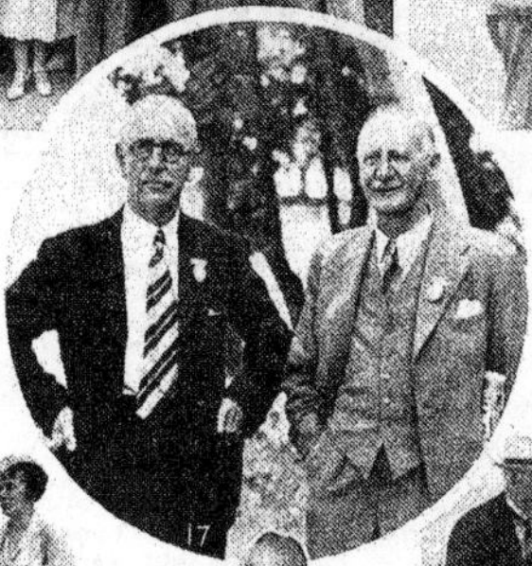

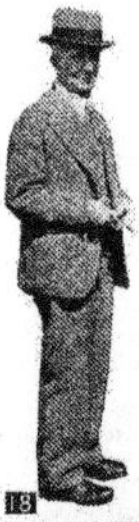

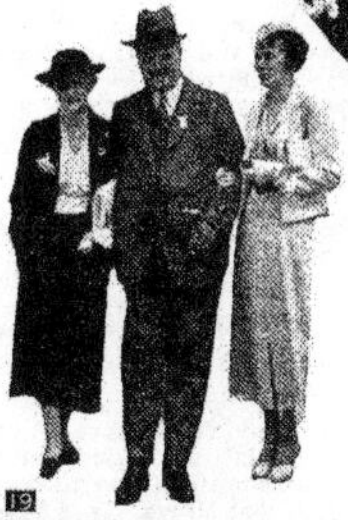

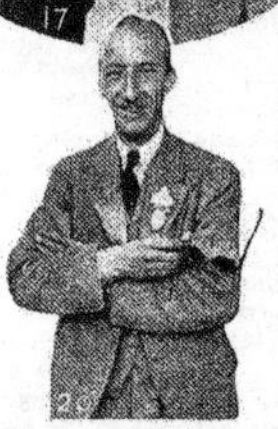

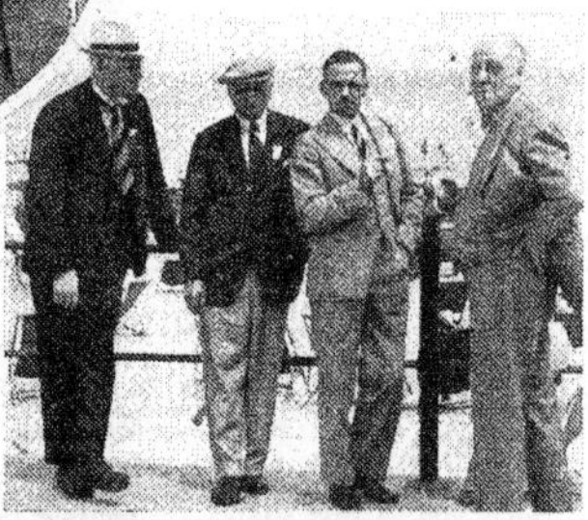

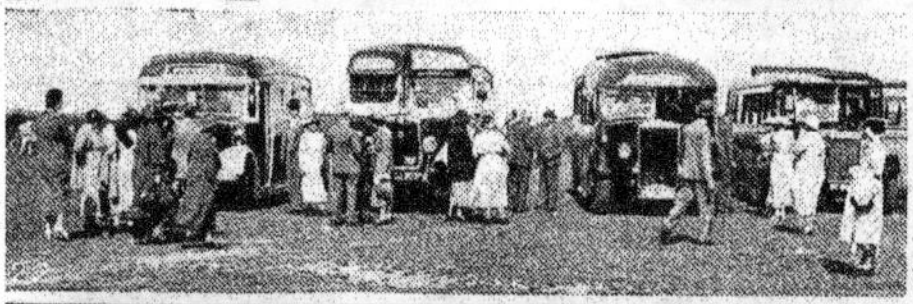

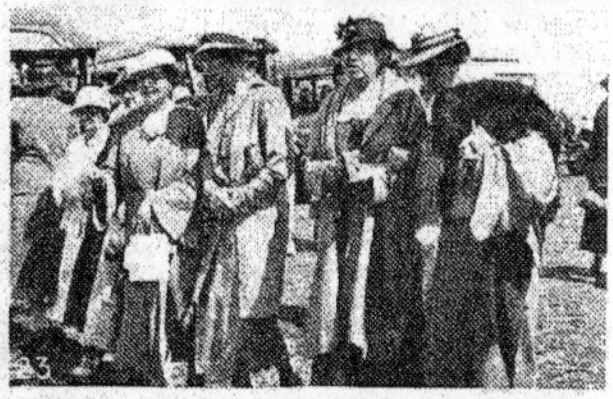

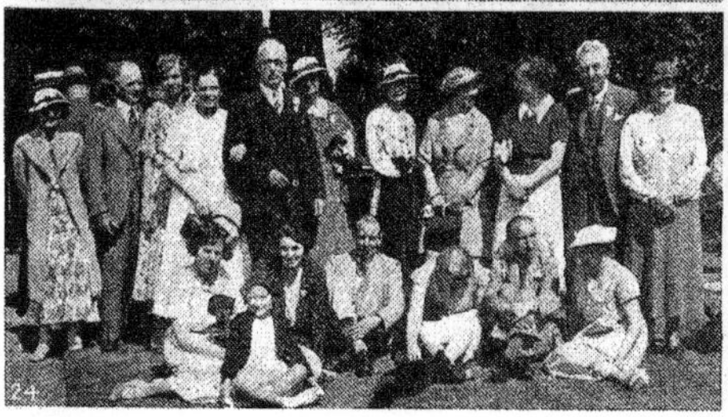

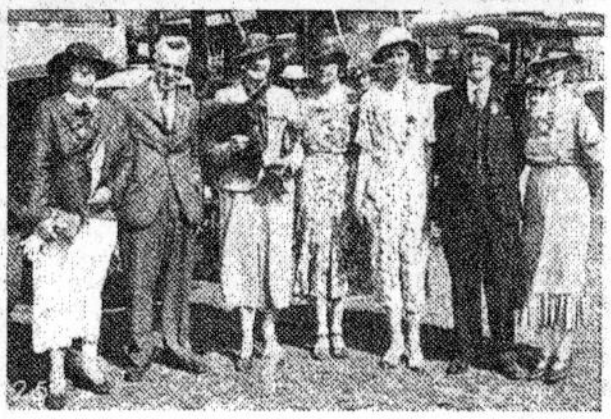

Trade Notes

PYREX SYRINGES.—We have to express our regret that the address of the General Surgical Co., Ltd., manufacturers of

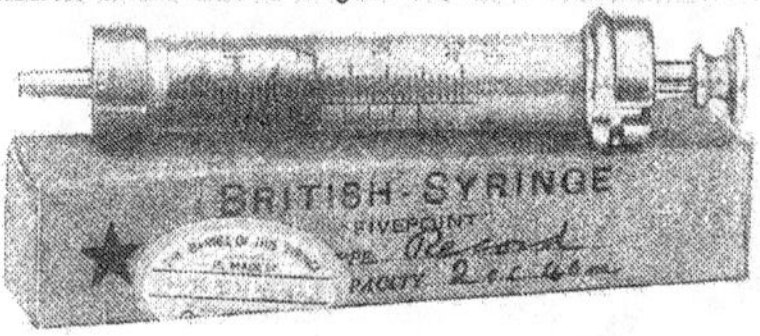

Pyrex syringes, was wrongly given in our Special Issue of June 27. The address of the head office and factory is as follows: Gensurco House, Rosebery Avenue, London, E.C.1.

VICK PRODUCTS.—J. C. Gambles & Co., Ltd., Blackfriars Road, London, S.E 1, have been appointed the sole distributors of Vick brand products.

DR. PAGE-BARKER'S SCURF LOTION.—A special large size of this preparation has been introduced. Full details may be obtained from Thomas Christy & Co., Ltd., 4-12 Old Swan Lane, London, E.C.

In the advertisement pages of our Special Issue of June 27 a former advertisement of Philip Josephs & Sons, Ltd., 90 and 92 St. John Street, Clerkenwell, London, E.C.1, was repeated in error. The present telephone number is Clerkenwell 4111, 4112.

COTY BEAUTY CREATIONS.—Coty (England), Ltd., 3 Stratford Place, London, W.1, have introduced a range of moderately-priced toilet preparations, including Avocado beauty milk and soap. An illustrated booklet giving details of these products will be sent on application.

VIGGORMALT.—It is stated that there is a constantly increasing demand for pure beer, ale or stout easily made at home by means of Viggormalt. Display stands may be obtained from the distributors, Fassett & Johnson, Ltd., 86 Clerkenwell Road, London, E.C.1, or from the manufacturers, Viggormalt, Ltd., Hove, Sussex.

BONUS OFFERS.—A bonus offer is made in connexion with Oculex during July. Details may be obtained from the usual wholesalers or from the proprietors.—E.N.T. Manufacturing Co., Ltd., Bristol, 7, offer during July for fourteen days' window display an extra cash discount on E.N.T. nerve powders.—Henry Tetlow Co., Ltd., 61 Eagle Street, London, W.C.1, are making a bonus offer in connexion with their Swan Down Complexion Milk. Particulars will be found elsewhere in this issue. This preparation is to be nationally advertised.

MAW'S CHEMISTS' CATALOGUE.—S. Maw, Son & Sons, Ltd., Aldersgate Street, London, E.C.1, have just published a new edition of their catalogue of medical and surgical sundries. As the list remains current for a considerable time, the plan of this issue differs in some respects from that of its predecessors. For example, there has been omitted from it lines of a seasonal nature which are liable to frequent change, and also articles such as hot water bottles and surgical dressings, which may not change in pattern, but which are very liable to considerable alteration in prices. For actual prices of such goods customers are referred to the special lists which will be published as occasion arises. Probably the most important alteration in the plan deals with surgical appliances. For many years past chemists have experienced the difficulty that they could not show the list to their customers without disclosing the wholesale prices. This difficulty has been met by gathering together, in one section, all lines of surgical appliances and such other items as the chemist could not be expected to stock, but which he would find it necessary to describe accurately to his customers The prices are quoted in the pages preceding this section. This re-grouping of goods should undoubtedly make the new catalogue of additional service.

STAFF OUTING.—Wright, Layman & Umney, Ltd., London, S.E.1, inform us that their factory, warehouse and offices will be closed on July 4, the date of the annual staff outing.

SUMMER LINES.—Potter & Clarke, Ltd., Artillery Lane, London, E.1, call attention elsewhere in this issue to a number of packed preparations which are in demand at this time of year.

KNAPP & Co., Essential Oils Manufacturing Co., Budapest, are the makers of synthetic Hungarian lilac oil for perfumes and toilet waters. The firm also manufacture Apricot brandy composition—a popular drink known as Hungarian speciality.

C. & D. COSMETIC HARMONY CHART.—In response to numerous requests, we are having THE CHEMIST AND DRUGGIST Cosmetic Harmony Chart (published in our Special Issue of June 27) reprinted on stiff cardboard suited to use in the pharmacy. The charts will be available early next week, price 1s. each or three for 2s. 6d., post free.

WINDOW-DRESSING COMPETITION.—The County Perfumery Co., North Circular Road, West Twyford, London, N.W.10, are conducting a window-dressing competition in connexion with Brylcreem from July 6 to August 1. Folders giving details of this competition have already been sent out, and any chemist who has not received one should write to the above address.

EXAKTA HANDBOOK.—Garner & Jones, Ltd., Polebrook House, Golden Square, London, W.1, have published a handbook (printed in English) dealing with the Exakta camera and its capabilities. Though primarily intended for users of this camera, there is a great deal of information in this publication which will be of interest to all photographers. The price of the handbook is 3s. 6d.

AMMOKET.—Boots, Ltd., Nottingham, have placed on the market under this name an elixir which is stated to be a most convenient way of administering mandelic acid, as the unpleasant taste of ammonium mandelate is covered by means of suitable flavouring agents. Ammoket is supplied in bottles containing 8 oz. and 16 oz., the latter being sufficient for eight days' treatment.

SELO FILMS.—Ilford, Ltd., Ilford, have introduced three new Selo films suitable for miniature cameras, and particulars of these are given in the company's advertisement in this issue. It should also be noted that Messrs. Ilford have adopted green duplex paper for all Selo panchromatic films in place of the red and black paper previously employed. The use of green paper should facilitate processing by ensuring handling of the films in the correct light.

MEGGESON & Co., LTD., New Church Street, Bermondsey, London, S.E.16, two of whose popular summer lines are illustrated below, have joined the Chemists' Friends scheme.

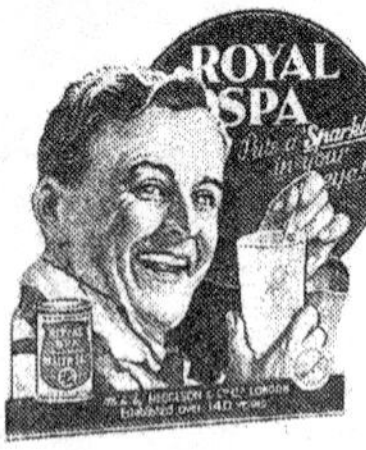

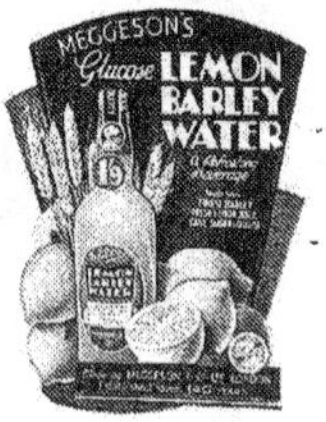

Apropos the barley water, a point of interest is that at the last dance at the Pharmaceutical Conference on June 25 Meggeson's glucose lemon barley water was supplied to guests from the running buffet.

Births

Notices for insertion in this column must be properly authenticated.

FEATHER.—On June 28, Joyce, the wife of R Campbell Feather, M.A., B.Sc. (director, Meggeson & Co., Ltd., London, S.E.16), of a son.

NICHOLSON.—At 5 Morningside Park, Edinburgh, on June 17, the wife of Hugh W. Nicholson, M P S, Tranent, of a son.

RATCLIFFE.—On June 27, Ena, the wife of John Clayton Ratcliffe, M.P.S., Cheadle, Staffs, of a daughter.

SHEPHERD —At the Bristol Maternity Hospital, on June 24, Joyce, the wife of Arthur Geoffrey Shepherd, M.P.S., 72 Shirehampton Road, Stoke Bishop, Bristol, of a daughter.

Marriages

DALTON—CORDINER.—At St. Michael's Church, Croston, Preston, on June 20, Robert Dalton to Edith, daughter of Mr. D. G. Cordiner, chemist and druggist, South Shields.

DANIEL—HUDSON.—At the Methodist Church, Delph, Oldham, on June 20, Arnold H. Daniel, chemist and druggist, Dukinfield, to Lucy Hudson.

FLEMING—SIMPSON.—At St. Kilda, Great King Street, Edinburgh, on June 27, Robert Fleming to Jean L. Simpson, chemist and druggist.

ORR—BLACK.—At St. Jude's Parish Church, Belfast, on June 9, by the Most Rev. the Lord Bishop of Meath (uncle of the bridegroom), assisted by the Rev. James Quinn, B.A., and the Rev. T. Maxwell Orr, B.A. (brother of the bridegroom), William H F., elder son of Mr. W. R. H. Orr, Ph.C., 165 Ormeau Road, Belfast, to Mary A. (Dollie), younger daughter of the late Mr. William Black and of Mrs. Black, 30 Ava Street, Belfast.

SHAW—GARRETT.—At St Nicholas's Church, Carrickfergus, on June 24, Gilbert Mains Shaw, Ph.C., to Rosemary Johnstone Garrett.

WILSON—HEBDEN.—At the Church of St. Bartholomew, London, recently, Clifford Wilson, M.D., first assistant to the medical unit of the London Hospital, to Kathleen, daughter of the late Mr. Harry Hebden, Ph.C., Halifax.

Deaths

BREMNER.—At Chilworth, Surrey, on June 11, Mr. Allan Hugh Bremner, retired chemist and druggist, formerly of Thurso and Glasgow, aged eighty-four.

CRAIL.—On June 25, ex-Bailie John Crail, J.P., 4 Fairfield Place, Annan, aged seventy-one. Mr. Crail, who was a native of Londonderry, went into business in Annan in 1893. He became a member of the Town Council in 1896 and a magistrate a few years later.

CULLWICK.—On June 17, Mr. George Hamar Jones Cullwick, chemist and druggist, 2 Market Square, Waltham Abbey, aged seventy-six. Mr. Cullwick purchased the business known as Wood's Cash Chemists after the war, and conducted it until his death. He was a former chairman of the local chamber of trade and a Past-Master of the James Terry Lodge of Freemasons.

EVANS.—At Portsmouth, on June 14, Mr. Daniel Evans, chemist and druggist, aged seventy-one. Mr. Evans was in business at Pen-y-Stryt, Rhos, near Wrexham, until 1916, afterwards removing to 167 Dover Road, Copnor, Portsmouth.

LOWTHER —At Mumbles, on June 26, Mr. Herbert Reginald Lowther, chemist and druggist, aged seventy-three. Mr. Lowther was in business at Mumbles for forty years.

HESLOP.—At 59 Overhill Road, Dulwich, London, S E 22, on June 7, after a brief illness, Mr. George Heslop, chemist and druggist, aged eighty-eight. Mr. Heslop was born at Newcastle-upon-Tyne, and was educated at the Royal Grammar School there. In 1865 he was apprenticed to the late Mr. J. C. Eno, then in business at 5 Groat Market. This term over, he became an assistant, and in 1874, after a period of special study at the South London College of Pharmacy, he passed the Minor Examination with honours and returned to the Groat Market in Newcastle At this time business in Eno's Fruit Salt was making vigorous growth, and in 1878 Mr. Eno decided to move the centre for its preparation to London. Mr. Heslop, in partnership with the late Mr John Walton, continued the Groat Market business, and later opened a second shop in Westgate Road. The Groat Market buildings were some 300 years old, and when demolition came that business was moved to No. 25. After some years the partnership was dissolved and Mr. Heslop retained the Westgate Road business. This he carried on till 1897, when Mr. Eno invited him to join the staff of the limited company then formed. In 1902 he became general manager and a director of J. C. Eno, Ltd. He retired in 1919. Mr. Heslop's tastes were of a quiet order, and he never took any active part in pharmaceutical politics. He read a great deal and was very fond of music: gardening was also a hobby of which he never tired.

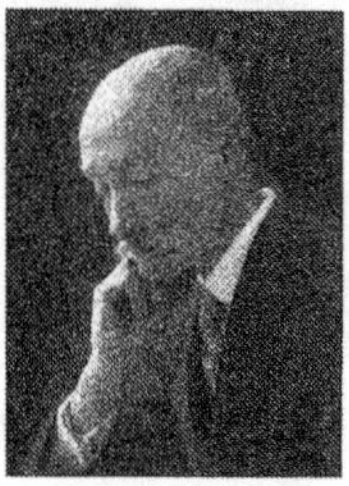

MR. GEORGE HESLOP

Personalities

MR. H. J. WHITEHEAD, M.P.S. (C. M Holmes, Ltd., chemists, London, E 5), was on June 30 inducted as president of the Rotary Club of Hackney.

THE South-West Lancashire and Cheshire Joint (Prescriptions) Committee has appointed Mr. William Haigh, Newcastle-upon-Tyne (recently of Exeter), to the post of superintendent and technical adviser to the Committee.

Wills

ALDERMAN WILLIAM GOWEN CROSS, J.P., 70 Mardol, Shrewsbury, chemist, twice Mayor, a former vice-president of the Pharmaceutical Society, died on March 10 last, aged eighty-seven, leaving £6,689, with net personalty £2,160.

MR. GEORGE BROOK PARKER, Hollins Close, Bolton, Bradford, Yorks, managing director of Brook Parker & Co, Ltd., wholesale chemists, of Ashfield, Bradford, died on March 21 last, aged sixty-five, leaving estate value £46,971, with, so far as can at present be ascertained, net personalty £42,978.

Coming Events

This section is reserved for advance notices of meetings or other events. These should be received by Wednesday of the week before the meetings, etc. occur.

Monday, July 6

Society of Chemical Industry, Liverpool. Annual meetings, concluding July 11.

Royal Sanitary Institute, Southport. Annual congress, concluding July 11.

Thursday, July 9

Pharmaceutical Society, Metropolitan Branches. Maw's Sports Ground, New Barnet, Herts, at 3 p.m Competition for Maw's challenge shield, Admission free.

Information Department

INFORMATION WANTED

Postal or telephone information with respect to makers or first-hand suppliers of the undermentioned articles will be appreciated.

S/30. Botipol
S/22. Blue for colouring swimming bath water
W/25. Guardian bandage
T/96. Inspro (for cleaning gas cookers)
H/30. Neogestin
F/25. Phosphofer (tonic syrup for dogs)
B/27. Quinalia (for washing gloves)
B/30. Watson's blister
B/29. Zilatone pills

THE
CHEMIST AND DRUGGIST
VOL. CXXV. July 4, 1936 NO. 2943

The Bournemouth Conference Meeting

The seventy-third annual meeting of the British Pharmaceutical Conference, held at Bournemouth last week and reported in our Annual Special Issue and the present issue, will long remain in memory as one of the most successful of recent years in general arrangement and smooth working, and as placing on record a series of monographs equalling or exceeding the average of the research papers presented year by year. The Local Executive Committee must be cordially congratulated on a highly successful piece of team work; and the somewhat formidable distances from point to point in the widely spaced town became of no account in the perfect weather prevailing. The address of the chairman (Mr. Harold Deane), which has a prescriptive right of recognition as the "high light" of the Conference, makes a further claim on careful reading as the pronouncement of an expert on a subject unquestionably his own. The particular importance of Mr. Deane's survey lies, we venture to suggest, in his indication of the need for research on the pharmacology of drugs, a subject in which, as he showed, current knowledge is very deficient.

By way of index to the twenty-two Conference papers, we give our usual brief mention of the subject-matter. *The Effect of Degree of Comminution on Extraction by Percolation* is examined in the cases of belladonna leaf, ipecacuanha and stramonium by A. W. Bull. James Coutts, in *Santonin in English and Welsh Artemisias*, extends the scope of the investigation he has previously made regarding the practicability of manufacturing santonin from British-grown plants. New light is thrown on the subject of sterilisation on a manufacturing scale in *The Penetration of Heat into Surgical Dressings*; the author of the monograph, R. Maxwell Savage, discusses in detail the effect of autoclave conditions on the material submitted. Kenneth Bullock, in *The Analytical Examination of Commercial Desiccated Hog Stomach Preparations*, gives reasons for the use of analytical data in controlling the manufacture of these products. Norman Evers and Wilfred Smith discuss *The Measurement of the Proteolytic Activity of Pancreatic Preparations*, and suggest an improvement on the B.P. method of determination. The same authors have worked out a modification of the official process for *The Determination of Strychnine in Easton's Syrup*, their process yielding satisfactory results with both new and old syrups. W. C. Peck examines various factors relating to the preparation of tinctures and extracts, and suggests improved methods for *The Extraction of Vegetable Materials*. A. T. Moorhouse has evolved a process for making *Dry Extract of Stramonium*. C. Gunn and P. F. R. Venables describe a method for the *Determination of Cod-Liver Oil in Cod-Liver Oil and Malt Extract*. The blue fluorescence given by rhapontic rhubarb is made the basis of examination by Sydney K. Crews into *The Detection of Rhapontic Rhubarb in Galenical Preparations*. Norman Glass discusses the variable composition of *Magnesium Trisilicate*. An approximate method of determining whether or not solutions are isotonic with the blood serum is described by F. Wokes in *Isotonic Solutions for Injection*; the same author describes *An All-Glass Bacteria-proof Filter*. G. J. W. Ferrey gives details of modifications that overcome the inaccuracies of the B.P.C. method of *The Determination of Manganese in Iron and Manganese Citrate*. In two papers entitled respectively *The Anomalous Viscosity of Mucilage of Tragacanth* and *The Standardisation of Tragacanth*, G. Middleton returns to the problem of obtaining a perfect mucilage from this gum, and offers suggestions. H. Brindle and C. E. Waterhouse review present methods and suggest a new procedure for *The Quantitative Determination of Mercury in its Compounds*. G. F. Hall and A. D. Powell discuss the effects of various factors on the solubility of acriflavine and the relative merits of determining its unmethylated constituents in *Acriflavine: Solubility and Diamino-acridine Content*. Bernard F. Howard calls attention to *The Standardisation of Tablets in the Swiss Pharmacopœia*, and suggests that corresponding standards should be officially adopted in the United Kingdom. Miss M. O. Barrie examines *The Effect on the Isolated Heart of the Preservative present in Insulin Solutions, B.P.* C. G. Lyons and F. N. Appleyard consider *The Determination of Official Preparations of Iron by Means of Ceric Sulphate*, and outline a method for *The Assay of Saccharated Iron Carbonate*. C. Morton and D. C. Harrod demonstrate that the presence of glucose renders inaccurate titrations with potassium dichromate but has no disturbing effect on those with sodium iodate in *The Assay of Saccharated Iron Compounds*.

The full text of these papers will, as usual, be available in due course: meanwhile we desire to call attention to a few with which chemists who realise the importance of following current developments of scientific thought and research will be wise to make themselves acquainted. Mr. R Maxwell Savage, under the title "The Penetration of Heat into Surgical Dressings," has contributed a valuable study of results obtained in sterilising various materials under selected conditions, and has gone far towards putting such processes on a definite basis. Dr. Kenneth Bullock has attacked the intricate problem of hog stomach preparations, which owes so much to the brilliant work of Dr. J. F. Wilkinson at the Manchester Royal Infirmary, from the analytical side, and has made certain definite advances in securing products of satisfactory activity. Mr. Norman Glass has further elucidated the difficulties in the way of obtaining magnesium trisilicate of constant chemical composition and physical properties. If this antacid fulfils the expectations of its chief sponsor, Dr. Nathan Mutch, it will probably supersede other alkaline remedies to a considerable extent in medical practice. Near the end of the list of monographs will be found one by Mr. Bernard F. Howard, which, ostensibly dealing only with the standardisation of tablets in the Swiss Pharmacopœia, raises (as was evident in the discussion that followed its presentation) the larger question of the desirability of laying down official standards for compressed tablets of potent substances, first with regard to weight and secondly as to rate of disintegration. We may add a brief comment on the new type of programme drawn up this year and referred to in our Annual Special Issue. The effect of the change will no doubt be reviewed by the Executive Committee in the light of experience thus obtained; it is obvious that more than one kind of Conference member has to be taken into account, and we trust that the claims of each will be sympathetically considered.

Pharmaceutical Society of Northern Ireland

Council Meeting

THE monthly meeting of the Council was held on June 19 in the Society's offices, 73 University Street, Belfast, the president (Mr. W. S. Taylor) in the chair. There were present also Messrs. W. C. Tate, H. F. Moore, S. H. Forrest, Charles Abernethy, J. F. Grimes, J P., James Glendinning, James McDowell, W. Martin and Dr. S. E. Acheson. Mr. D. L. Kirkpatrick (secretary) was in attendance. Apologies for absence were received from Messrs. S. Gibson (vice-president), John Grey, R. I. Edwards and J. T. Nicholl.

Arising out of the minutes MR. TATE said he had been reported as having stated at the last meeting that he would have liked some provision made in the regulations so that their B.Sc. graduates might be available for posts of examiners, but that this did not seem to be feasible. What he did say was that if these regulations were passed it would not be possible.

CORRESPONDENCE

The Pharmacy Board of Victoria and South Australia, the Ontario College of Pharmacy and the Pharmacy Board of Queensland wrote acknowledging receipt of the Register.

An application was received from Louis Heath Valentine Longmore, Christchurch, N.Z., for registration under the reciprocity agreement.

THE SECRETARY said that Mr. Longmore was the son of a pharmacist in Dromore. He was a student in Queen's University, Belfast, and would only be here for a time. The applicant's papers were all in order.

On the motion of DR. ACHESON, seconded by MR. ABERNETHY, the application was granted.

The Ministry of Labour wrote forwarding a copy of a letter issued by the Department to firms in Northern Ireland who make or supply first-aid boxes in compliance with Section 26 of the Workmen's Compensation Act (Northern Ireland), 1923, and Regulations and Welfare Orders under the Factory and Workshop Acts. The letter referred to the use of the white or silver cross on a red ground, and stated that in the meantime the factory inspectors were being instructed not to take any objection to the absence or deletion of the cross on first-aid equipment in factories and workshops provided that the cupboards and boxes are distinctly marked.

EXAMINATION RESULTS

The secretary read the results of the June examinations as follows:—

Preliminary Scientific Examination.—A. W. Gamble, H. G. Gwynne, A. G. Kerrigan, J. J. Knox, J. F. Lowry, J. J. McMichael, Miss E. W. Press, A. M. Stevenson.

Final Qualifying Examination.—W. A. Beggs, J. M. S. Bingham, H. G. Campbell, R. Frew, W. B. Hewitt, A. J. Howard, Miss H. L. Mackenzie, F. A. Mackey, M. D. Moore, T. McFadden, D. O. Pinkerton, W. H. Poulter, N. Sanderson, R. J. F. Saunderson, O. A. Wasson, W. Wilkinson, R. E. Young

THE SECRETARY said that in Part I sixty-six students sat for the examination; sixty-five completed and one apologised for presenting himself to the examiners for an examination he knew nothing about. Eight passed in the Preliminary Scientific, twenty-eight failed and thirty were referred. It was a deplorable pass list for Part I, but Part II was a great deal better. Forty-two entered, thirty-nine completed, seventeen passed, four failed and eighteen were referred. The three passes up for the first time were all from the country—from Coleraine, Ballyclare and Londonderry.

THE PRESIDENT said there was something wrong with the teaching somewhere.

MR. TATE: What is the slaughter in?

THE SECRETARY: Everything. Proceeding, Mr. Kirkpatrick said fourteen failed and fourteen passed in Part I in botany and chemistry. In botany alone there were seven failures; in botany and physics seven failed, and in chemistry and physics two failed. In the Final Qualifying examination seventeen passed, five were new and the others were referred candidates.

THE PRESIDENT said there was a lot of bad failures. There had not been anything drastic in the marking.

MR. GRIMES asked if the papers were beyond the mentality of the boys with ordinary reasonable study.

THE PRESIDENT said many of the boys had long hours to work.

MR. FORREST.—They had to work longer twenty years ago with fewer facilities for study.

MR. GRIMES maintained that the papers were too difficult.

THE PRESIDENT: You have an excess proportion of pharmaceutical chemists. It is not so much in the Final they are coming down as in the Preliminary Scientific.

MR. FORREST said they should have to take the Preliminary Scientific before they began apprenticeship at all.

THE PRESIDENT: Where will you get apprentices then?

THE SECRETARY, in reply to Mr. Tate, said that for the Final examination there were nineteen new candidates, and for the Preliminary Scientific thirty-four were new. He also reported that at the Preliminary Scientific in Queen's twenty-five candidates went up and only two got through. Replying to Mr. Moore, he said that in England apprentices only did two years' apprenticeship.

MR. ABERNETHY said he thought that when many boys got the Preliminary they slacked off.

MR. GRIMES: It comes back to this: you must restore the Registered Druggist examination.

MR. McDOWELL suggested going into the matter with some of the teachers.

In the result the whole question was referred to the Education Committee, THE PRESIDENT saying they would have to go into the matter very seriously.

It was also agreed that an effort be made after the holidays to arrange a conference with the principal of the Belfast Municipal College of Technology.

HOME OFFICE MEMORANDUM

A memorandum on pharmacy administration for the year ended September 31, 1935, was submitted from the Ministry of Home Affairs. It was as follows:—

REGISTRATION.—The number of names on the Registers on December 31, 1933, 1934 and 1935, respectively, was as follows:—

	1933	1934	1935
Pharmaceutical chemists	817	856	876
Superintendents of bodies corporate (Ph.C)	59	66	73
Chemists and druggists	11	11	10
Registered druggists	140	140	138
Superintendents of bodies corporate (R.D.)	—	—	1
Certified assistants	6	6	7
Apprentices	546	558	578

Twenty-three apprentices qualified by examination as pharmaceutical chemists, and registered as such during the year. In addition, two persons availed themselves of the provisions of Section 7 (1) (*a*) of the Pharmacy and Poisons Act (Northern Ireland), 1925, and were registered as pharmaceutical chemists, and one person was registered as a certified assistant.

ISSUE OF LICENCES.—The number of licences issued in respect of the years ended December 31, 1933, 1934 and 1935, respectively, was as follows:—

	1933	1934	1935
Pharmaceutical chemists	444	455	467
Registered druggists	43	42	43

Of the total number of pharmaceutical chemists' licences eighty-five were issued to bodies corporate, and nine to executors of deceased pharmaceutical chemists. Three of the registered druggists' licences were issued to the executors of deceased registered druggists, and one to a body corporate.

LICENCES FOR THE SALE OF POISONS USED IN AGRICULTURE AND HORTICULTURE.—On December 31, 1935, there were 147 agricultural poison licences in force, compared with 149 on December 31, 1934.

INSPECTIONS.—During the year under review the Pharmacy Inspector carried out regularly visits of inspection to pharmaceutical chemists, chemists and druggists, and registered druggists, agricultural poison licence holders, methylated spirit retailers other than pharmaceutical chemists, chemists and druggists and registered druggists. He also paid numerous visits to traders suspected of selling poisons. In addition many visits were paid to street markets and fairs.

METHYLATED SPIRITS.—The fact that offences by pharmaceutical chemists, etc., in connexion with the sale of methylated spirits continue to increase is a matter which is causing much concern. It is most regrettable that although the attention of persons holding licences under the Pharmacy and Poisons Act, 1925, has repeatedly been drawn to the necessity for the most rigid observance of the regulations governing the sale of methylated spirit, offences for breaches of these regulations continue to increase, and, while this report deals with the year 1935, it is even now evident that records for 1936 will show an even greater number of convictions than in previous years.

In the discussion which followed MR. GLENDINNING said that in a certain store methylated spirit could be bought for 6d. disguised as eau de Cologne.

DR. ACHESON said that was not methylated spirit.

MR. GRIMES said there were people in his town selling the thing without any restrictions at all.

In reply to Mr. Abernethy, THE SECRETARY said there had been a conviction against a person other than a chemist in one case that he knew of.

THE PRESIDENT said that if unregistered persons sold the spirit it was a matter for the police.

MR. GLENDINNING said this business was gradually being filched from them through negligence. There were inspectors for this and that, but no other business was bothered.

MR. TATE said that if the term "personally known" were defined it would save a lot of trouble.

THE PRESIDENT agreed. To have a ruling on "personally known" would be a great help. Chemists who broke the law only got the whole body into disrepute.

Insurance Act Dispensing

Record of matters concerning Chemists' interests in the National Health Insurance Acts.

ENGLAND AND WALES

Blackburn.—Discussing a letter from the Ministry of Health regarding a rise in the cost of prescribing, a member said dispensing costs had been much higher during recent months than for some years; the increase was general throughout the country. The Minister in his letter declared his decision, as a precautionary measure, to reduce advances for dispensing fees as from April 1, 1936, to ninety per cent of such fees.

Rochdale.—For the third successive year the tests of drugs and appliances supplied to insured persons in the area of the Rochdale Health Insurance Committee have shown not a single case of inaccurate dispensing. On behalf of the chemists, Mr. Etherington declared that insured people secured the best possible medicine and service.

Warwickshire.—"Considerable inaccuracy" in the ammon. carb. content of mist. expectorans in two prescriptions was reported to a recent meeting of the county Pharmaceutical Committee, but the matter had not at that time been referred to the subcommittee concerned. Little change was discernible in the prescription costs in 1935 compared with 1934. At a meeting of the Insurance Committee Alderman Charles Davis, chemist and druggist, Leamington Spa, was appointed *Vice-Chairman*. Mr. Davis has been a member of the Committee since its inception.

Wigan.—The annual report of the Insurance Committee states that during the year 169,660 prescriptions were dispensed by chemists at a cost of £5,388. No complaints of incorrect dispensing had to be considered during the year.

Warts Treated by Suggestion

IN a reply in its "Queries" column, "The Journal of the American Medical Association" recently gave (106, 3, 235) an informative account of Bruno Bloch's investigation into the possibility of curing warts by suggestion. Authenticated details, according to this reply, commence in or about the year 1862, when Heim, afterwards a Swiss geologist, saw his father cure the warts on the hands of his little sister by pointing to them and saying for each, "This one goes away." Years later, when his son was afflicted and the warts did not yield to caustic treatment, Professor Heim attempted suggestion and was successful. He first treated the warts on one hand. As they disappeared in four days he treated the warts on the other hand, and in four days the warts on the face. After that he treated many people with a good measure of success. One resistant person he had to hypnotise in order to cure. He always felt that unless he could embarrass the patient he would not obtain a cure. Stupid children he could not cure. After the age of sixty he gave up the attempt as the effort was too great. Bonjour, a neurologist of Lausanne, treated warts by this method and reported no failures.

Professor Bloch, a dermatologist of Zurich, became interested and treated many cases. His success with this method was as great as with any other method, medical or surgical. There were 179 cases in his series in which follow up was possible. Of common warts he was able to cure 44 per cent., of the flat juvenile variety 88.4 per cent. Forty-three per cent. of the cures occurred in the first month, 39 per cent. in the second month and 18 per cent. after two months. Most of these cases had been treated by other methods without success. In one case the mother reported that all the warts swelled up a few days after the treatment and that some of them still showed blood crusts when observed by the physician. In four weeks all were gone except a few filiform ones on the lips and about the nostrils. These disappeared during the second month. Professor Bloch devised a more complicated procedure than that used by Professor Heim. After carefully examining the wart he blindfolds the patient and leads him into an adjacent room, where he places him with his hands spread out, if the hands are involved. He then draws an outline of the hand, drawing in each wart life-size. Then he starts a machine, which produces some noise but makes no connection with the patient. He then paints each wart with some vivid colour, red, green or blue, leads the patient back to the consultation room, removes the blindfold, and orders that the colour be not removed from the warts or the treatment will be less effective. The patient is asked to return in two weeks and is kept under observation for several months. One patient treated by Professor Bloch was a neurologist who was told that he would be treated by suggestion. He was indignant and expressed his disbelief in any such treatment but submitted because of his great desire to lose the warts. In spite of his disbelief and to his great astonishment, all the warts disappeared in two weeks. Bloch proposes and answers the following objections:—

(1) That the series is too small to prove anything. He answers that, because of the large percentage of cures, it is large enough.

(2) That the colouring matter may have exerted a chemical effect. Several different colours were used intentionally to overcome this objection. None is known to have any direct effect.

(3) That a part of the cases were cured. As many as by any other method.

(4) That the cures were due to spontaneous healing. There is such a thing as spontaneous healing of warts. Everyone knows that, but there could not be so high a percentage at any one time. If, after any treatment, warts that have been present for months or years and have been treated in many ways without effect disappear within two to eight weeks, one is logically bound to grant a causal connection between the treatment and the cure. There are no statistics on spontaneous cures.

Memmesheimer and Eisenlohr found that about as many untreated cases were well in six months as in the series of treated cases. The facts of the suggestive therapy seem to make a strong case in favour of the reality of such a process.

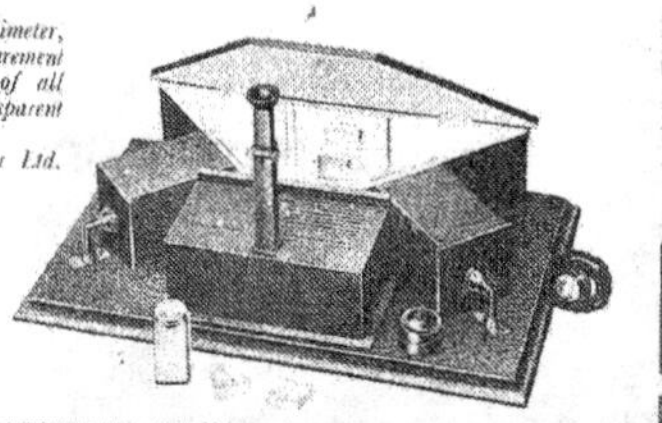

Complete Colorimeter, for precise measurement of the colour of all substances, transparent and opaque.—
Tintometer Ltd.

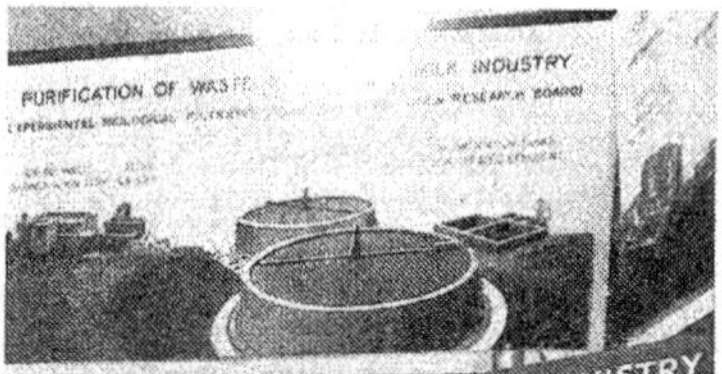

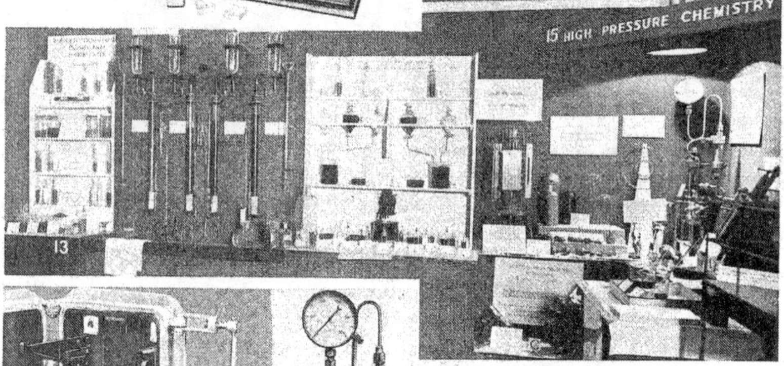

"High Pressure Chemistry."—
Department of Industrial and Scientific Research.

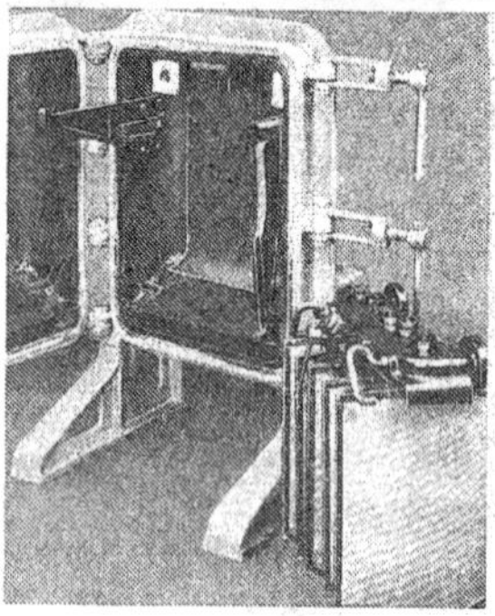

Vertical Leaf Filter.—
Manlove, Alliott & Co., Ltd.

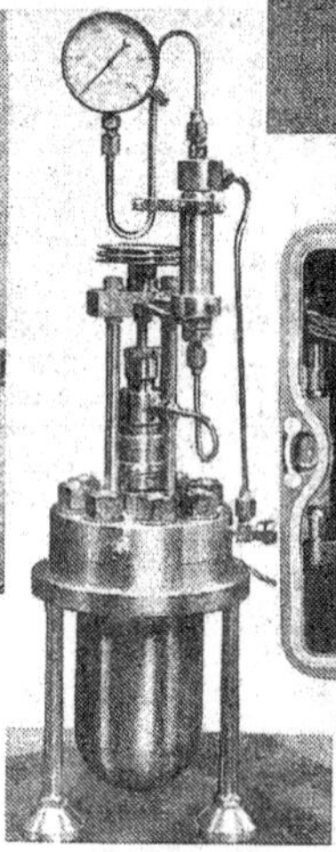

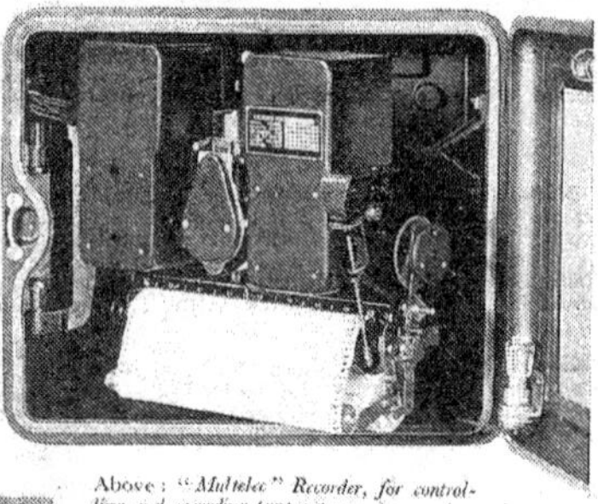

Above: *"Multelec" Recorder, for controlling and recording temperatures, etc.*—
George Kent, Ltd.

Left: *Autoclave (2 litres capacity) for temperatures up to 450° C. and 250 atmospheres pressure.*—*Hadfields, Ltd.*

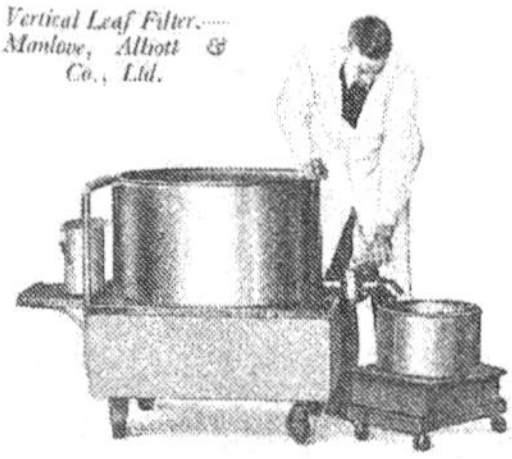

Monel metal equipment for cod liver oil industry.—
The Mond Nickel Co., Ltd.

Some of the Exhibits at the British

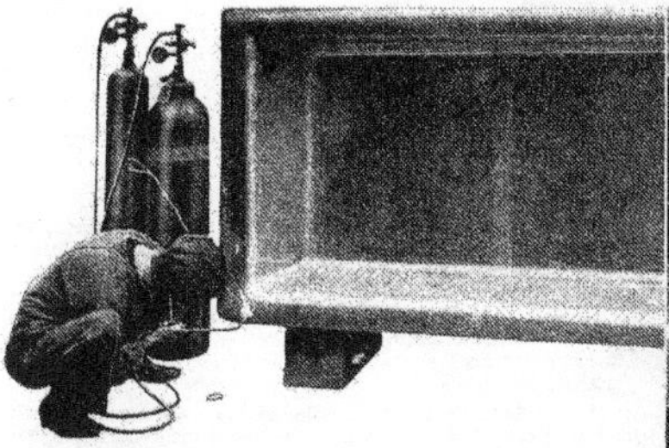

Welding an aluminium storage tank.—The British Oxygen Co., Ltd.

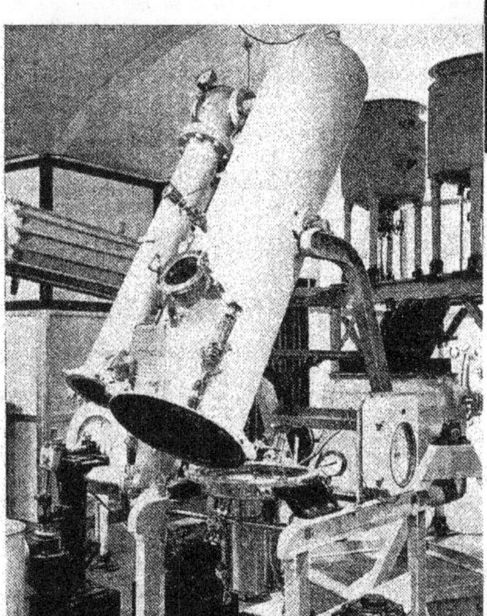

Forced circulation Evaporator for pharmaceutical extracts, etc., working under high vacuum.—George Scott & Son (London) Ltd.

Chemical Plant Exhibition

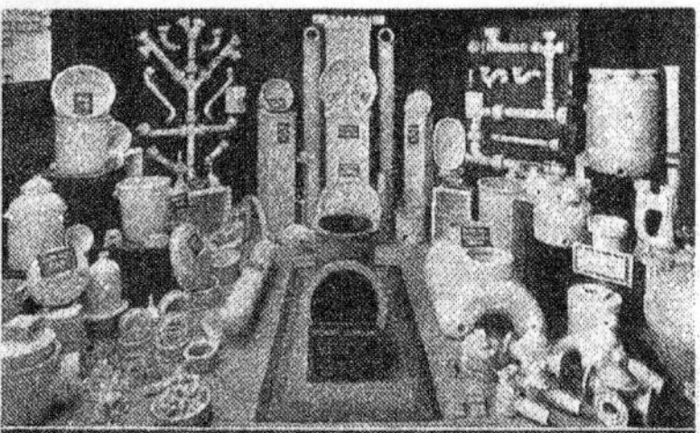

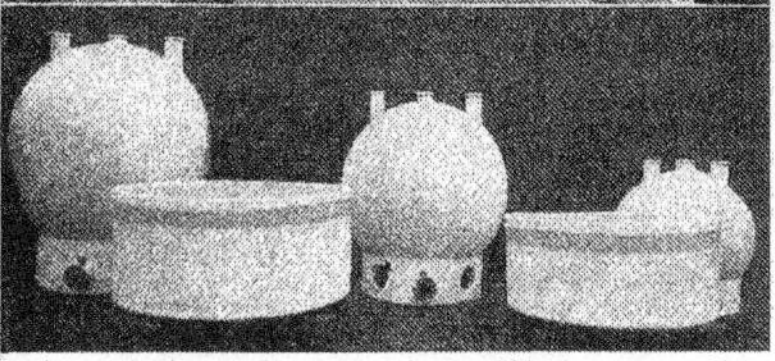

Top: *Unglazed and cream glazed acid resisting Stoneware.—George Skey & Co. Ltd.*

White Stoneware Vacuum Vessels and Filters.—Hathernware, Ltd.

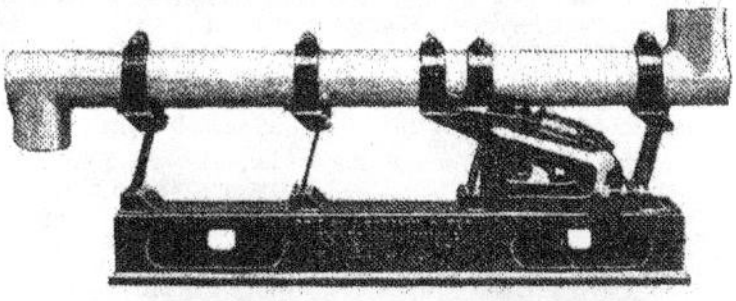

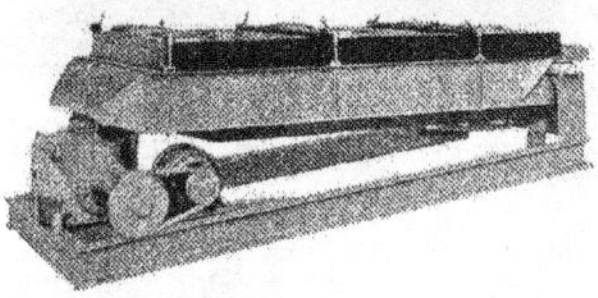

Above: *Rotex Screener, balanced gyratory motion, dust-tight, and low consumption electric Conveyor.—Lockers (Engineers) Ltd.*

Below: *Representative group of "Staybrite" Steel Tanks for fine chemicals.—Firth-Vickers Stainless Steels.*

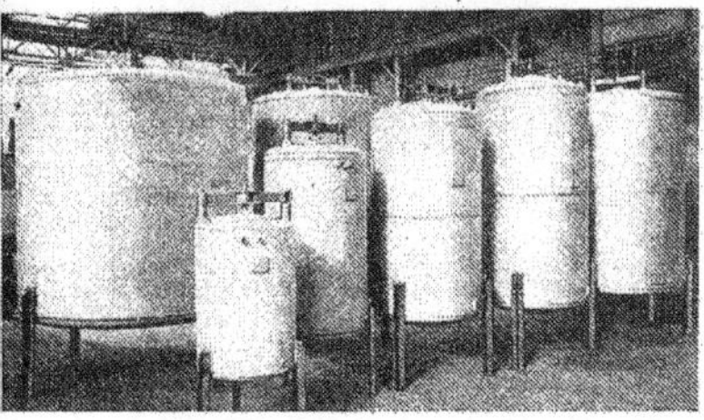

Pharmaceutical Latin in 1685

RECORDS of the life of Richard Browne, a physician well known in England in the last quarter of the seventeenth century, are extremely scanty. It is believed that he was educated at Queen's College, Oxford, became a licentiate of the London Royal College of Physicians in 1676, and obtained the M.D. degree of Leyden University. Beyond these details, the titles of five books constitute almost all that is known about him. One of these books is of perennial interest to pharmacists and medical men, as it purports to teach the pronunciation of Latin words used in medicine and is, as far as we are aware, the first work of its kind written in English. Its title is: "*Prosodia Pharmacopœorum*: OR THE *APOTHECARY'S* PROSODY. SHOWING The exact Quantities, in the Pronunciation of the Names of Animals, Vegetables, Minerals and Medicines, and of all other words made use of in Pharmacy, many of which have been hitherto pronounced false."

The pronunciation of Latin, as Browne acknowledges in his prefatory remarks to "the Reader," was not a new subject in 1685. He records his indebtedness to the "Lingua Pharmacopœorum" of Olaus Borrichius (1670), of which his book is substantially a translation, with additions. He proceeds to justify his undertaking by citing as parallels the syntax of Linacre (1524) and the prosody of Smetius (1635). The last-named is a monument of industry, comprising, in addition to the usual trimmings, 648 closely printed pages filled with words arranged alphabetically, each one being illustrated by a quotation from a Latin author. Browne is full of the importance of his subject; he writes:—

> "Now if in any Art proper Pronunciation be of moment, it must be so in Physick; but in Pharmacy especially, wherein Man's Life is more nearly concerned, and where a *Sibboleth* may encrease the number of the Slain. . . . It will, I hope, be granted me, that this undertaking may be of use to Youth, when they come to the Apothecaries Trade; though for a man after he has made *Diachylon* Plaster forty Years, to be then taught how to call it, sounds a little odd."

After his own remarks to the reader, Browne translates those of Borrichius to "the candid and uncorrupt reader." Borrichius refers to the strictness of Latin speakers in keeping their rules of prosody: he tells us that an actor who made a slip in the quantity of a vowel in Rome was hissed off the stage, and he professes to base his own system on the usages of the Latin poets The latter part of his address to the reader is occupied by a discussion of the penultimate (or penultima, as it was then called). A general statement leads to a more detailed exposition:—

> "But some will judge it supervacaneous for me to go about to show the quantity of the penultima in those words that are short by A vowel before a Vowel"; [then follows a list of about ninety examples. The author continues:] "But . . . not every Vowel before a Vowel is short, . . . we cannot always safely trust this Rule, as not being general: for example, aristolochia, cadmia, centaurium, mithridatium, mumia, scordium, make long the penultima; bysimachia and cichorium have their penultima doubtful . . . But as the number of Pharmaceutick Words is almost infinite, so we are not solicitous for the quantities of Dissyllabes, nor for those words, whose penultima is long by Position or Diphthong."

About fifty words are given as illustrations of this apparent latitude, the reason for which immediately follows: "For Boyes come to the Apothecaries Shops sufficiently instructed in the common Rules of Grammar, how to pronounce all these with a due Pause." But the "boyes" are not, after all, so advanced as we may have been led to expect; the next sentence reads.—

> "Among other Polysyllables, which are judged by the plain Authority of the Antients, and by invincible Analogy, there are many, which at this day are otherwise pronounced in the Shops, than Reason and the Practice of the Antients do perswade."

About forty examples follow; and Borrichius comments: "The young Beginner will sweat, and he also, who has got beyond his Rudiments, will be puzzled, how to express these and the like words in their due Accents, unless"—unless, of course, he is guided by "some Aridnæan Clew," in other words, by the book before him. With two lines from Horace we are launched on the Prosody.

The Author's Method

The arrangement of the work is ostensibly alphabetical, but the author's discursiveness leads him into various breaches of continuity A short paragraph will disclose his method of treating the subject:—

> **Colcŏthar**, burnt Vitriol It is an Arabian word, and makes long the penultima by position: For Aviceuna calls it Kolkhotthar, whose first original, without doubt, came from the chalcitis of the Greeks.

On the whole, Browne's quantities and accents are not widely different from those now in use. A few of his preferences may be quoted · Aconitum and cubeba he pronounces with the short penultimate; diachylon and diascordium with the long; diarrhodon and elleborus with the short; hypericum with the long; storacis with the short. Under the heading "asarum" Avicenna receives some hard knocks:—

> "If any one object, that Asarum in Avicenna makes long the penultima, for he calls it atsârum . . .; I answer, that we are not bound to Avicenna's Laws in measuring of Greek Words, but we must stand to the judgment of the Greeks, of whom Avicenna borrowed these same words, and wrested them a little into the similitude of a strange sound, after the manner of the Arabian tongue. . . . But where the Greek and Latin are silent, whether we must appeal to the accent of the Arabians, in Words which the Apothecaries Shops owe to the Arabick School, would prove a Controversie perhaps too tedious."

Our author, in spite of his desire to avoid being tedious, nevertheless occupies three pages of his book with "asarum" and the disquisition arising from it Browne's principal claim to remembrance is his methodical survey of Latin pronunciation from a medical and pharmaceutical point of view, a field in which, as we have indicated, he was a pioneer.

Treatment of Ringworm

GOOD results in the treatment of ringworm of the face, neck and arms are reported in a recent issue of "The Journal of the American Medical Association" (106, 18, 1563) by Dr. M. Molitch. The treatment consists chiefly in the application of an ointment containing 0.5 per cent. of dihydroxyanthranol. At first the author tried a 0.1 per cent. ointment and found it non-irritating but only feebly effective. He then tried the 0.5 per cent ointment and found it both non-irritating and effective. One application caused, within a few hours, a light purplish discoloration of the lesion and of the skin adjacent to its border. The next day the skin crinkled, and on the third or fourth day it desquamated. No scars or other complications resulted in the twenty-four boys (aged from nine to fourteen) treated. As not one additional new case appeared during the past six months, it appears that the one application of the 0 5 per cent. ointment was sufficient to sterilise the lesion and thus prevent the infection of other children. The author points out that dihydroxyanthranol differs from chrysarobin chemically by the absence of the methyl group.

STUDENTS' MAGAZINE.—Number three of the "Pharmimag and P.S.A. Record," the organ of the Pharmacy Students' Association of Bristol Merchant Adventurers' College, is chiefly remarkable for a cartoon-like essay in photo-montage, entitled "The Student's Nightmare." Humorous prose is another main feature of its forty-four pages.

A CRIME-DETECTION COURSE IN THE U.S.A.—The most recent curriculum of the Philadelphia College of Pharmacy and Science, Pennsylvania, includes the curriculum of a course in "Scientific Methods of Crime Detection." The subjects include forensic science, forensic analysis, finger-printing and identification, ballistics, analytical chemistry, bacteriological chemistry, biology and applied microscopy.

Trade Report

Where possible scales of prices of chemicals are given for bulk down to small quantities. Prices recorded for crude drugs, essential and fixed oils and coal tar products are for fair sized wholesale quantities. Qualities of chemicals, drugs, essential and fixed oils, etc., vary, and selected brands or grades would be at higher values

28 Essex Street, W.C.2, July 2

A RATHER BRIGHTER TONE is reported in most markets, with a fair business being done. The steadier feeling in Continental rates of exchange has had a good effect. In the PHARMACEUTICAL CHEMICALS markets business has moved along well up to average, and all the recent price changes are being steadily maintained. Where any isolated competition is noted, the makers of IODIDES are meeting it. Rumours have been on the market that the scales of prices for SALICYLATES and ASPIRIN were to be adjusted, possibly to slightly lower levels: we have made full inquiry in appropriate quarters and are assured that, while the position on the Continent may be somewhat obscure, British makers have no intention of revising their prices.

Crude Drugs

Inquiry for these products continues fairly good and prices in many instances are firm at current good figures; scarcity of supplies continues a common feature of this market. Still no shipment offers of Cape ALOES. The spot market for BARBASCO ROOT has been quiet and is rather easier. Spot prices for remaining bales of BUCHU continue to advance. A parcel of Duckwari CARDAMOMS has just been landed. Values for CASCARA SAGRADA, spot and new peel for shipment are firm. Final fishing and oil figures for Norwegian COD-LIVER OIL are to hand, the oil crop being substantially short Sudan GUM ACACIA is steady on quotation; business quiet. Matto Grosso IPECACUANHA is slightly cheaper on spot LYCOPODIUM is scarce and dear on spot. MENTHOL has remained quiet. Spanish-Italian MERCURY is cheaper for shipment. Prices for PIMENTO show a recovery. Fair sales of RHUBARB on spot, mostly in rough round quality. Quite a fair demand on spot for SENEGA at full prices. All grades of TRAGACANTH are firmly held as quoted on spot, with the white grades again dearer; source reports purchasing difficulties will restrict shipments. WAXES are steady but rather quiet.

Essential Oils

There has been a little more life in the markets this week, and business has been better Quotations for a number of oils on spot are very irregular, the variation being generally due to difference in quality. ANISE (STAR) is dull and easier forward. All the SICILIAN OILS are in very quiet demand on spot; supplies in dealers' hands appear to be moderate. Quotations from the source for these oils for shipment when sanctions are raised vary considerably, but they are all on a higher level and reports to hand suggest conditions are strong and likely to remain so At the moment, however, there is no indication of interest in the offers, either from merchants or consumers. The deciding factor in these markets from now up to the new crop oils will be the weight of demand, and we are of opinion most consumers have well covered their requirements for this season. CASSIA is dull; some off-quality material offering here Madagascar CLOVE firm for shipment and scarce. Californian cold-pressed LEMON has been advanced again this week; distilled unchanged. French Guinea ORANGE is steady but in quiet demand; shipment nominal, nothing offering Californian ORANGE is quoted dearer. Fair spot business in Japanese PEPPERMINT; the advances in the American NATURAL OIL are fully maintained, and the source indicates a strong position PETITGRAIN is being quoted at attractive figures on spot.

Exchange Rates on London

THE following is a list of the chief Continental and other exchange rates at the opening on Thursday morning:—

Centre	Quoted	Par	July 2	Value of the £
Amsterdam	Fs. to £	12·107	7·36½	12/2
Berlin	Mks. to £	20·43	12·43	12/2
Brussels	Belgas to £	nominal	29·67½	16/11½
Copenhagen ...	Kr. to £	18·159	22·40	14/8
Lisbon	Esc. to £	110	110¼	19/11¾
Madrid	Ptas. to £	25·22½	36⅝	28/10¾
Milan	Lire to £	92·46	63 13/16	13/9¼
Montreal	Dol. to £	4·86⅔	5·03¾	20/8
New York	Dol. to £	nominal	5·02 11/32	20/7¾
Oslo	Kr. to £	18·159	19·90	21/11
Paris	Fr. to £	124·21	75⅞	12/2½
Prague	Kr. to £	164·25	120¼	12/2¼
Stockholm	Kr. to £	18·159	19·39½	21/1¼
Warsaw	Zloty to £	43·38	26⅝	12/2¼
Zurich	Fr. to £	25·2215	15·33	12/2¼

Bank rate 2 per cent.

Pharmaceutical Chemicals, etc.

THE market continues generally steady with routine business moving. Prices for acetone, B.G.S., are reduced. Bromides are steady. Makers of iodides are meeting competition. Salicylates are unchanged.

ACETANILIDE.—Values steady, market quiet: B.P. crystals and powder, 1s. 5½d. to 1s. 8d. per lb., as to quantity.

ACETONE, B.G.S.—The scale of prices has been reduced to £54 to £56 per ton, in drums, as to quantity.

AMIDOPYRINE.—Market dull, competition keen: crystals, five cwt., 18s. 0¾d.; two cwt., 18s. 5½d.; less than two cwt., 18s 10½d per lb., with powder 2½d. per lb. extra.

AMMONIUM ICHTHIOSULPHONATE.—Steady business in small quantities. one cwt., 1s 6½d., in 14-lb. tins; 1s. 8d., in 1-lb tins; 1s. 10½d., in 8-oz. tins, and 2s. 1d. per lb., in 4-oz. tins

ASPIRIN.—Makers' scales of prices fully maintained: home trade, ten cwt., 2s. 7d., five cwt., 2s 8d.; one cwt., 2s. 8½d.; 28 lb., 2s. 9d; 14 lb., 2s. 10d; 7 lb., 3s; 4 lb., 3s. 2d.; 1 lb., 3s. 4d. per lb. Bulk packing free, net, carriage paid Contracts: Over twelve months, minimum one ton; over six months, less than one ton.

BARBITONE.—Remains dull and unsteady: spot, two cwt., 15s 3½d.; 56 lb., 15s. 8d.; small parcels, up to 16s. 3d. per lb.

BENZOIC ACID (B.P.).—Fair inquiry, market fully steady: quantities, ex works, 1s 9½d.; spot parcels, 1s. 10d. to 2s. 3d. per lb., as to quantity.

BISMUTH SALTS.—Makers' scales of prices are steady, fair demand: Carbonate, B.P., one cwt., 6s. 6d; 28 lb., 6s. 9d; 8 lb., 7s 3d.; less than 8 lb., 8s. 6d per lb., with rebates on contracts for larger quantities

BROMIDES.—Makers' and dealers' scales of prices continue at the recent advance. The home trade prices are: Potassium B.P., not less than five cwt., 1s. 7d.; not less than one cwt., 1s. 8d; not less than 28 lb., 1s. 11d; 14 lb., 2s. 1d. per lb Sodium, B.P., not less than 5 cwt., 1s. 9d; not less than 1 cwt., 1s. 10d.; not less than 28 lb., 2s 1d.; 14 lb., 2s 3d per lb. Ammonium, B.P., not less than 5 cwt., 1s. 10d.; not less than one cwt., 1s. 11d.; not less than 28 lb., 2s. 2d; 14 lb., 2s. 4d. per lb., net. 28 lb., parcels and one cwt cases free. Distributors' prices for quantities less than 14 lb. would be at higher figures. Scales of prices for export, quoted f.o.b. London for prompt shipment, are as follows: POTASSIUM, 5 cwt., 1s 1½d.; one cwt., 1s. 2d. SODIUM, 5 cwt., 1s. 2½d., 1 cwt., 1s 3d. Ammonium, 5 cwt., 1s 4d; one cwt., 1s 4½d. per lb. Contracts over a period are not being booked

BUTYL CHLORAL HYDRATE.—Market quiet, quoted unchanged: spot, 14 lb., 8s.; 7 lb., 8s. 3d.; 1 lb., 8s. 6d. per lb., in 1-lb. bottles.

CAFFEINE.—Continental makers' agreed prices: pure alkaloid, two cwt., 7s. 10d; one cwt., 8s.; 56 lb., 8s. 2d.; smaller quantities, 8s. 4d. per lb., delivered, 5-lb. tins free, smaller packing extra. Citrate, two cwt., 5s. 5½d.; one cwt., 5s. 6½d.; 56 lb., 5s. 7½d.; smaller quantities, 5s. 8½d. per lb., delivered. British material: pure, 56 lb., 8s 4d.; less, 8s. 6d per lb. Citrate, 56 lb., 5s. 9d; less, 6s. per lb.

CALCIUM LACTATE.—Moderate business at former prices: spot, one cwt., 1s. 0¾d.; 56 lb., 1s. 1½d.; 28 lb., 1s 2½d; smaller quantities, up to 1s. 6d per lb.

CHLORAL HYDRATE.—Makers' prices steady in home market: duty-paid crystals, in 14-lb. free containers, five cwt., 3s. 1d; one cwt., 3s. 2d; 28 lb., 3s. 3d.; 14 lb., 3s. 4½d. per lb; 28-lb. jars one penny per lb. extra.

CHLOROFORM.—Makers' prices are as follows: two cwt., 2s 5½d; one cwt., 2s 6d; 56 lb., 2s 6½d; less, 2s. 7½d per lb., in w-quarts of 8 lb. Packed in drums, ½d. per lb. less. Small bottles extra, from 5d per lb for ½-lb. bottles to 1d for 2-lb. bottles Carriage paid on minimum cwt. lots

CITRIC ACID (B.P. CRYSTALS).—Seasonal demand, quoted unchanged: British material quoted at 1s per lb., less 5 per cent. discount, nominal and without engagement. Dealers' prices for imported material are competitive.

CREAM OF TARTAR.—Fair demand, market steady: British material, 99 to 100 per cent., 79s per cwt., less 2½ per cent discount. Dealers' prices for foreign material competitive.

GUAIACOL CARBONATE.—British and imported material is being quoted on spot in the region of 9s per lb., as to quantity.

HEXAMINE.—Makers' prices for bulk quantities are competitive: fair business: B.P. powder, from 1s. 3d. to 1s. 4d; free-running crystals, from 1s. 6d to 1s 8d. per lb., carriage paid, for bulk lots. Dealers quoting free-running crystals, two cwt., 1s 6d; one cwt.,

1s. 6½d ; 14 lb , 1s 10d , smaller parcels, up to 2s. per lb , carriage paid.

IODIDES.—Makers' recent reduction in the scales of prices for these salts, as follows: POTASSIUM IODIDE, B.P , for quantities not less than one cwt., 4s. 6d.; 28 lb , 4s. 8d.; 14 lb., 4s. 10d.; 7 lb., 5s. 4d.; 4 lb , 5s. 10d ; smaller quantities, 6s 6d. per lb SODIUM IODIDE, B P., for quantities not less than 28 lb , 5s. 6d ; 14 lb., 5s 8d ; 7 lb., 6s 2d ; 4 lb , 6s. 10d.; smaller quantities, 7s. 10d. per lb. IODINE, B P., resublimed, for quantities not less than one cwt., 5s. 6d.; 28 lb., 5s. 8d., 14 lb., 5s. 10d.; 7 lb., 6s. 4d.; 4 lb., 7s.; smaller quantities, 7s 11d. per lb IODOFORM, B P., crystal, precipitated or powder, for quantities not less than 28 lb , 8s , 14 lb , 8s 2d ; 7 lb., 8s. 10d ; 4 lb., 9s. 8d., smaller quantities, 10s 8d. per lb. Sales terms . Contracts for one cwt or more (assorted if required) with " Fall Clause," for delivery over four months. No rebate now applies. Packages . Tins, 28-lb jars and one-cwt. cases, free. Bottles extra or returnable within three months, carriage paid. Delivery : Carriage paid on all quantities. Re-sale : It is a condition of sale that buyers undertake not to re-sell at prices below or on terms other than those ruling at the time of re-sale.

LACTIC ACID (B.P) —Moderate inquiry, market steady . quantities in carboys, 1s. 4½d. to 1s. 5d ; in winchesters and bottles, 1s 5½d. to 1s. 10d per lb., as to quantity.

MERCURIALS.—Makers' prices for the salts are keeping steady : Chloride, B.P., not less than one cwt , 4s 11d ; less than one cwt , from 5s. per lb. upwards, as to quantity.

METHYL SALICYLATE.—Market is dull : spot, ten cwt., 1s. 2½d ; five cwt , 1s. 3d.; one cwt., 1s. 3¼d.; less than one cwt , 1s 3½d ; small quantities, in bottles, up to 2s. per lb

METHYL SULPHONAL —Market dull and unsteady : two cwt., 19s. 3¼d , one cwt., 19s. 9¼d ; 56 lb , 20s. 2¾d ; small parcels, 20s 8d. per lb.

PARALDEHYDE.—Average business, market competitive : 1 w-quart, 1s. 9d ; 6 w-quarts, 1s. 7½d.; 12 w-quarts, 1s 5½d.; 36 w-quarts, 1s. 4½d. per lb., carriage paid on minimum 6 w-quarts ; one demijohn, 1s. 1d. per lb., carriage paid.

PHENACETIN.—Limited business, market steady as quoted : crystals or powder, bulk quantities, 2s. 6d. to 2s. 7d.; smaller parcels, 2s. 7½d. to 2s. 10½d. per lb., as to quantity.

PHENAZONE.—Market is dull and very irregular : crystals, five cwt , 8s 9½d.; two cwt., 9s. 0½d., and less, 9s 3d. per lb , with powder 2½d per lb. extra.

PHENOLPHTHALEIN.—Not much business moving, quoted unchanged : two cwt , 2s. 9d ; one cwt , 2s 10d ; 28 lb., 3s ; 14 lb , 3s 1d.; 7 lb , 3s. 2d.; smaller parcels, up to 3s 6d. per lb.

PHENYL ETHYL BARBITURIC ACID.—Average small spot business : quoted from 25s. to 26s. per lb., in 2-lb bottles.

PHOTOGRAPHIC CHEMICALS.—AMIDOL —28 lb , 7s. 6d.; 14 lb., 8s. 3d ; 7 lb , 9s.; under 7 lb., 11s. 9d per lb , in 1-lb. bottles. CHLORQUINOL. —1-lb. bottles, 21s. per lb. GLYCIN —7 lb , 10s. 6d ; 1-lb. bottles, 13s 6d. per lb HYDROQUINONE.—56 lb., 4s 10½d.; 28 lb., 5s.; 14 lb., 5s 3d., 7 lb , 5s 6d , 1-lb. bottles, 6s. 6d per lb. METOL.—28 lb., 9s. 6d.; 14 lb , 9s. 9d., 7 lb., 10s. 9d ; 3 lb , 11s. 6d.; 1-lb. bottles, 12s 6d per lb ALUM (PHOTOGRAPHIC QUALITY).—1 cwt , 21s. per cwt. 28 lb. for 6s GOLD CHLORIDE.—15-grain tube, 52s. 6d. per doz. MAGNESIUM POWDER.—10s. per lb. PARAMIDOPHENOL HYDROCHLOR.—8s 6d. per lb. POTASSIUM FERRICYANIDE.—14 lb., 2s. 3d ; 7 lb , 2s. 6d.; 1 lb., 2s 9d per lb POTASSIUM METABISULPHITE.—One cwt , 7½d ; 28 lb 8d ; 14 lb., 9d.; 7 lb., 11d.; 1 lb., 1s. per lb. PYROGALLIC ACID —28 lb., 6s. 9d.; 14 lb , 7s. 6d.; 7 lb., 8s. 3d.; under 7 lb., 8s 9d per lb SODIUM CARBONATE (RECRYST) —5 cwt., 12s. 6d. per cwt ; 1 cwt , 15s. 6d. per cwt ; 56 lb. for 11s. 6d.; 28 lb. for 6s. SODIUM HYPOSULPHITE, CUBES, CRYST —5 cwt., 16s 3d.; 1 cwt., 18s. 6d. per cwt ; 56 lb. for 11s. 6d ; 28 lb. for 6s. SODIUM SULPHIDE (PURE).—7 lb , 1s 3d ; 1 lb , 1s. 6d. per lb.

POTASSIUM PERMANGANATE (B P.).—Dealers doing average business in smallish quantities : quantities in drums, 8¾d. to 9½d.; druggists' parcels, from 10d. to 1s. per lb , as to quantity.

POTASSIUM SULPHOGUAIACOLATE.—Market is dull and competitive : quoted in the region of 6s. 3d. per lb.

QUININE SALTS.—Convention prices were advanced as follows from June 8 : sulphate, 2s. 2d.; bisulphate, 2s. 2d ; ethyl carbonate, 2s. 9½d ; salicylate, 2s 10½d ; hydrochloride, 2s. 8½d.; bihydrochloride, ; hydrobromide, 8½d.; bihydrobromide, 3s.; valerianate, 3s. 8d.; hypophosphite, 4s.; alkaloid, 3s. 0½d. per oz , carriage paid on bulk quantities ; 100-oz. tins free, smaller packages extra.

RESORCIN.—Modest business. British material : crystals, one cwt , 4s 11d.; 56 lb , 5s.; 28 lb , 5s 1d ; 14 lb , 5s. 3d.; 7 lb., 5s. 6d.; less than 7 lb., up to 6s per lb.

SALICYLIC ACID (B.P.).—Market remains dull, quoted unchanged : five cwt , 1s. 7d.; one cwt , 1s. 7½d ; 28 lb , 1s. 8d.; 14 lb., 1s. 9d ; 7 lb., 1s 10d.; 4 lb., 2s per lb.

SALOL.—Fairly steady, market quiet : spot, crystals, two cwt., 3s.; one cwt., 3s. 0½d.; 56 lb., 3s. 1½d.; smaller parcels, 3s. 2d. to 3s 6d. per lb.; powder, 2½d per lb. extra.

SANTONIN.—Dealers' quotations for outside parcels now quoted at about £21 to £22 per kilo. No change in first-hand prices : not less than 50 kilos., £35 12s. 6d ; not less than 25 kilos., £36 1s.; not less than 10 kilos., £36 9s.; not less than 3 kilos., £36 17s.; not less than 1 kilo., £38 13s. 6d ; less than 1 kilo , £39 13s. 6d. Special prices are in operation for export to all markets

SODIUM SALICYLATE (B.P.).—Business quiet, quoted unchanged : home trade, crystals or powder, five cwt., 1s. 8½d.; one cwt., 1s. 9d ; 28 lb , 2s.; 14 lb., 2s. 2d.; 7 lb , 2s 3d.; 1 lb., 2s. 6d. per lb.

STRYCHNINE SALTS.—Makers' prices are steady :—

	Under 16 ozs.	16 ozs.	35 ozs
	Per oz. s. d.	Per oz s. d.	Per oz. s. d.
Alkaloid cryst.	2 8½	2 7	2 6½
Alkaloid powder	2 7½	2 6	2 5½
Bisulphate	2 2½	2 1	2 0½
Hydrochloride	2 4½	2 4	2 3½
Nitrate	2 3½	2 2	2 1½
Sulphate cryst.	2 4½	2 3	2 2½

25-oz. containers, free ; 1-oz. bottles, 2½d.; 2-oz. bottles, 3½d. Other conditions as usual. Lower prices for bulk quantities. Wholesale distributors' prices for small quantities would be dearer.

SULPHONAL —Dealers' prices continue keen, business slow : crystals or powder, two cwt., 15s. 5½d.; one cwt , 15s. 10½d , 56 lb , 16s. 1d.; smaller parcels, up to 16s 9d per lb.

TARTARIC ACID (B P. CRYSTALS) —Seasonal demand, with quoted values steady : British makers quote at 1s. per lb , less 5 per cent. discount. Dealers offering foreign materials at competitive prices.

THEOBROMINE.—Continental material ; pure, two cwt., 7s. 10d.; one cwt., 8s ; 56 lb , 8s. 2d.; smaller quantities, 8s. 4d. per lb. Sodium salicylate, two cwt , 6s 3½d ; one cwt , 6s 4½d.; 56 lb., 6s. 5½d.; smaller quantities, 6s. 6½d. per lb., delivered, 5-lb. tins free, smaller packages extra.

THYMOL.—Business remains rather slow ; fine white, two cwt., 5s. 10d.; one cwt., 6s.; 56 lb., 6s. 4d.; 28 lb., 6s. 9d.; smaller parcels, 7s. 6d. per lb.; ex ajowan seed, one cwt., 8s. 7d ; 56 lb., 8s. 10d.; 28 lb , 9s. 4d.; 14 lb , 10s. per lb.

VANILLIN —Market has been rather quiet, steady : ex clove oil or guaiacol, five cwt , 12s. 9d.; one cwt., 13s.; 56 lb., 13s. 3d., less, 13s. 9d per lb.

Crude Drugs, etc.

ACONITE ROOT.—Dealers continue to quote spot Napellus root at about 67s. 6d per cwt. for small parcels.

AGAR.—Market is about steady, business not of much importance : spot, Kobe No. 1, 2s. 7½d ; No. 2, 2s. 5d ; Yokohama No. 1, 2s. 4½d. per lb ; shipment, Kobe No. 1, 2s 5d ; No. 2, 2s. 5d.; Yokohama No 1, 2s. 2d. per lb., c i.f.

ALKANET ROOT.—Some inquiry on spot with holders quoting small parcels at about 45s. per cwt.

ALOES.—Plenty of inquiry for Cape, but nothing offering forward. On spot the few boxes are firmly held. Cape, spot, firm at 63s ; shipment, nominal. Curaçao, spot, 97s. 6d. to 110s., as to quality ; shipment, from origin, 87s. 6d. per cwt , c.i f.

ANTIMONY.—Chinese crude is now quoted for July shipment at £24, c.i f. English regulus at £66 10s. to £67 10s. spot.

ARNICA FLOWERS.—Not very much business moving. Spot is quoted at 1s. per lb.

ASAFETIDA.—Dealers are quoting cases of sticky blocked tear at 87s. 6d. to 90s. per cwt., spot.

BALSAMS.—Continue steady, business moderate : *Tolu*, 1s. 9d.; *Canada*, 2s. 9d.; *Peru*, 5s. 4d. per lb , spot.

BARBASCO ROOT.—Market has been rather dull : spot, material 1s. to 1s. 3d., as to test. Shipment, July, 10½d. per lb., c i f.

BELLADONA.—Dealers continue to do some fair business ; leaves, 60s ; root, 50s. per cwt., spot.

BENZOIN —Some inquiry continues for Siam, which is in short supply and firm : pea size, £22 ; small peas, £20 ; blocky seed, £17 per cwt Sumatra in free supply : middling small almonds, 86s.; fair almonds, £5 5s. to £6 7s. 6d. per cwt.

BUCHU.—At the further sharp advances the market is firm Only about six bales arrived last week and supplies continue very small. Green rounds, 2s 5d to 2s. 7d. for fair to good. Ovals, rather stalky, firm at 2s 2d per lb. One holder is not selling rounds under 3s.

BURDOCK ROOT.—Dealers are quoting small spot parcels at about 45s. per cwt.

CAMPHOR.—Values about steady, business in small spot parcels : Japanese, spot, tablets, 2s 5d.; powder, 2s. 3d.; slabs, 2s 2½d. per lb , ex store Shipment, tablets, 2s. 1½d.; powder, 2s. 0½d ; slabs, 1s 11½d per lb , c i f. English refined is unchanged ; flowers, 1 cwt.,

3s 1d.; 28 lb., 3s. 2d.; small lots, 3s. 3d per lb. Transparent tablets, 4 oz., 8 oz. and 16 oz., 3s. 4d; 1 oz and 2 oz., 3s. 5d.; ½ oz., ⅓ oz. and ¼ oz., 3s. 6d. per lb.; special prices for contracts and bulk quantities.

CANTHARIDES.—Not much inquiry on the market. Russian, 6s; Chinese, 1s. 11d.; shipment, 1s. 6d. per lb.

CARDAMOMS.—The spot market continues fully steady with Indian seeds at 4s. 3d. per lb. A parcel of Duckwari is now being landed, containing the usual selection, and it is understood they will be put up for auction in due course.

CASCARA SAGRADA.—The spot market is firm, tending to advance, and inquiry has been good. 1933 peel, 57s. 6d. to 60s.; 1935 peel, 55s. and upwards asked. A few shipment offers are being received for new peel with the figure for car-load lots 44s. per cwt, c.i.f., and more for less.

CHAMOMILES.—Moderate inquiry with holders of last season's flowers quoting 90s. to 110s. per cwt., as to quality.

CLOVES.—Market continues steady. Zanzibar, spot, 7½d.; shipment, July-August, 7⅜d. per lb, c.i.f. Madagascar, in bond, 6⅝d.; shipment, July-August, 6⅜d. per lb., c i.f.

The landings of Zanzibar in London during the week ended June 27 were 100 and the deliveries 149, leaving a stock of 1,728. From January 1 to date the landings of Zanzibar have been 2,234 and the deliveries 1,581. Landings of Madagascar for the week ended June 27 were *nil*, and the deliveries 14, leaving a stock of 1,876. From January 1 to date landings of Madagascar have been 1,756 and the deliveries 1,442 packages.

COCOA BUTTER—Market is steady at recent better values Prime English, 10½d. to 11d. per lb.; foreign 9¾d. to 10½d. per lb., as to quantity.

COCONUT (DESICCATED).—Values tend to be on a slightly lower level on spot: spot, fine, 23s. 3d.; medium, 22s. 9d per cwt.; shipment, halves, July, 20s. 9d per cwt, c i f.

COD-LIVER OIL—Bergen reports fishing has concluded; final figures are: 137,112 tons of cod and 64,147 hectol of oil, compared with 116,670 tons of cod and 69,050 hectol. of oil last season and 143,870 tons of cod and 85,254 hectol. of oil in the 1934 season. Shipment market very quiet Finest Lofoten steam refined non-freezing medicinal oil, 84s. per barrel, c i f. London: spot, in small lots, 126s. per barrel, ex store, duty paid. Newfoundland non-freezing medicinal oil, about 130s per barrel, ex store. British non-freezing medicinal oil is quoted at 100s. per barrel, London, duty free, while quotations from another home source are at higher figures.

COLCHICUM.—Dealers are offering spot supplies at about 42s. 6d. per cwt. for small parcels.

COLOCYNTH.—The firm shipment conditions continue with the figure at 2s., c.i.f., for U.S.P. quality pulp. On spot, the price is firm at 1s. 10d. per lb, in bond.

CUTTLE-FISH BONE—Market is still on the quiet side, with fair East Indian at 6½d to 10½d. per lb, spot.

DAMIANA LEAVES.—At current prices quoted a fair quantity of business has been done. spot, 8d. to 9d. per lb, as to quantity.

DANDELION ROOT—Dealers are quoting spot supplies of foreign root in the region of 80s. per cwt., as to quantity.

DERRIS ROOT.—Market has remained quiet: spot, 1s. 3d. to 1s. 4d. per lb., as to ether extract; shipment, July-August, 10¼d. to 10½d.; per lb., c.i.f., basis 17 per cent. ether extract.

DIGITALIS LEAVES.—Origin reports values are dearer, but does not mention a figure.

DRAGONS BLOOD—A quiet demand for reboiled, fair to good, quoted at £23 to £24 per cwt Medium, £21 to £22 per cwt.

ERGOT.—Some bold Russian on the spot is available at 4s, with Hamburg offering at 3s. 6d, c i.f Portuguese and Spanish are nominally unchanged on spot at 6s 9d. One Portuguese shipper has suggested that business in new crop might be booked at 3s 9d. per lb, c.i f, for a bulk quantity, but does not offer firm at this figure.

GENTIAN.—Dealers report steady inquiry, with spot from 37s. 6d. to 40s. per cwt., as to quantity.

GINGER—Spot quiet and slightly easier for West African; shipment unchanged· West African, spot, 60s; for arrival, 56s per cwt, c.i f. Jamaican, spot, sold in barrels, 86s to 90s; small grinding, 62s. 6d to 65s per cwt, in bags, ex store

GUAIACUM.—Market has been rather quiet, with fair to good glossy sorts at 1s. 7d to 1s. 8d and good bright refined at 1s. 9d. per lb.

GUM ACACIA—Values are being maintained, but business remains slow: spot, Kordofan cleaned sorts, 42s. 6d., bleached No. 1, 110s.; extra, 120s. per cwt, shipment, Kordofan cleaned sorts, 40s. per cwt, c.i f.

HENBANE—Spot supplies are available in small parcels at about 80s. per cwt. Market quiet.

HENNA—Dealers are offering good green Egyptian leaves at about 37s 6d. and brown leaves at 30s. per cwt., in small parcels.

HONEY.—Inquiry rather slow· quoted values steady: Jamaican, spot, 32s. to 42s. 6d. for dark liquid manufacturing to pale set Haiti, 32s 6d to 40s for dark to pale, duty paid. Mexican, 35s. per cwt, duty paid. Canadian, 42s. 6d to 45s. per cwt. for pale to good.

HYDRASTIS—Values maintained, business moderate: spot, 9s. 6d.; shipment, 9s. 3d. per lb, c i.f.

IODINE.—The Convention price for crude continues at the recent reduction at 8s. per kilo, with usual rebates for bulk quantities.

IPECACUANHA.—With more arrivals there has been some pressure to sell, and the spot market is slightly easier: Matto Grosso, B.P., 5s. 4½d. to 5s. 6d. per lb, as to quantity; shipment, 4s. 10d. per lb, c.i f.

LIQUORICE ROOT.—Some supplies of natural root are available in the region of 12s. 6d. per cwt.

LYCOPODIUM.—Very scarce indeed on spot and firmly held at the high figure of 5s. 6d per lb. No shipment offers.

MENTHOL—Market has been on the quiet side, only a limited spot business moving: K/S brands, 13s. 1½d; in bond, 11s 9d. Japanese shippers quote July-August at 11s. 4½d. to 11s. 7½d., with re-sellers at 11s. 3d per lb., c.i f. The October-December position remains neglected, with a seller at 10s. 10½d., c.i f.

MERCURY.—The Spanish-Italian group report their shipment quotation is cheaper at 60 dollars per bottle, f o.b. Continent: spot, £12 2s. to £12 2s. 6d. per bottle, ex store.

MYRRH.—Some parcels of fair Aden sorts quoted steadily at £6 10s. per cwt, ex store.

OPIUM—Average small spot sales. spot, 1s. 3½d. to 1s. 4d. per unit, landed and duty paid.

ORRIS ROOT.—A few small parcels of Florentine are quoted firmly up to 75s. per cwt. Business negligible.

PEPPER—Quoted fractionally easier, market dull· Lampong, in bond, 2⅜d.; shipment, July, 2$\frac{7}{16}$d.; August-October, 2$\frac{7}{16}$d., c.i.f. Tellicherry, spot, 4⅜d.; shipment, August-October, 36s, c.i f. Aleppy, spot, 4⅜d.; shipment, August-October, 35s. 6d., c.i.f. White Muntok, in bond, 4¾d; shipment, July, 4$\frac{3}{16}$d.; August-October, 4$\frac{3}{16}$d. per lb., c i f.

PIMENTO.—Quoted values have recovered sharply, market steady: spot, 7⅜d per lb.; shipment, July, 67s 6d. per cwt, c.i.f.

PSYLLIUM SEED—French seed reported dearer at origin. Some recleaned seed on spot is available at about 8d. per lb.

QUASSIA CHIPS—A moderate inquiry is being received, with small parcels quoted up to 21s. per cwt.

QUILLAIA BARK.—Dealers are offering spot supplies of crushed bark at about 35s. per cwt., in small parcels.

RED ROSES—New crop, to arrive, are being offered at about 4s 6d. per lb.

RHUBARB.—A few cases of poor selection of Shensi available on spot and quoted at 4s 6d to 4s 9d. Some Shensi pickings are available at 2s. 9d. to 3s. per lb. Offers of rough round, high dried, all pinky quality for shipment, the price being 1s 2½d. per lb., c.i.f. On spot values steady at 1s. 5½d. to 1s 6½d. per lb, as to quality.

RUBBER.—Fair business has been done this week and the market is steady: Standard ribbed smoked sheet, spot, 7⅝d.; July, 7⅝d; August, 7⅝d.; September, 7$\frac{11}{16}$d; October-December, 7¾d.; January-March, 7$\frac{13}{16}$d; April-June, 7⅞d. per lb.

SAFFRON.—Small business, quoted unchanged: spot, B.P., 1898, prime, 43s, extra, 40s 6d; super, 37s. 6d. per lb., and less for bulk quantities.

SARSAPARILLA—Occasional demand, market steady as quoted: spot, Jamaican grey, 1s. 2d to 1s 3d; native, mixed colours, 10d. to 11d per lb, as to quantity, spot.

SEEDS.—ANISE—Spot, duty paid, Spanish, 57s 6d; Bulgarian, 29s 6d. CARAWAY.—Dutch, on spot, 38s, sellers, duty paid. CORIANDER.—Spot, Morocco, old crop, 21s 6d., duty paid; new crop for July-August shipment, 12s., c i.f., quoted. CUMIN.—Spot, Morocco, 43s., duty paid; Malta, 43s. 6d.; Morocco, for shipment, new crop, July-August, offered at 30s 6d, c.i f. FENUGREEK.—Morocco, spot, 13s 6d, duty paid; new crop, for shipment, quoted at 11s., c i f MUSTARD.—English, 20s to 31s per cwt., according to quality.

SENEGA.—Quite a fair business reported on spot, with the price well held at 1s. 5d New crop has been done at 1s. 4d. and the quotation is now fully steady at 1s. 4¼d. per lb., c i f.

SENNA.—The market for Tinnevelly leaves continues steady, with good green parcels offering on spot as follows: prime bold at 7½d; No 1 at 6d; No. 2 at 4¼d; No. 3 at 3d. per lb. Off-coloured leaves are available at slightly cheaper prices. Best quality hand-picked pods are scarce and prices up to 5d. per lb. have been paid for good greenish, with lower qualities offering down to 3⅜d. per lb. Alexandrian. Recent arrivals of hand-picked pods have fallen off considerably and the quality of the recent importations shows a much lower grade. Holders of the early shipments of best pods are now requiring higher limits, but ordinary qualities are commanding little attention: spot values as follows:—bold No. 1, 5s. to 5s. 6d.; No. 2, 3s. to 4s; No. 3, 1s 2d to 2s 6d. per lb, according to quality.

SHELLAC.—Rather quiet but steady: spot, standard TN orange, 54s to 59s.; fine orange, 65s. to 135s; pure button, 65s. to 70s. per cwt., spot. For delivery, TN, August, 64s.; October, 55s. For arrival, TN, July-August, 51s. per cwt, c i.f.

SLIPPERY ELM BARK.—Small demand on spot: five-pound wired bundles, 1s. 2d. per lb.; grinding grades, about 7½d. per lb.

SQUILL.—One or two small lots of fair white are reported available on spot at about 55s. per cwt.

STRAMONIUM—Some parcels of good green leaves are available at about 45s. per cwt., in small lots.

TONKA BEANS.—Rather quiet on spot, with fair frosted Para beans very steady at 4s. 3d New crop, for shipment, 2s 9d. per lb., c.i f.

TRAGACANTH.—The spot market continues firm, particularly for the white grades, for which higher prices are again recorded. The source continues to advise difficulty in making purchases. White ribbon is now up to £33. Medium white grades, £18 to £25. Textile grades are being inquired for and quoted from £5 upwards per cwt.

VALERIAN ROOT.—Dealers are quoting small spot parcels at about 37s. 6d. per cwt, business slow.

WAX—BEES'—Market is steady, spot and forward, business moderate. Calcutta, bleached, spot, 135s.; afloat, 130s; shipment, 122s. 6d., c i f Abyssinian, spot, 120s; in bond, 108s; shipment, 106s., c.i f.; Benguella, spot, 120s.; shipment., 106s., c i f, Conakry, spot, 107s. 6d.; shipment, 107s per cwt., c i f. Dar-es-Salaam, spot, 120s.; shipment, 117s per cwt., c.i f. CARNAUBA.—The spot market is rather quiet; shipment quotations steady. Fatty grey, spot, 157s. 6d.; afloat, 150s; shipment, June-July, 148s, c.i f Chalky grey, spot, 160s; shipment, June-July, 150s, c.i.f. Primeira, spot, good quality, 212s. 6d; afloat, 205s.; shipment, June-July, 196s, c i f. Mediana, spot, 205s.; shipment, 192s. 6d. per cwt., c i f.

Essential Oils, etc.

RATHER more business reported this week, with the trade spread over most items Anise (Star) is easier forward. Shipment quotations for all Sicilian oils are sharply dearer, but business has so far been negligible. Japanese peppermint steady; the American oil is firm at the advance Petitgrain is quoted keenly on spot

ALMOND—Fair business in small parcels. English-made, cwt. lots, 2s. 2½d.; smaller parcels, up to 2s 6d. per lb; foreign, cwt. lots, 2s. 3½d.; smaller parcels, up to 2s. 7d. per lb French, bitter, 6s. 3d per lb

ANISE (STAR).—Market is slow on spot and shipment offers are easier: spot, leads, 2s. 6d.; tins, 2s. 4d; drums, nominal, per lb., ex store; shipment, leads, not quoted; tins, 1s. 9½d.; drums, 1s. 8½d per lb., c.i f.

BAY—Dealers report some small business: 49 to 50 per cent, 4s. 7d. to 4s. 9d; 59 to 68 per cent, 4s. 10d. to 5s per lb, as to quantity

BERGAMOT—There is very little inquiry on spot, with holders asking from 8s. 3d. to 10s. 3d per lb, as to brand, quantity and seller The position at the source is reported strong, with quotations for shipment upon the raising of sanctions from 7s 10½d. to 8s. 9d per lb, c i.f., but actual business has so far been negligible.

BOIS DE ROSE—Occasional business of modest size: spot, Brazilian, 5s. to 5s. 3d.; shipment, about 4s. 10d per lb., c i.f.

CAJUPUT.—Some small spot business: B P., 1s. 9d. to 2s. 1d. per lb, as to quantity.

CANANGA—This market continues unsteady and dull: shipment is not more than 7s 4½d, with spot in the region of 8s. 4½d to 8s. 6d. per lb

CARAWAY—Values quoted are unchanged, market quiet. Dutch rectified, 9s to 9s 1½d., crude, 8s 6d to 8s. 9d. per lb., landed and duty paid.

CASSIA—Shipment offers at about 2s 6d., c i f., drums, and spot prices 3s 2d. to 3s 3d per lb, as to quantity.

CEDARWOOD—The African oil continues to be quoted keenly on spot at about 1s. for drums and up to 1s 4d. for small parcels. American, spot, drums, 1s 1½d.; smaller parcels, up to 1s. 4½d per lb.

CINNAMON LEAF—The market has been dull and is slightly easier. Ceylon oil, spot, drums, 2s. 11d.; smaller parcels, up to 3s. 2d; shipment, 2s 7½d. per lb, c.i f, in drums.

CITRONELLA—Business in the Ceylon oil has been very moderate on this market. The Java oil is quoted unchanged, with inquiry small: Ceylon, spot, drums, 1s. to 1s. 1d; smaller parcels, up to 1s. 4½d.; shipment, drums, 8½d. per lb, c i.f. Java, spot, drums, about 1s 3d; smaller parcels, 1s 4d. to 1s. 7d., shipment, drums, 1s. 0½d. per lb, c.i f

CLOVE—The Madagascar oil is firm for shipment and very few offers are being made: Madagascar, spot, drums, 3s. 3d. to 3s. 4d; smaller packings up to 3s. 6d. per lb; shipment, if available, 2s. 8d. per lb., c i f. English oil, 4s. 2d. per lb.

EUCALYPTUS—Market continues very firm, with spot values tending to advance: Australian, 70 to 75 per cent, 1s. 2d. to 1s. 2½d.; 80 to 85 per cent., 1s 3d to 1s. 3½d. per lb, landed; higher prices for small lots on spot. Spanish, 70 to 75 per cent., 1s. 3½d. per lb., ex store.

GERANIUM.—Business has remained quiet: Bourbon, spot, 21s. to 21s. 6d; shipment, 19s. 9d., c.i.f.; Algerian, spot, 21s. to 22s.; shipment, 20s. per lb., c.i.f.

GRAPE-FRUIT.—Dealers quote spot parcels of hand-pressed from about 15s. to 16s. per lb.

HO (SHIU).—A moderate business is reported, with prices slightly steadier: spot, from 1s. 6½d. to 2s. 1½d. per lb., as to quality and quantity.

JUNIPER BERRY.—Suppliers are finding some modest business, with prices ranging from 2s. 10d. to 3s. per lb., as to quality.

LAVENDER—Market remains dull and irregular on quotation. The source reports that with the recent rains the plants are well developed and, with plenty of sun during the next few weeks, the flower crop should be good: 50 to 52 per cent., 29s. 6d.; 48 to 50 per cent., 27s.; 40 to 42 per cent, 22s; 38 to 40 per cent., about 20s.; 36 to 38 per cent., 18s. per lb., landed, for good brands. Lavandin is quoted 11s. to 12s. 6d. per lb.

LEMON.—The very limited quantities of Sicilian hand-pressed oil in dealers' hands are held for about 7s. 9d to 9s. 6d., as to brand and quantity, but business seems to have been of no great account recently. At the source, according to advices, the position is firm and still higher prices are being mentioned for shipment when sanctions are raised, the figures ranging from 6s. 9d. up to as much as 7s. 6d., c i f.; at these prices there is not likely to be a rush of business, although it seems possible that high values may be maintained up to the end of the summer. A further advance in the Californian cold-pressed oil is notified, and the supplies to become available are extremely small. Distilled, regular quality, small drums, 3s 9d.; large drums, not offering; cold-pressed now 5s. 4½d. per lb., c.i.f.

LEMONGRASS.—A few orders for shipment reported at cheap prices. shipment, 1s. 6d., c.i.f.; spot, 2s. to 2s. 2d. per lb., as to quantity.

MANDARIN.—Any genuine oil on spot would be about 31s. per lb. For shipment still higher prices are now being quoted, the average being about 19s. to 20s. per lb., c i.f., for shipment when sanctions are raised.

ORANGE.—Sicilian sweet on spot is nominal. The source reports a very strong position and suggests shipment values are now in the region of 12s to 14s per lb, c i.f, for post-sanctions shipment. These prices are of little interest at the moment. The demand on spot for French Guinea oil has been small this week, with sellers of drums from 3s. 3d. upwards; practically nothing offered for shipment, with the price nominal and firm at 3s. 3d. per lb., c.i.f., in drums. The Californian oil has been advanced, as follows: one case, 4s.; two or more cases, 3s. 10d.; small drums, 3s. 9d. per lb, c.i f

PALMAROSA.—There has been a marked lack of business for this oil. Spot, about 6s.; shipment, 5s. 6d. to 5s. 9d. per lb., c i.f.

PATCHOULI.—Market has remained rather dull. Good quality Singapore oil is steady at 16s. per lb. Seychelles oil on spot, about 12s. to 12s 3d. per lb.

PEPPERMINT.—Moderate spot business continues, with values about 5s. 10½d to 6s. Japanese shippers quote July-August at 5s. 9d. to 5s 10d., with re-sellers at 5s. 8d, c.i f. Speculative business in the end-of-the-year position quiet, with buyers at 4s. 6d. and sellers at 4s. 8d per lb, c i f. Japanese shippers quote October at 5s. 6d. and October-December at 5s. 3d. per lb., c i.f., with very little interest shown The source reports a strong position in American natural oil, stating that the plantations, although of normal acreage, are very poor and thin, due to dry and cold weather. It is suggested that the oil crop will therefore be well below former tonnage. Shippers now asking 2 dollars 20 to 25 cents for 50 per cent. menthol oil and 2.10 to 2 15 for 46 per cent menthol content, c.i.f., in drums.

PETITGRAIN—New arrivals are quoted cheaply on spot: spot, 3s. 6d. for cases up to 3s. 10½d. for smaller packings; shipment, about 3s. 4d. per lb., c.i.f.

ROSEMARY.—Limited inquiry on the market: Spanish, good quality oil, about 2s. 3d per lb, with some offers well under this figure.

SANDALWOOD—Genuine East Indian Mysore, 19s. per lb., in one-case lots on spot; practically no second-hand offerings. English-made East Indian, 22s. 6d. to 25s per lb, as to quantity. English-made West Indian, cwt. lots, 5s. 10½d.; 56 lb., 6s. 1½d; 14 lb., 6s 4½d. per lb Australian oil continues steady at the recent reduction: 5 cases, 14s. 6d.; one case, 14s. 9d; 7-lb tins, 15s 3d. per lb.

SASSAFRAS—A little more inquiry reported. Natural oil quoted from 3s. 7d to 3s. 9d. per lb, as to quantity. Artificial oil at cheaper prices.

SPIKE.—Business has been limited in volume, with good quality Spanish oil at about 3s. 8d. to 4s per lb. Inferior oils at cheaper figures.

VETIVERT.—A few small parcels of Bourbon on spot are quoted at 37s. 6d. per lb.

WORMSEED.—Market is steady but quiet· U.S P. oil, spot, 9s.; shipment, 8s 7½d per lb, c i f.

Correspondence

Letters should be written on one side of the paper only. Correspondents may adopt an assumed name, but must in all cases furnish their real name and address to the Editor

Chemists' Friends Scheme

SIR,—An analysis of the patents section of a small pharmacy undertaken to ascertain the most profitable patents to display reveals the following approximate percentages of patents showing 33⅓ per cent. profit or over on turnover:—Of medicinal patents stocked, 15.8 per cent. of total number; of toilet patents stocked, 52.7 per cent. of total number. Razor blades, tooth powders, etc., are counted as toilet patents, and total numbers represent various sizes, shades, etc , each size or shade counting as one. Direct orders are included at buying prices. The remaining 84 per cent. of medicinal patents and 47 per cent. of toilet patents do not show a profit reaching 33⅓ per cent. on turnover—probably the majority show about 25 per cent. and quite a number much less Shall we assume average overhead expenses to work out at 20 per cent. of turnover? They will be more or less, of course, but 20 per cent. may be taken as a reasonable basis. What inferences arise?

(1) Patents showing 20 per cent. on turnover give neither gain nor loss—percentages over 20 show direct gain and those below direct loss.

(2) Even allowing for the greater volume of medicinal patents it obviously pays to display more toilet patents.

(3) Displays of patents showing less than 20 per cent. gross become free advertisement for the manufacturer without counting in loss of time, energy and space.

(4) The beauty specialist, hairdresser, etc , can make a higher percentage profit on toilet patents than can the chemist on medicinal patents: should this be so?

(5) If the C.F. scheme is to be of practical use, profits also must be taken into account. Of what use is a C.F. line unless it pays to display it?

(6) If any "doubting Thomases" still question the necessity for the C.F. scheme, let them study a wholesaler's list and analyse a section of patents taken at random.

(7) Distributing wholesalers should be roped into the C F movement (to avoid leakages), as they stand to benefit.

These seven inferences do not by any means cover the whole ground, but each one gives scope for thought and, I trust, action.—Yours, etc ,

EVERY DOG TO HIS BONE (19/6).

The Chemist's Dilemma

SIR,—"B. Practical," in your issue of June 27 (p. 788), longs for an era of high pharmacy yet is fearful of the regulation of apprenticeship. Could the lack of system of recent years be expected to produce any other result than the one it has? When a pharmacist during his lifetime turns out thirty apprentices he makes thirty competitors, for the 75 per cent. who are refused registration must needs attempt to carry on without it. If outside competition is not desired, the pharmacist must cease to create it and take less apprentices, and they must be given more than a one-in-four chance of registration. All governments have some regard for equity, and none would grant "pharmacy for the pharmacist" on less than those terms.—Yours faithfully,

ECO (27/6).

The Conference Chairman's Address

SIR,—The chairman's address at the Bournemouth Conference, given by Mr. Harold Deane (*C. & D.*, June 27, p. 719), was a departure from the usual kind, and therefore perhaps the more interesting; and although the title was given as "The Cultivation of Drugs," the matter contained many features of interest to pharmacists apart from this. The quotation from the first presidential address is a point to be noticed: in spite of the prosperity of those present at the Conference there are still to-day many chemists in small businesses whose whole lives are spent in scraping a scanty pittance. In regard to the remarks on modern medical practice, are we not really reviving some of the ancient ideas in a modern dress (vitamins, hormones, and so on) which were prescribed in a much cruder form by the old practitioners? On the other hand, in the case of potent drugs such as alkaloids the tendency seems to be to revert to the use of the whole drug, it being found that the isolated principle is not so effective, thus getting back to the use of herbs. As Mr. Deane pointed out, vegetable drugs are more largely used on the Continent than in England; there every pharmacy shows packets of herbs for the making of tisanes or teas, and in some of the country parts the women and children can be seen collecting herbs at the proper seasons, especially lime. Even in this country I can remember when people used to collect dandelion and elder to make their own preparations or to bring them for sale to the country pharmacy; and I have more than once been offered newts and snakes with the idea that they were used in medicine. I can also remember as a boy being taken on a visit to a relative who had a pharmacy in Lincolnshire, and he grew his own peppermint, hyoscyamus and belladonna, distilled his own oil and made the green extracts. I think it will be many years hence before the public relinquishes its belief in drugs and herbal remedies —Faithfully yours,

IMMUNITY (30/6).

Subscribers' Symposium

For interchange of opinion among "C. & D." readers and brief notes on business and practical topics.

The C. & D. Special Issue

My hearty congratulations on a particularly fine production which surpasses even the excellent issues of previous years. The advertisements are artistic, colourful and attractive to an extent which enhances their business appeal. The literary sections, too, so rich in illustration, provide interest and information of permanent value. A publication to be enjoyed and retained.—*Beta* (29/6).

I want to thank you for the Special Issue this week. I think it is the best issue you have ever done. The advertisements are especially attractive. The editorial matter is also good; the colour chart for powder and cream was fine and fascinating, bringing this part of pharmacy into a proper scientific method of grading. I have often thought that these productions were the limit of what could be done, but this shows that there is always room for some advance.—*W. T. G.* (30/6).

"It is not so good as it used to be" is a phrase which certainly cannot apply to the 1936 Annual Special Issue of the *C. & D.* I have read and re-read all the Special Issues for more years than I care to count, and I may say "every year and in every way they grow better and better." It must be a marvel to many, as it is to me, how you can gather together such a wealth of material on so many subjects, all dealing directly or indirectly with pharmacy. A week-end is much too short a period in which to explore such a treasure-house of literary art, so I have promised myself many hours of well-occupied leisure. Nor shall I overlook the advertisement pages, in which I am always keenly interested; and undoubtedly the whole issue is colourful. In expressing my appreciation I am but voicing that of numerous subscribers in Scotland.—*Scotia* (29/6).

In the wonderful selection of matter which you have provided in your Special Issue the article which is of special interest to me is the one describing "The Oldest Pharmacy in Europe" (p. 784), as during my various visits to the Continent I have visited many old pharmacies. With regard to the pharmacy at Dubrovnik, it is stated that the precise date of foundation is not certain, although it was in existence before 1318; it is a pity this cannot be ascertained exactly, as there are other pharmacies which extend back to the same period. For instance, there is the Pharmacie du Cerf at Strasbourg, which I described in some notes on a visit to that town (*C. & D.*, August 23, 1930, p. 256), and which was illustrated in further notes (*C. & D.*, August 24, 1935, p. 256). This pharmacy is known to have been open continuously from 1268.—*Pharmatoura* (29/6).

Miscellaneous Inquiries

When samples are sent particulars should be supplied to us as to their origin, what they are used for, and how. We do not undertake to analyse and report upon proprietary articles nor to publish supposed formulas for them.

M. J. (26/66).—SOFTENING SEA WATER.—So far as we are aware there is no economical method of rendering sea water soft and suitable for toilet and domestic use, and we think the best way out of the difficulty would be to use a special sea-water soap.

L. D. C. (30/66).—DEXTRIN PASTE.—The following recipe is from among those given in "Pharmaceutical Formulas," Volume II:—

Dextrin	3 lb.
Borax	6 oz
Glucose	5 oz.
Water	42 oz.

Dissolve the borax in the water, mix well with the dextrin and glucose, and heat till solution takes place. Set aside for three or six months to ripen.

W. P. (26/66).—POISON FOR MOLES.—Liquid extract of red squill has been found to be an efficient substitute for strychnine. The bait should be prepared as follows:—

Meal	250 gm.
Shredded meat	210 gm.
Liquid extract of red squill	212·5 gm.

Divide the material into 150 baits, two of which should be inserted in each hole.

Another method of killing moles is to place pledgets of cotton-wool soaked in carbon disulphide in the animals' runs and cover up the holes again.

F. B. (25/66).—SUPPLIES TO DOCTOR'S N.H.I. PATIENTS.—In a rural area where an insured person has difficulty in obtaining drugs and appliances from a chemist's shop, the doctor who provides treatment may be required by the local Insurance Committee to supply any medicines that are needed. In such circumstances the regulations require that the practitioner shall provide all necessary drugs and appliances to what are known as his "dispensing patients" and he is specially paid a sum calculated to cover the cost of these. It is quite wrong, therefore, for a practitioner to obtain any special appliances that he may not keep in his surgery, such as plaster of Paris or elastic adhesive bandages, from an insurance chemist in a neighbouring town by means of the ordinary insurance prescription made out in the name of the patient, and then supply those himself to the patient. In that way the chemists' fund bears the cost of a prescription for which payment will be made by the Insurance Committee to the doctor. Intimation of the fact that a practitioner adopts this practice of issuing Insurance prescriptions for his dispensing patients should be sent to the Insurance Committee for the area through the local Pharmaceutical Committee. The Insurance Committee is able to check the prescriptions against the list of insured persons in their possession and can take any necessary disciplinary action without the name of the local chemist being brought into the matter.

C. W. M. (25/66).—(1) SAL MARIENBADENSE.—The usual method of taking this is to dissolve a small quantity, say as much as will lie on the point of a knife, in three-quarters of a tumblerful of soda water filled up with warm water. This should be taken in sips. Four to six glasses should be taken per day.—(2) SAL PHYSIOLOGICUM.—Hager's formula is given in P.F.1, p. 504, and is as follows:—

Calcium phosphate	40 gm.
Potassium sulphate	2·5 gm.
Sodium phosphate	20 gm.
Precipitated sulphur	5 gm.
Sodium chloride...	60 gm.
Magnesium phosphate	5 gm.
Artificial Carlsbad salt	60 gm.
Silicic acid	10 gm.
Calcium fluoride...	2·5 gm.

A. G. (57/6).—REGISTERING A TRADE MARK.—You will find particulars of the registration of trade marks in *The Chemist and Druggist Diary*, 1936, p. 323. We cannot undertake search, and for this purpose you should employ one of our advertisers who specialise in this class of work.

S. S. (28/66).—FERTILISERS.—The following recipes are given in "Pharmaceutical Formulas," Volume II:—

For Roses

Calcium superphosphate	57 parts
Fine bone meal	96 parts
Potassium sulphate	38 parts
Ammonium sulphate	28 parts
Ferric oxide	5 parts

For Carnations

Calcium superphosphate	44 parts
Fine bone meal	34 parts
Potassium sulphate	14 parts
Ammonium sulphate	20 parts

S. D. (29/66).—PHOTOGRAPHS ON WALLS.—The photo-mural process of decoration is being undertaken commercially. In carrying out the process, the surface of the wall is first treated and then sprayed with a photographic emulsion. Then at night exposures are made by means of an enlarger, the subsequent developing, washing and fixing also being carried out by means of spraying apparatus. As in ordinary photography, the scale and size of the picture is limited only by the sharpness of the negative and the size of the wall space available. The methods, spray guns and composition of the emulsion are covered by patents. This photographic process is a step beyond the previous method of making photo-murals by enlarging on paper, which is then pasted or nailed on to the walls. The latter process was the one used by certain exhibitors for decorating their stands at the British Industries Fair.

J. E. W. (27/66).—EARWIG PEST.—The following are formulas for poison-baits:—

I

Sodium fluoride	1 lb.
Molasses	64 oz.
Water	1½ gall.
Wheat bran	16 lb.

II

Sodium fluoride	1 oz.
Molasses	5 oz.
Glycerin	5 oz.
Water	5 oz.
Ground oat hulls ... ... about	1 lb.

Dissolve the sodium fluoride and then the molasses in the water. Add the bran (or oat hulls) last. The second preparation does not dry up so quickly as the first, and is perhaps more suitable for late summer dressing. The bait should be scattered over the ground and small quantities placed in the crotches of trees or at intervals along fences and walls. Sodium fluoride is poisonous to human beings, but death from it is rare. Soluble calcium salts may be given as an antidote.

Retrospect of Fifty Years Ago

Reprinted from "The Chemist and Druggist," July 3, 1886

Vichy Lozenges

Some time since the Seine-et-Marne pharmacists, organised as a syndicate, prosecuted Puisais, a grocer of Provins, for selling the Vichy lozenges manufactured by the company managing the mineral springs of the same name. The syndicate contended that the lozenges, being a medicinal preparation, could only be sold by pharmacists, and such was the decision of the Court of Provins. But on appeal the Paris Court has reversed the judgment, holding that Vichy lozenges are not medicinal, but scarcely anything more than a hygienic product, like orange-flower water, which anyone is at liberty to sell. The fact, adduced by the syndicate, that the lozenges were recognised and described by the French Codex, was held by the Court to be of no value, as the same authority treats in the same manner rice powder, Cologne water and such preparations.

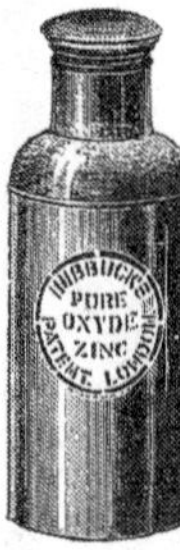

Hubbuck's Pure Oxide of Zinc

is made by sublimation and is warranted to contain upwards of

99·9 PER CENT.

of pure oxide; in fact, the impurities are not traceable

Thos. Hubbuck & Son, Ltd.

ESTABLISHED 1765

24 Lime Street, London, E.C.3

MANUFACTURERS OF WHITE LEAD, WHITE ZINC, PAINT, OILS, COLOURS, VARNISHES, &c.

Australian Office: 34 *Queen Street, Melbourne*

Sold by the following Wholesale Druggists in Boxes of **7** *lb. and* **14** *lb. stamped by the Manufacturers: also in* **1**-*lb. Boxes and* **1**-*lb. Glass Bottles:*

Allen & Hanburys, Ltd.
Ayrton, Saunders & Co., Ltd.
Bell, Jno., & Croyden
Bell, John, Hills & Lucas, Ltd.
Bleasdale, Ltd
Boots Pure Drug Co., Ltd.
British Drug Houses, Ltd.
Brook, Parker & Co., Ltd.
Burgoyne, Burbidges & Co., Butler & Crispe Ltd.
Cockburn & Co., Ltd.
Dakin Brothers
Duncan, Flockhart & Co.
Evans, Gadd & Co., Ltd.
Evans Sons Lescher & Webb, Ltd.
Ferris & Co.
Gale & Co.
Glasgow New Apothecaries Co
Goodall, Backhouse & Co.
C. R. Harker, Stagg & Morgan, Ltd.
Harkness, Beaumont & Co., Ltd.
Hatrick, W. R., & Co.
Hurst, Brooke & Hirst
Hodgkinson, Prestons & King
Horner, L. A., & Sons
Huskisson, H. O., & Co.
Lofthouse & Saltmer, Ltd.
Mackay, Jno., & Co., Ltd.
May, Roberts & Co., Ltd
Oldfield, Pattinson & Co.
Pinkerton, Gibson & Co., Ltd.
Potter & Clarke, Ltd.
Raimes & Co
Raimes, Clark & Co., Ltd.
Rankin & Borland
Silversides, R. B. G.
Smith, T. & H., Ltd.
Southall Bros. & Barclay, Ltd.
Sumner, R., & Co.
Taylor, Jas. (Trongate), Ltd.
Thompson, John, Ltd.
Wilkinson & Simpson, Ltd.
Willows, Francis, Butler & Thompson, Ltd.
Woolley, Jas., Sons & Co., Ltd.
Wright, Layman & Umney, Ltd.
Wyleys (Lim.)

Barry, E. J., New York
Finlay Dicks & Co., New Orleans
E. Fougera & Co., 90-92, Beekman Street, New York
Chas. L. Huisking & Co., Inc., 155, Varick St., New York
Lehn & Fink, Inc., N. York
McKesson & Robbins, Inc., New York
Muth Brothers & Co., Baltimore
Palmers, Ltd., Montreal
S. B. Penick & Co., Inc., New York
Roller & Shoemaker, Philadelphia
Schieffelin & Co., Inc., New York
Shoemaker & Busch, Philadelphia

SOLAZZI

The Chemist's Brand

LIQUORICE JUICE

SOLAZZI JUICE IS GUARANTEED TO CONSIST ENTIRELY OF THE CONDENSED EXTRACT OF FINEST CALABRIAN LICORICE ROOT **WITHOUT ANY ADMIXTURE WHATEVER**

Should any enquiry as to the composition of SOLAZZI be received from the public, Chemists are asked to emphasise the fact that SOLAZZI is not included in the category of Secret Remedies, and that the accompanying guarantee obtains with every parcel.

Chemische Fabrik

JOH. A. BENCKISER, G.m.b.H., LUDWIGSHAFEN-ON-RHINE

TARTARIC ACID IN POWDER CRYSTALS and GRANULATED

GUARANTEED IN STRICT ACCORDANCE WITH B.P.'32

ACID PYROPHOSPHATE OF SODA

Quality in all respects equal to Cream of Tartar, especially as regards stability of Baking Powder

MARKETING in INDIA

"Open for Agencies on Indent &/or Stock basis"

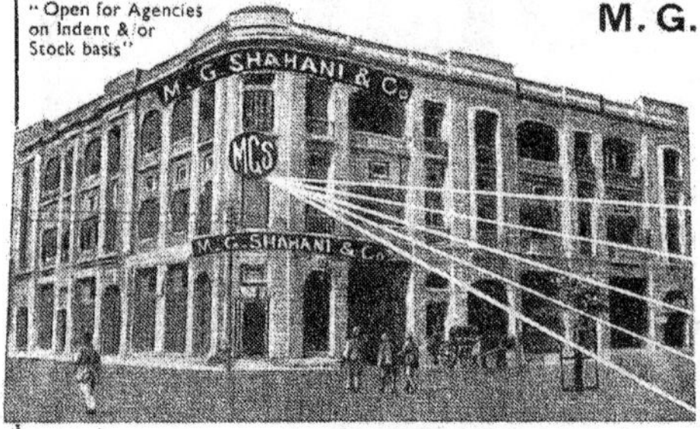

M. G. SHAHANI & Co.

Offer a complete Marketing, Selling & Distributing Organisation of many years' reputation and standing in

- KARACHI (Head Office)
- BOMBAY
- CALCUTTA
- DELHI
- MADRAS

M. G. SHAHANI & Co

Sole Agents for **COTY** (ENGLAND) **LTD.**

KARACHI.

TO PHARMACISTS OF THE NORTH WE OFFER

PROMPT SERVICE: KEEN PRICES: SOUND QUALITY, AND FREQUENT MOTOR VAN DELIVERIES IN THE TYNE, WEAR AND TEES AREAS.

For fuller particulars consult page 66
THE CHEMIST & DRUGGIST DIARY AND YEAR-BOOK, 1936

BRADY & MARTIN, Ltd. Northumberland Rd., NEWCASTLE-ON-TYNE

A. & M. ZIMMERMANN
Petri Bros. Ltd. Proprietors

CHEMICALS
Pharmaceutical
Technical
Chlorophyll
all
Grades

CHEMICALS DRUGS ESSENTIAL OILS

COD LIVER OIL
Medicinal
and Cattle
Marseilles Soap

3 LLOYDS AVENUE LONDON. E.C.3

HOPKIN & WILLIAMS LTD.

MANUFACTURERS OF

PHARMACEUTICAL CHEMICALS

FINE CHEMICALS for RESEARCH and ANALYSIS

INDICATORS & MICROSCOPIC STAINS

16 & 17 CROSS ST., LONDON, E.C.1

NIGROIDS for the Throat and Voice

Registered Trade Mark.

Sold in tins 4½d. and 1/6 each.

WHOLESALE TERMS ON APPLICATION

Sole Makers: **FERRIS & CO. LIMITED, BRISTOL**

The
CHEMIST AND DRUGGIST SUPPLEMENT

This Supplement is inserted in every copy of The Chemist & Druggist

28 ESSEX STREET, LONDON, W.C.2

JULY 4, 1936

ADVERTISEMENT TARIFF

ALL ADVERTISEMENTS are PREPAID, so that remittance must accompany instructions in each case. If it be necessary to telephone or telegraph an urgent announcement this may be done, provided the money is telegraphed at the same time.

BUSINESSES WANTED and for **DISPOSAL, PREMISES TO LET** and **FOR SALE, PREMISES WANTED, PARTNERSHIPS, GOODS** for **SALE** and **AGENCIES**—6/- for 50 words; every additional 10 words or less, 6d. (Box No., 1/- extra.)

SITUATIONS OPEN—6/- for 40 words; every additional 10 words or less, 6d. (Box No., 1/- extra.)

SITUATIONS WANTED—2/- for 18 words; every additional 10 words or less, 6d. (Box No., 1/- extra.)

LEGAL NOTICES, TENDERS, AUCTIONS, and all specially-spaced announcements, 1/3 per nonpareil line (12 lines = 1 inch single column). (Box No., 1/- extra.)

MISCELLANEOUS (Wholesalers') Section for odd and second-hand lots—10/- for 60 words; 1/- for every additional 10 words or less. (Box No., 1/- extra.)

EXCHANGE COLUMN (for Retailers, etc.)—**Twopence** per word, minimum 2/-. (Box No., 1/- extra.)

REPLIES FROM ADVERTISERS—1/- per line; 3 lines 2/6.

THE CHEMIST & DRUGGIST, 28 Essex St., Strand, London, W.C.2
Telephone: Central 6565 (10 *lines*). *Telegrams: "Chemicus, Estrand, London."*

CLOSING FOR PRESS

All advertisements intended for insertion in this Supplement must reach us not later than **FIRST POST THURSDAY MORNING**

ERNEST J. GEORGE & Co.

Bank Chambers, 329 High Holborn, London, W.C.1
Telephone Nos.: Holborn 7406 & 7407 (2 lines)

15 Bridge Street, Walsall Telephone: Walsall 3774

Lancashire and District Representative: Mr. E. BROWN, 21 Davenport Road, Hazel Grove, Stockport. Telephone: Great Moor 2405

Correspondence, mutually confidential, is invited from prospective purchasers of the following businesses at present available for purchase.

(C1) CORNWALL.—Good family business, which during the past few years has shown a rapid increase; turnover for last financial year, £3,102; net profit approximately £550; rent £155; price about £1,150; immediate sale desired as Owner is moving North; exceptional opportunity to acquire sound proposition at "bargain" figure.

(C2) LONDON, S.W.—Attractive middle-class Pharmacy showing steadily increasing returns, which are now at the rate of approximately £2,350 per annum, and should undoubtedly reach an early £3,000, consequent upon building extensions now in course of process; premises situated in congenial area; reasonable overheads; price asked £1,500, or very near offer; nothing less entertained; please supply bankers' references.

(C3) HAMMERSMITH (NEAR).—Middle-working class cash business with no near opposition; turnover approximately £1,850 per annum; good scope for considerable further development; rent and rates (lock-up shop only), £105 per annum; lease 14 years; living accommodation above might be available if required; price £900 or near offer.

(C4) CHESHIRE (RETIREMENT VACANCY).—Old-established business with living accommodation; no immediate opposition; turnover upwards of £1,250 per annum; net profit £375; very low rental; large N.H.I.; price £850, including stock and fixtures estimated at £540.

(C5) FINSBURY PARK.—Old-established business occupying prominent position in busy main thoroughfare; present returns approximately £25 weekly, with excellent scope for increase under personal proprietorship; rent £100 per annum; flat above at present sub-let for 25s. weekly; long lease; reasonable purchase price, part of which might remain.

(C6) CLACTON-ON-SEA (NEAR).—Drug Store offering excellent scope for substantial increase under qualified proprietorship; turnover for 1935–36, £1,042; rent and rates, £60; sub-let £52; premises held on lease; price £485 all-at, subject to value of stock, which can be reduced if so desired.

(C7) LANCS.—Old-established unopposed country Pharmacy, with good living accommodation; turnover for last financial year, £1,147; net profit £339; good panel; rent £52; population to draw upon approximately 3,000; stock and fixtures estimated at £500; price for quick sale £700.

(C8) CHISWICK (NEAR).—Good-class business showing steady and consistent increase; present returns approximately £2,000 per annum; lock-up shop; low rental; excellent scope; price approximately £1,100.

(C9) BRIGHTON.—Excellent opportunity for chemist, with limited capital to purchase an old-established business not of a seasonal character, with living accommodation; now doing in the region of £20 per week; main-road situation; reasonable rental; price £450–£500 or first reasonable offer accepted.

(C10) CROYDON (NEAR).—Main road business with up-to-date self-contained flat above; average returns approximately £27 per week; excellent scope for further increase; very reasonable rental; no near opposition; price approximately £950.

(C11) CHISWICK.—Established retail business occupying prominent main-road position, now doing at the rate of £18/£20 per week, but these figures are capable of considerable augmentation; rent £180 p.a. less sub-lets £100; price all-at £500, representing approximate value of stock and fixtures only; near offer considered for quick transaction.

(C12) EDGWARE ROAD (NEAR).—Lock-up Pharmacy with steadily increasing turnover; returns for last year, £1,364; rent and rates approximately 22/- per week only; reasonable purchase price, part of which might remain under approved circumstances.

(C13) LONDON, E.—Recently-established lock-up Pharmacy, with good optical connection, and other profitable side-line; combined turnover for first complete year approximately £1,850; good scope for considerable further increase; no near opposition; price £650/£700, including stock approximately £400, part of which might remain.

(C14) KENT.—Established retail business, occupying good position; owing to ill-health has not been adequately exploited during the past few years, but scope exists for early resuscitation under energetic proprietorship; turnover for last financial year, £1,386; good living accommodation, including garden; low purchase price.

(C15) WOODFORD (NEAR).—Progressive lock-up Pharmacy, the turnover of which has increased during the past three years from £1,600 to over £2,100 per annum; rent £100; good scope for further development; price £1,100 all-at, including stock £650.

(C16) EPPING FOREST (NEAR).—Drug Store, with excellent scope for increase under qualified proprietorship; present returns approximately £20 weekly; rent £80 per annum, including living accommodation; price all-at £450.

(C17) GLAMORGAN.—Good family business with full wine licence; turnover for last financial year upwards of £1,600; net profit £400; genuine scope for considerable further increase; price £750, including stock £400; excellent opportunity.

(C18) HAMMERSMITH.—Old-established retail and dispensing business for disposal owing to retirement; turnover for 1935 financial year, £1,120; gross profit, £499; rent £65, including living accommodation; lease 20½ years unexpired; no near opposition; excellent scope for increase under energetic proprietorship; price by negotiation.

Valuations for transfer, probate, income tax, etc., promptly executed at economical rates. Agency for locums, managers, etc.

THE ASSOCIATION OF MANUFACTURING CHEMISTS, LIMITED

(Business Agency, Transfer & Valuation Department)

KIMBERLEY HOUSE, Holborn Viaduct, LONDON, E.C.1 *and at* EXCHANGE CHAMBERS, 2 Bixteth St., LIVERPOOL.

PARKIN S. BOOTH, Valuer. *Tels.: CITY* 3691 (4 lines).

VALUATIONS. SALES OF BUSINESSES. STOCKTAKINGS.

Enquiries Invited.

S. F. CLARK, F.N.A.A.

'Phone: Prospect 3366

CHEMISTS' VALUER & TRANSFER AGENT

34 Marksbury Avenue, Richmond, Surrey

I have, *for exclusive disposal,* a number of attractive businesses, and invite correspondence from buyers. Vendors desiring sales by private direct introduction to purchasers, are advised to adopt my PERSONAL and CONFIDENTIAL SERVICE.

Stocktaking, Insurance and Mortgage Departments.

INTERNATIONAL MEDICAL AGENCY & ESTATES, LTD.

MEDICAL TRANSFER BUSINESS of every description undertaken.

PARTNERSHIPS ARRANGED. INSURANCES AND CAPITAL ADVANCED.

Further particulars forwarded on application to—

WALTER HOUSE, 418-422 STRAND, W.C.2

Phone: Temple Bar 3769

THE PHOTOGRAPHIC CHEMIST. Price 3s. 6d., by post 3s. 8d.

THE C. & D. PRICE LIST FORMULARY, "P.L.F." Price 2s. 6d. post free.

PROVINCIAL HOSPITAL PHARMACOPŒIAS. Price 3s. by post 3s. 2d.

"THE CHEMIST AND DRUGGIST," 28 Essex Street, W.C.2

Practical Books for Everyday use

PHARMACEUTICAL FORMULAS (P.F., Vol. I)

Price 15s. by post 15/6

The tenth edition of this, the most complete pharmaceutical formulary in the English language, is devoted to the official and semi-official preparations of practically every country in the world. This volume (published 1929) contains 1146 pages. Invaluable to the busy pharmacist. One of the most useful and handiest reference books in the trade.

PHARMACEUTICAL FORMULAS (P.F., Vol. II)

Price 15s. by post 15/6

Published 1934. Supplementary to Vol. I, and known as "The Chemist's Recipe Book." Contains formulas for adhesives, beverages, cleaning materials, culinary and household requisites, horticultural and agricultural preparations, inks, lozenges, perfumes, photographic preparations, polishes, soaps, toilet articles, varnishes, veterinary preparations, etc., including numerous descriptions of practical methods employed in their manufacture, and other information of use to pharmacists and manufacturers. Over 1000 pages.

No business library is complete without these books. They are time savers and money makers.

You can order through your usual Wholesaler or direct from The Publisher

THE CHEMIST & DRUGGIST

28 Essex Street, London, W.C.2

Branch Offices: 4 Cannon St., Manchester 3; 54 Foster's Buildings, High St., Sheffield; 19 Waterloo St., Glasgow; and at Paris, France; Auckland, N.Z.; Melbourne and Sydney, Australia.

BUSINESSES FOR DISPOSAL.

6s. for 50 words or less ; 6d. for every additional 10 words or less, prepaid. (Box No., 1s. extra.)

BOLTON DISTRICT.—Established Working-class Business; average for last 3 years about £19 weekly at good profits; Panel averages 600 per month; rent and rates 21s. per week; owner requires larger business and will sell for value of stock and fixtures (£500); turnover can be increased by one used to type of business. 24/25, Office of this Paper.

CORNWALL.—Dispensing, Photographic and Toilet Business for immediate disposal; Rexall, Ucal, Kodak; opening for Optics. 24/5, Office of this Paper.

HOVE.—Rapidly-growing Chemist's Business for Disposal (owing to illness); good district; well fitted and good saleable stock; main-road position. Apply 24/11, Office of this Paper.

LIVERPOOL.—Chemist, buying larger business, desires to sell branch; splendid opportunity for owner management in densely populated working-class district; corner shop and flat; rent £1, rates 10s.; lease; about £350 or valuation terms; part can remain. 30/21, Office of this Paper.

LIVERPOOL.—Old-established Business; main road; well fitted and compact; moderate clean stock; working-class district; will be improved under town planning; present hands 24 years; good house; rent low; scope for increase; no reasonable offer refused; worth seeing. Apply 67 Netherfield Road South, Liverpool.

LIVERPOOL (residential suburb).—Excellent prospects for Pharmacist with capital; unique position; pleasant surroundings; freehold property; monopoly site; present returns below average, ample scope for increase; business £550; property £1,650; substantial mortgage transferable; if rented, 50s. per week; shop, double-fronted, private entrance, garden, garage; reasonable offers entertained. "Celeritas," 24/6, Office of this Paper.

LONDON.—Well-established Chemist's Business for Sale; well stocked and fitted; Kodak and Ucal Agencies; scope and accommodation for Optics; value of stock and fittings for quick sale £450-£500; genuine reasons for disposal. 30/32, Office of this Paper.

LONDON (Ilford).—Old-established Retail Chemist's Business, with living accommodation, at present tenanted; good position; well populated district; lease 9 years; N.H.I. and Kodak Agency; excellent opportunity for owner proprietor; fullest investigation invited; owner retiring; goodwill £350; stock at valuation. Apply 24/4, Office of this Paper.

LONDON, S.W.—Good-class Family suburban Business, in busy main-road position; returns under management £45 weekly, good profits; owner-proprietor would clear £450 to £500; stock and fixtures worth about £1,200; price £1,550 cash. Apply to sole agents, Berdoe & Fish, Chemists' Valuers, 41 Argyle Square, King's Cross, W.C.1.

LONDON, W. (near Hammersmith).—Good-class Business for Sale immediately (illness); turnover over £2,000 per annum, steadily increasing; rent £75; 12½ years' lease; scope increase; heavy Photo and very good Toilet Trade; goodwill, fittings, fixtures, etc., £600; s.a.v. (about £500); easily run; all Photo Agencies; interview to genuine buyers only. 24/3, Office of this Paper.

MANCHESTER.—Excellent Modern Shop, both exterior and interior, for Disposal; well stocked; main road; thickly populated; doing good middle-class trade and N.H.I.; Kodak, Selo and Rexall Agencies; average takings £40 weekly; excellent house part; rent £70 p.a. Only genuine inquirers write to 30/7, Office of this Paper.

MIDDLESEX.—Well-established Retail and Dispensing Business for immediate disposal; owner retiring through age and ill-health; returns average the last 3 years over £30 weekly; full audited accounts; commodious shop, large house, garden and side entrance; rent £120 on lease; upper portion could be let off for 30s. week if not required; spacious accommodation and good opening for Optical; the business is particularly adaptable for partnership or a limited company, as its fine position close to 2 banks and cinema offers immense future possibilities with up-to-date methods and energetic management; nearest multiple store shop 2 miles away; price extremely low, £650; s.a.v. Fuller particulars at interview, for address only "Z.," 30/28, Office of this Paper.

MIDDLESEX TOWN.—Established Good-class Business, with increasing Optical practice; situate in premier position of main street; turnover last year £3,200; accountant's figures available; long lease; good living accommodation, side entrance, garden; if conducted under personal management is capable of development; good reasons for disposal. 283/261, Office of this Paper.

SOUTH COAST.—Chemist Business; N.H.I.; Kodak; corner position; double-fronted freehold property; living accommodation; shopping centre, main road; turnover £2,000 under management; plenty of scope; fittings, fixtures, stock, goodwill all at £3,500 or near offer. Also lock-up corner shop, main road; low rent; lease arranged, 7 to 21 years; turnover £500; stock, fittings, fixtures, goodwill all at £400 or near offer; plenty of scope (accounts audited); dissolving partnership. 30/33, Office of this Paper.

SOUTH COAST.—Drug Store for Sale in popular South Coast resort; lock-up shop in busy food market; rent £52 per annum, inclusive; neglected through illness; price £200 or near offer for quick sale. 25/2, Office of this Paper.

SOUTH DEVON.—Owner retiring; well-established business with large sale of own proprietaries; central position; turnover £2,100 under management, accounts audited, gross profit £850; own property; will grant 21 years' lease; no N.H.I. or Photo touched; price £1,500, £500 can remain. Apply to sole agents, Berdoe & Fish, Chemists' Valuers, 41 Argyle Square, King's Cross, W.C.1.

SOUTH DEVON (popular seaside resort).—Drug and Photographic Store for disposal; Kodak, Selo, Ensign Agency; definite scope for Qualified Chemist to add Dispensing; good position; no immediate opposition; genuine reason for disposal; stock, fixtures, etc., about £650; long lease, or property can be purchased. 24/15, Office of this Paper.

STAFFS.—Unopposed Village Business; turnover 1935, £1,300; low rent and rates; house and garden attached; genuine opportunity for young Qualified; price wanted for business £650. 24/26, Office of this Paper.

SURREY (9 miles out).—Owing to ill-health; sound business, no near opposition; rent £70, lease 13½ years; good living accommodation; returns £1,200 at good profits; stock and fixtures about £550 and very small sum for lease and goodwill; rapidly developing district; 200 flats being erected at present. 30/27, Office of this Paper.

YORKSHIRE COAST.—In time for high season, good-class Business, Photo, Toilet and Light Retail; smart shop, best position; returns £2,000; good profits and prospects; price, valuation of stock and fixtures, plus £300 for lease and goodwill; owner retiring; full particulars at personal interview, by appointment. 24/24, Office of this Paper.

AN Excellent opportunity occurs for one to acquire a Chemist Shop (well established) in main road in thickly populated working-class area (West Ham); stock and fittings need not be purchased; excellent shop premises, with 6 rooms above (side entrance) and garage at rear; rental £150 p.a., exclusive of which £78 is collected from tenants; lease 21 years (or premises can be purchased freehold); special reasons for disposal; premium £100. 283/269, Office of this Paper.

CHEMIST'S and Druggist's in busy suburban high road; beautifully fitted; self-contained flat over; must be sacrificed as owner is unable to supervise; at present under management; takings £33 per week; has been taking £36 per week; unique opportunity. P.C.B. 209/23, Office of this Paper.

LARGE Modern Pharmacy for Disposal; beautifully fitted and stocked; main road; good residential district; turnover £2,000, with great scope; a genuine bargain to a man of initiative and worker; first deposit secures; price £1,250. "Chemist," 104 Grove Road, Chadwell Heath, Essex.

OLD-ESTABLISHED Chemist, Drug Stores; same proprietor 40 years; Wines and Spirits; no opposition; now under Unqualified management; good opening for N.H.I.; takings £1,600 per year, accountant's figures. 26/2, Office of this Paper.

OLD-ESTABLISHED Pharmacy, Light Retail, Dispensing, Photography, with up-to-date living accommodation, for disposal, in residential area of good seaside town, South Wales; sells profitable own specialities; net profit last 3 years over £500 per annum, accountants' figures; reasonable rent; price £850 for long lease, fixtures and goodwill; stock approximately £800 on valuation; banker's reference must accompany first letter. 30/53, Office of this Paper.

PREMISES TO LET.

EWELL, SURREY.—Main-road double-fronted Lock-up Shop in parade of eight; good opportunity for Chemist, &c.; rapidly developing district, with advantage also of being well established; rent only £60 p.a. Adams, 12 Surbiton Hill Park, Surbiton, Surrey.

NEAR EAST GRINSTEAD.—Wonderful opening Chemists, monopoly trade in block of six shops with no opposition; only one left and reserved for this trade; £100 p.a.; modern shop and living accommodation, 3 bed, bath, sitting-room, kitchen, etc. Powell & Partner, Ltd., Forest Row. Tel. 204.

PORTMAN SQUARE (close to).—Shop, Parlour and Basement; also first-floor flat (if required); ideal opening for Chemist; rent only £175 per annum; no premium. Keys with Sole Agents, Payne & Ekin, 4 Bryanston Street, Portman Square, W.1. (Wel. 2231.)

BUSY Main-road Shop to Let; good opening for Chemist; few doors from factory employing thousands, near cinemas, etc.; rent £2 weekly; no premium; lease 3/21 years. Apply to 56/66 Stoke Newington Road, N.16. Telephone: Clissold 2373-4.

CHEMIST.—Shop to Let, 18 ft. by 50 ft., with smart front fitted; close to Tube Station; rent £200, no premium. Sole Agents, Douglas Martin, Ltd., adjoining Tube Station, Hendon Central, N.W.4.

MULTIPLE POSITION.—Live Traders wanted for unique New Parade of Shops, 50 ft. deep, to Let; separate entrances to upper parts; view 123-129 Essex Road, N.1; thousands of shoppers here. Apply "T.," 48 Menelik Road, N.W.2.

PREMISES.

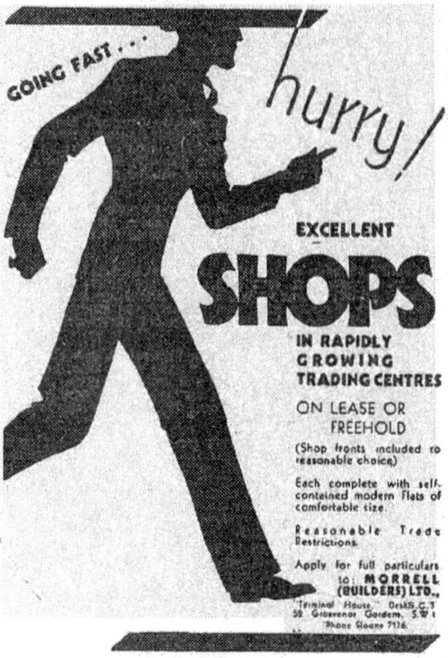

GOING FAST . . .
hurry!
EXCELLENT
SHOPS
IN RAPIDLY GROWING TRADING CENTRES
ON LEASE OR FREEHOLD
(Shop fronts included to reasonable choice)
Each complete with self-contained modern flats of comfortable size.
Reasonable Trade Restrictions.
Apply for full particulars to: MORRELL (BUILDERS) LTD.,
"Terminal House," Desk S.C.3
52 Grosvenor Gardens, S.W.1
'Phone Sloane 7176.

SALE BY AUCTION.

Removed from Hackney for Convenience of Sale.

5 LITTLE BRITAIN (close to G.P.O.), CITY.

Excellent well-made Mahogany CHEMISTS' SHOP-FITTINGS, Drug Runs, Perfumery and other Wall Show-cases, Plate-glass Counters, Mirrors, National Cash Registers, Office Furniture, Safes, Typewriters.

B. NORMAN & SON

will Sell by Auction, without reserve, WEDNESDAY NEXT, JULY 8, at Noon.

Catalogues on application. Telephone: NAT. 6463.

PARTNERSHIPS.

ADVERTISER requires active Partnership; for the past 15 years has been Chief Chemist and Works Manager in a well-known firm manufacturing Druggist specialities, Toilet articles and soap; small capital available. P.C.B. 210/2, Office of this Paper.

CONTINENTAL Chemist, planning to manufacture in United Kingdom an effective range of Original Cosmetic Preparations (prov. patented), seeks a Partner who would invest about £500; might suit established Pharmacist having some space available. Write Box 710 at Horncastle's, 103 Cheapside, E.C.2.

PARTNERSHIP entertained or will sell small modern factory, Cardiff district; equipped steam, gas, electricity; ground for expansion; low overheads; excellent nucleus; connection amongst Doctors and Chemists with proprietaries and general products from North to South England and capable of great expansion. 30/52, Office of this Paper.

AGENCIES.

LONDON.—Experienced Sales Manager, now working on own account, with staff of travellers covering London suburbs, and own warehouse and delivery service, requires lines suitable for the Grocery trade. Nash, 45 Perth Road, Ilford.

AGENTS.—If you are a Line Agent anywhere in England, know your job and can sell well-advertised Toilet articles, send full particulars to 283/270, Office of this Paper.

BUSINESS OPPORTUNITIES.

THE Manufacturers of a quite unique line of high-class Health and Beauty Products (comprising Creams, Face and Dusting Powders only), recently put on the market and most favourably commented on by the Press and users, are anxious to get in touch with a really first-class organisation distributing a non-competitive but similar line; correspondence from principals only. Write 283/271, Office of this Paper.

APPRENTICES.

THERE is a Vacancy for one Apprentice in a good-class Dispensing-Pharmacy in Bournemouth; a fine Dispensing and General Retail Pharmaceutical training and experience are assured. Apply "Ph.C.," 28/12, Office of this Paper.

SITUATIONS OPEN.

RETAIL (HOME).

6s. for 40 words or less; 1s. for every additional 10 words or less, prepaid. (Box No., 1s. extra.)

BIRMINGHAM.—Qualified Assistant; good Salesman, smart Window-dresser; able to take control; permanency. Apply, with full particulars, stating when free and commencing salary required, Hedges (Chemists), Ltd., 10 Dale End, Birmingham.

BRISTOL.—Immediately; Qualified Assistant and also a Junior Assistant. Apply by letter, with copies of testimonials, giving experience and salary required, 24/47, Office of this Paper.

LEICESTER.—Reliable Qualified Assistant wanted at once to take charge of Dispensing Department and assist in general Counter trade in a middle-class Pharmacy; permanency. State usual particulars and salary required to "Drugs," 36 Vicarage Lane, Belgrave, Leicester.

LONDON.—Junior Assistant (male), Qualified preferred, Dispensing and Retail, wanted at once. Apply Garner & Pope, Ltd., 244 Haverstock Hill, N.W.3.

LONDON.—Qualified Assistant, also Temporary Assistant (Qualified preferred, but not essential), for Holiday Relief work until end of September; middle-class trade and N.H.I. Dispensing; give full particulars of experience, names of references, when disengaged and salary expected. Apply (letter only) Chemist, 37 Sydner Road, London, N.16.

LONDON.—Qualified Lady for smart modern shop; easy berth; moderate salary to commence; state age, experience, when free. P.C.B. 210/11, Office of this Paper.

LONDON, EAST (near City)—Qualified Assistant for Dispensing and Shop Routine; permanency; full particulars and salary required. Apply 30/24, Office of this Paper.

LONDON, E 10.—Qualified Lady required July 25; permanency; Dispensing and Counter. Apply, stating age, salary required, references and photograph (returned if stamped addressed envelope enclosed), 28/10, Office of this Paper.

LONDON, N.W.—Qualified for branch, immediately; either sex; would suit elderly male; easy hours. Give full particulars to Chemist, 29 Ellington Street, N.7.

LONDON, S.E.—Locum, from August 17 to 31; lady or elderly gentleman; Qualified; moderate salary; honest, reliable; recent references. 30/39, Office of this Paper.

LONDON, S.W.—Assistant, Qualified or Unqualified, gentleman, from July 6 to September 19, for holiday relief. Apply, with particulars of experience and salary required, to Wilkie, 28 Hildreth Street, Balham, S.W.12.

LONDON, S.W.—Junior Unqualified Assistant, male, required for good-class Dispensing business; good prospects; full particulars, age, height, experience and salary expected. 283/264, Office of this Paper.

LONDON, W.1.—Qualified Senior Assistant required at once (gentleman) (age about 30); outdoors; no Sunday duty; give full particulars in first letter, stating salary required, but do not send photo or references, as personal interview will be necessary. 29/19, Office of this Paper.

MANCHESTER.—Locum required, Qualified, August 2 to 8. Apply "M.P.S.," 5 Clive Terrace, George Street, Manchester, 8.

SHEFFIELD.—At once, Qualified (male), for Counter, quick cash trade, Photography; outdoors; no Sunday duty. Full particulars, experience (letter only), salary required, and enclose photo, H. G. Williams, 118 The Moor.

SOUTH-EAST COAST.—Qualified Lady Assistant (M.P.S.) wanted to commence duties at once. Apply with usual particulars to 24/49, Office of this Paper.

SURREY.—Qualified Assistant Manager required; apply by letter, stating age, experience, when free, salary required; also photo if possible. 283/275, Office of this Paper.

SURREY.—Qualified Lady Assistant, M.P.S.; permanent position; good locality; must be smart Saleswoman and Window-dresser; state wages and full particulars in first letter. Also part-time Locum, lady or gent. 31/2, Office of this Paper.

SUSSEX COAST.—Unqualified Lady or Gentleman Assistant required for season, middle of July for 2 months; with good Counter experience, chiefly Toilet and Photographic. Apply, stating age, salary required, experience and full particulars, with photo if possible, to Lindsay, Arcade, Littlehampton.

WALSALL, Birmingham.—Qualified Branch Superintendents wanted (3) immediately; permanencies. Also several Unqualified Assistants, either sex; good prospects with progressive firm; send fullest particulars first letter; photo, to be returned. 30/50, Office of this Paper.

WEST OF ENGLAND.—Qualified Chemist, M.P.S., with Optical qualifications (male) (aged 30 to 40), for Works Dispensary; give full particulars of experience, salary required, recent testimonials, whether married or single, etc. 30/42, Office of this Paper.

A.A.A.A.—UNQUALIFIED wanted immediately for Middle-class Business, with large N.H.I.; Unqualified Assistant; either sex; must be a quick and accurate Dispenser. Apply Arnett & Co., 317 Lillie Road, Fulham, S.W.6.

A.—QUALIFIED Assistant (young) for Dispensing and Counter; capable of taking charge when required; suburbs of London; permanent and improving position for suitable young man; please state age, height, usual references and salary required. 24/37, Office of this Paper.

A CAPABLE Unqualified Assistant (20-25) required middle of August for middle-class business; permanent and progressive post for the right man. Write A. Stallard, Chemist, West Drayton, Middlesex.

A SMART Young Lady Assistant immediately, Unqualified or Qualified; must be keen and conscientious worker; efficiency at Sales essential and capable of creating new business; Birmingham district; Typing an asset; full particulars, age, experience, salary expected. 24/45, Office of this Paper.

AN Unusual Opening occurs in London Retail Shop for Qualified (either sex); applicant has no Dispensing to do, but Superintends generally; no Sunday work; age 25-35 and tall; must have excellent reference; used to busy Counter and capable of control; send full particulars first letter, also photo if possible. 27/4, Office of this Paper.

ANDERSON & VIRGO, of Worcester, have a vacancy for a Gentlemanly Assistant, principally for Counter work; must have had good all-round experience; qualification not essential; permanency to suitable man. Send full particulars to the above address.

PHOTOGRAPHS, TESTIMONIALS, &c.

When answering advertisements in this section applicants are strongly advised not to send (unless specially requested) ORIGINAL TESTIMONIALS or VALUABLE PHOTOGRAPHS. As can be readily understood, when an advertiser receives from 100 to 150 replies the task of returning photographs, testimonials, &c., is one of some difficulty.

ASSISTANT (about 24); July to October; capable Salesman, Window-dresser; experience in Photographic Sales essential. A. V. Ison, 5 West Cliff Road, Bournemouth.

AT ONCE.—Young Lady Assistant, Qualified, good Saleswoman, required for West-End Chemists. Reply, stating experience and salary required, 283/262, Office of this Paper.

CHEMIST.—Fully Qualified Man required to manage Drug and Dispensing branch under Superintendent Chemist. Applications in writing, stating age, qualifications and experience, with wages required, endorsed "Chemist," to be addressed to Birmingham Co-operative Society, High Street, Birmingham, 4.

COMPETENT Lady Assistant (Qualified preferred); start Monday, July 6; for good-class Retail and Dispensing business; also Photography; good appearance and address. Full particulars, age, height, experience, etc., to J. G. Kirkby, Belmont, Sutton, Surrey.

ELDERLY Qualified Dispenser wanted; easy duties. 89 Lever Street, London, E.C.1.

ELDERLY Registered Chemist; small, light, easy suburban; Manchester 6 miles; will stand very moderate salary only; good living accommodation if required; gentlemanly, civil, obliging; good references; or young Qualified Lady. Nowell, 70 Parrin Lane, Monton, Eccles, near Manchester.

EXPERIENCED Unqualified Assistant (25-30) required; single; salary £3 5s.; accurate Dispenser, capable Counterman essential; permanency. Reply, giving full particulars of experience, also height, photo if possible, 24/36, Office of this Paper.

FULL-TIME Qualified Dispenser and Caretaker of Surgery; to live on premises, rent, fuel and light free; commencing August 20, 1936; state age, experience, recent testimonials and salary required. Drs. Lyle, Hall, Anderson & Bow, 1 West End Terrace, Stockton-on-Tees.

JUNIOR Assistant, either sex, required; some experience of Dispensing; South-West London; state age and salary required. 30/8, Office of this Paper.

JUNIOR Assistant, Unqualified, wanted as soon as possible for Dispensing and Counter. Apply by letter, stating full particulars, age, height, salary required and when disengaged, to J. W. Rumsey & Son, 535 Lordship Lane, S.E.22.

JUNIOR or Improver (either sex); must be used to quick trade, Counter and Dispensing; Liverpool and Chester district. All particulars, including salary expected, to 283/273, Office of this Paper. N.B.—If applicants receive no reply within 7 days kindly understand not successful.

LADY Assistant, experienced Toilets, required for season; £2 10s. weekly; hours 8.30-7, less meals; state age, height, experience, enclose photograph and copies references. Bayley's, Chemists, Frinton-on-Sea.

LADY Assistant, Unqualified, required for light Retail Business. Please send full particulars (with photo or snapshot if possible) to Croasdale & Sons, Chemists, Bury St. Edmunds.

LADY Assistant, Unqualified (18-26). Turner, Chemist, Tamworth.

LADY, Qualified, as Assistant, in good-class Family and Dispensing Business in S.E. London; comfortable permanency. State age, experience and salary required, to Bernard Philips, Ltd., 27 Northcote Road, Clapham Junction, S.W.11.

LADY, Qualified, for N.H.I.; competent Dispenser essential; congenial post for suitable applicant. State age, past experience and salary required to Alleston, Ltd., Chemists, 191 Ilford Lane, Ilford.

LADY wanted for D. & P. Photographic work, at once, for several months; state age, experience and salary required. Wootton & Webb, 20 George Street, Luton.

LADY with Hall qualification for Dispensing and Counter. Co-operative, Worcester.

LOCUM, Qualified; at once; lady or gent.; for one month at least; state salary and references. H. E. Graham, Ltd., 22 Burlington Street, Bolton.

LOCUM, Qualified, August 4 to August 22. Also Locum, Unqualified, for August 31 to September 12. Apply by letter only, giving full particulars, to A. W. Craig, Chemist, 283 Regent Street, W.1.

LOCUM, Qualified, August 17 to 22 inclusive; Somerset; duties light; suit elderly gent.; state terms, age, etc. 283/266, Office of this Paper.

LOCUM, Qualified, for July 13-25 inclusive. Terms, Marshall & Co., 51 Pimlico Road, S.W.1.

LOCUM, Qualified, lady or gentleman, wanted now, for 3 weeks; London. Full particulars to 29/14, Office of this Paper

LOCUM, Qualified, required for fortnight commencing August 30. Particulars and salary required to Large, 149 Broad Street, Dagenham.

LOCUM, Qualified, required immediately; active and of good address and reliable; until August 29. 'Phone Ravenbourne 2336.

LOCUM, Unqualified, young, required from July 13 to 25. Please apply, full particulars, to Venables, 246 North End Road, Fulham, S.W.6.

MANAGER required; used to good-class Retail and Dispensing Business; state salary required. Apply A. R. Hewish, 8 Oakhill, Orpington, Kent.

M.P.S., LOCUM required July 20, for one week, lady or gentleman. Apply Hay's Drug Stores, Ltd., 77 Carlton Vale, Maida Vale, N.W.6.

QUALIFIED Assistant or Locum required immediately; permanency for suitable applicant; experience not essential; youth an advantage. Write, forwarding full particulars, including salary required, Ileys, Ltd., Ryhope, near Sunderland, Durham County.

QUALIFIED Assistant, Registered; at once; single; progressive salary and commission. Full particulars to Fereday, Cheslyn Hay, Nr. Walsall, Staffs.

QUALIFIED Assistant required at once; capable of taking charge of new medium-class Retail, with N.H.I.; knowledge of Photographic and Window-dressing. Apply with full particulars, age, name of references and salary required, to be based on results, to Lewis, 53 Kirby Road, Portsmouth.

QUALIFIED Assistant wanted at once; must be good Counterman. Full particulars as to age, height, experience, references, salary, to Venables, Chemist, 260 Upper Tooting Road, S.W.17, or 'phone Streatham 2443.

QUALIFIED Assistant wanted for permanency in good-class Retail and Dispensing Business. Apply with fullest particulars re experience, age, salary required to Tilley, Droitwich Spa.

QUALIFIED Assistant (25-30) required for good-class Pharmacy in S.W. London; permanency. Write, stating age, salary required, etc., to 30/55, Office of this Paper.

QUALIFIED; for small branch in West Country; lock-up shop; light Retail; moderate salary and commission. State age, height, salary and experience, and when at liberty, to 24/29, Office of this Paper.

QUALIFIED Lady Assistant required; smart appearance and alertness most essential; interview desired; no Sunday duty. Modern Chemists Ltd., 231 Westminster Bridge Road, S.E.1 (opposite County Hall). 'Phone: Waterloo 4445.

QUALIFIED, lady or gent; North London. Please send full particulars in first communication to "Chemist," 1 South Street, Islington, N.1.

QUALIFIED Lady wanted; permanency or locum; about July 15-31; state age, when Qualified, experience, etc. Also Unqualified Lady. S. M. Morris, Ltd., 143 Broadway, W.7.

QUALIFIED Locum required immediately; please state full particulars and salary required. Letter only, Williams, Portland Road, Hove.

QUALIFIED Locum wanted for 2 weeks from July 20. Particulars, Jones, Chemist, 100 Dalling Road, Hammersmith, W.6.

QUALIFIED, male or female, for one or two months; easy duty; no Sunday business; state age, experience and salary (moderate) required; near London. 30/19, Office of this Paper.

QUALIFIED Manager for branch; working-class district; N.H.I. Dispensing. Please write, giving full particulars, to Bewells' Ltd., 19/21 Pitfield Street, N.1.

QUALIFIED Young Lady Assistant required for Good-class Family Dispensing and Photographic Business, S.W. London; good Dispenser and preferably some Counter experience; apply stating experience and salary required; letters not answered in week respectfully declined. P.C.B. 210/9, Office of this Paper.

UNQUALIFIED Assistant (under 25), with knowledge of Photography, required for season, mid-July to September; state height and wages required and enclose references. Withers & Son, Chemists, 45 Rosemary Road, Clacton-on-Sea.

UNQUALIFIED Gentleman wanted for evenings, 5-8; to commence July 13; easy berth. Apply 283/274, Office of this Paper.

UNQUALIFIED Junior required immediately. Reply, giving particulars of age, experience, references, salary required, when disengaged, and if possible enclosing photograph, to W. Bates & Co., Ltd., 50 Oxford Street, Southampton.

UNQUALIFIED.—Wanted, Temporary Assistant, lady or gentleman, from August 24 to September 19; one accustomed to ordinary Retail Business; knowledge of Photography preferred. Apply, stating experience and salary required, to W. Gowan Cross and Son, Pharmaceutical Chemists, 70 Mardol, Shrewsbury.

WANTED for two weeks, Qualified Locum (male); Dispensing and light Retail; good Prescriber essential; for July 13 or 20. A. J. Hall, 97 High Street, Maidenhead.

WANTED, Locum, Qualified, for one week, July 20-25 inclusive. Terms and references, Findlay, Oakleigh Pharmacy, Hillingdon Heath, nr. Uxbridge, Middlesex.

WANTED, Qualified and Unqualified Assistants; good Counter personality, Window-dressing, etc. Also Assistant for Photographic Department. Apply, with full particulars, photo, age, salary, or interview Murray, Chemist, Electric Parade, Clacton-on-Sea.

WANTED.—Qualified Assistant, either sex; used to quick N.H.I. Apply O. Tobin, Ltd., 49 Harford Street, Mile End, E.1.

WANTED.—Qualified Manager; easy distance London; £5 per week and commission; good prospects for smart man (25-35). All particulars to 24/30, Office of this Paper.

WANTED.—Qualified Manager for Stockport district; must be well recommended and experienced. Also Qualified Locum for 2 or 3 weeks commencing September 7. Apply Dutton, 1248 Ashton Old Road, Manchester.

WANTED.—Unqualified Assistant for Holiday Relief for six weeks from July 20; usual particulars in first letter, please. Litchfield, South Farnborough, Hants.

WANTED.—Unqualified Locum from July 31 to August 15, inclusive. State terms to H. Jowett, 125 Pasture Street, Grimsby, Lincs.

WANTED.—Young Qualified Assistant, either sex. Also Chemist-Optician; London suburbs, W.; full particulars. Apply 24/32, Office of this Paper.

YOUNG, recently Qualified Assistant; good appearance; used to quick Counter and N.H.I.; for London, W.C.1; state salary and send photo if possible. Apply in first instance, Walkers (Holborn), Ltd., 240 High Holborn, W.C.1. 'Phone: Euston 1789.

NAMES AND ADDRESSES.

When sending advertisements for any of the sections in this Supplement, advertisers—as a guarantee of good faith and not necessarily for publication—should always give their names and addresses. It sometimes occurs that this rule is not followed and delay and disappointment ensue. Strict attention to this detail will be appreciated.

YOUNG Unqualified Male Assistant required immediately for City Pharmacy; Counter and Windows; please state full particulars, age, and salary required. 283/268, Office of this Paper.

WHOLESALE.

NORTH London Rubber Manufacturers require Traveller for Hot Water Bottles, Sponges and other Toilet requisites. Write, stating age, experience, 283/267, Office of this Paper.

FOR SCOTLAND.

REPRESENTATIVE.—Wanted, Young Man of good appearance to call on members of the Medical Profession, one capable of presenting his proposition in a dignified manner and of obtaining the interest and subsequent recommendation of the Doctors, for a well-known proprietary commodity of outstanding dietetic value. The man appointed will also be required to form liaison with the Retail trade, thereby bringing his propaganda to a successful issue. Age, experience and past earnings to 283/272, Office of this Paper.

MANUFACTURING Chemists require Young Assistant (Unqualified) in Cosmetics Department; reliable and energetic; one accustomed to preparing Stock Mixtures and Dispensing would suit; excellent opportunity to suitable applicant; experience in Cosmetics an advantage; state full particulars and wages required. P.C.B. 210/7, Office of this Paper.

MEDICAL Propaganda Representative required for West End of London; write, giving particulars of experience, age, height and qualifications; knowledge of Glandular Products an advantage. 282/250, Office of this Paper.

ONE or Two Medical Representatives required, calling on Hospitals, Institutions and Medical Men, by well-known Continental Laboratory; Biological Products, Sera and Vaccines; remunerative commission. Write, indicating present connection, 30/37, Office of this Paper.

PHARMACEUTICAL ADVERTISING.—Opportunity occurs in London firm for Pharmacist, with experience in advertising or with literary ability; Unqualified man with trade experience would be considered; full-time position; state age, experience and salary. 283/263, Office of this Paper.

PHARMACEUTICAL organisation marketing nationally-known proprietaries will shortly have a vacancy on their representative staff. Applications will be considered from Qualified Chemists resident in London, single and with previous experience of detailing the trade and profession. Particulars of age, business experience, etc., should be sent in complete detail to 283/260, Office of this Paper.

PROPAGANDA Representative required by well-known firm of Manufacturing Druggists; able to drive car, and intimate connection with chemists in outer London area essential. Write giving full details, past experience and references. 28/14, Office of this Paper.

REPRESENTATIVES, preferably with car, wanted on salary, bonus and commission, with connection amongst Hairdressers, for Packed and Bulk Toilets in South Wales, South Coast, Middlesex, Cambridge and Bedford; competitive lines; existing connection. Send details of experience to 31/3, Office of this Paper.

REPRESENTATIVES wanted, calling on Chemists, Ladies' Hairdressers and Stores; to carry an additional line; easy seller; to work on liberal commission basis. 30/51, Office of this Paper.

SMART young Salesman wanted by house of repute, to sell well-known proprietary to Chemists; experience and good sales record essential; state salary required, references, full personal particulars, 283/265, Office of this Paper.

TWO First-class Representatives required for the following territories: Cornwall, Devonshire and Dorset; Northumberland, Durham, Cumberland and Westmorland; excellent commission basis only; first-class opportunity for men with good connection amongst Chemists and Druggists; preferably with own car. Apply 283/276, Office of this Paper.

VETERINARY.—Two Representatives with good personal connections, calling on Qualified Veterinary Practitioners in Wales and Scotland, required by distributors of Veterinary Sera and Vaccines; good commission offered. Write, giving full details of present lines, 30/370, Office of this Paper.

SITUATIONS WANTED.

RETAIL (HOME).

2s. for 18 words or less; 6d. for every additional 10 words or less, prepaid. (Box No., 1s. extra.)

A.A.A.A.—QUALIFIED (35); smart appearance; good personality; all-round Managerial and West End experience; good Window-dresser and real Salesman; open for Locum. "M.P.S.," 2A Mount Ephraim Road, S.W.16.

A.A.A.—UNQUALIFIED (28); 3 years' West End experience; competent Dispenser, Salesman, Photographics; also Veterinary experience; expert Window-dresser; highest references; London or South Wales preferred. Jenkins, 162 Colum Road, Cardiff.

AN Assistant, Unqualified (26), desires change; permanent; 8 years' all-round experience London and Provinces. 29/4, Office of this Paper.

ASSISTANT; experienced Dispenser and Counterman; Photography; single, active, elderly, Unqualified; moderate salary. "Statim," 42 Fenton Road, Lockwood, Huddersfield.

ASSISTANT (25), lady; German qualification; Dispensing, Counter, Photography; English-, French-, German-speaking. Simonis, 53 Belsize Avenue, N.W.3.

ASSISTANT (27), Unqualified; good, all-round experience Dispensing, Counter, Window-dressing; London. "Advertiser," 44 Turneville Road, W.14.

ASSISTANT (24); 10 years' all-round Pharmacy experience, 3 years Optics, Part I S.M.C.; capable Refractionist; 5 years Window-dressing; honest and reliable; London, S.E. preferred. P.C.B. 209/18, Office of this Paper.

CHEMIST (50), fully Qualified, well up in all branches of Pharmacy, desires position as Manager or Superintendent; locum or permanent. "Chemist," 41 Leyton Road, London, E.15.

F.S.M.C. OPTICIAN, Unqualified Chemist (35), experienced, seeks permanency; West London or Middlesex; would start Optical Department; own equipment. 24/20, Office of this Paper.

LOCUM, free; Unqualified; good all-round Dispenser, Counter, Photographic; 25 years' experience. 29/2, Office of this Paper.

LOCUM; free until July 27 and September 1 onwards; London only; experienced; unregistered. Harries, 24 Brixton Road, S.W.9.

LOCUM; one or two weeks free between July 6 and 18; highest references; Unqualified. "E.," 43 South Street, Reading.

LOCUM, Qualified; experienced, trustworthy; disengaged August 3 to 8 and from August 31. Harris, 10 Claremont Road, Maida Vale, W.9.

LOCUM, Qualified, experienced (38); moderate terms; from July 6. "Chemist," 30 Bark Place, London, W.2.

LOCUM.—Unqualified (45); free July 11; experienced all branches; excellent references. "A. B.," 2 Walham Grove, Fulham, S.W.6.

LOCUM work required September 21 to October 3; Unqualified; all-round experience; excellent references. Barnes, 49 Rother Street, Stratford-on-Avon.

LOCUM (44; height 5 ft. 8 in.); Unqualified; Counter, Dispensing; take charge; abstainer; well recommended; now disengaged. Mack, 18 Aycliffe Road, W.12.

LOCUM (27), Qualified; July 27-August 1; London or suburbs; state wages. "Chemist," 33 Creffield Road, Ealing, W.5.

LOCUM (34), Unqualified; smart, active, thorough all-round experience; free immediately until August 1; anywhere. "Leon," 9 Spinney Rise, Birstall, Leicester.

M.P.S. (37) seeks permanency; 10 years' varied experience as Manager; married; free soon; London or near preferred. 30/10, Office of this Paper.

PERMANENCY or locums till suited; experienced, energetic Assistant (45); tall; Unqualified; keen Salesman, quick Dispenser, Photo, Windows, Agricultural, etc.; conscientious and trustworthy; disengaged. Haigh, 25 Hetley Road, Shepherd's Bush, W.12.

PHARMACIST (35), married, desires permanency as Branch Manager, preferably with living accommodation; all-round experience; present position (branch manager) 10 years. 22/1, Office of this Paper.

QUALIFIED Manager (27), Scot, married, seeks permanency, London or near; Manager or Assistant, with prospects; capable; experienced; reliable; excellent references. 29/11, Office of this Paper.

QUALIFIED, Scottish Square-trained, 1932 B.P., young, tall, live Salesman, seeks position, home or abroad, as Manager or Represent firm of repute; all-round high-class experience; London and Provinces; quick, accurate Dispenser; excellent references; interview any time; free immediately. Strang (Mr.), Bel Air Esplanade, Guernsey.

QUALIFIED (37), single, tall, reliable, excellent experience, as Manager, Superintendent or Senior; East Coast or South preferred; free end July; moderate salary for comfortable position. 32/1, Office of this Paper.

SEPTEMBER.—Assistant (26); tall; efficient Counterman, Dispenser and Window-dresser, Prescribing; quick, clean and accurate; desires permanency in good-class Pharmacy; London or suburbs; not afraid of work. Write "Chemist Friend," 77 Woodberry Avenue, N.21.

TEMPORARY Assistant (21); July 27 to October, or part; Salesman, Photo, Dispensing, Windows; East Anglia preferred; excellent references. 30/25, Office of this Paper.

UNQUALIFIED Assistant requires situation; anywhere if convenient R.C. Church; hard worker and capable (age 32). 24/46, Office of this Paper.

UNQUALIFIED Lady Assistant (20) requires post, London, central part preferred; salary £2; excellent references; interview any day until July 18. 27/3, Office of this Paper.

UNQUALIFIED (29), good Salesman, Window-dresser and Dispenser; clean habits and appearance; pleasing personality; Streatham district; free; £3 10s. K. Thompson, 65 Ena Road, S.W.16.

UNQUALIFIED (27) seeks post in Chemist's or Drug Stores (8 years); S. London preferred. 47 Palace Road, Bromley, Kent.

YOUNG Lady, experienced in Pharmacy, Toilet and Window-dressing; slight Dispensing; London districts preferred. 28/15, Office of this Paper.

WHOLESALE.

A PHARMACEUTICAL Chemist (29), Scot, with exceptionally good references, seeks opening with scope for advancement in Works, Laboratory or Hospital; proceeding to A.I.C.; keen and loyal. Box No. D.426, "Efficiency Magazine," 87 Regent Street, London, W.1.

A THOROUGHLY experienced and reliable Representative; very strong connection whole of London, Chemists, Hairdressers and Stores; exceptional credentials; own car. 30/31, Office of this Paper.

ADVERTISER desires Representative or Inside Post; lengthy Retail and some road experience; South; own car; ref. Sales Manager, Hop 0707; available now. F. J. M., 57 Huxley Road, Welling, Kent.

EXPERIENCED Representative (36), fully trained Pharmacy, Retail and Wholesale—15 and 5 years respectively; live connection London; desires change; join reputable firm; Drugs, Toilets, Sundries, Packed Goods or Specialities;. scope financial interest later; business builder; highest references; own car. 30/40, Office of this Paper.

EXPERIENCED Traveller of highest integrity (M.P.S., F.B.O.A. (Hons.)), desires represent really good house (Drug and Sundries), Commission basis; Perth to Thurso (own car), with Aberdeen as centre, where have stockroom and staff; bankers' refs. State commission. 282/252, Office of this Paper.

LADY (33), Qualified, seeks post other than Retail; Yorkshire preferred; Wholesale, Institution, Representative; conscientious worker; some Wholesale experience. 28/13, Office of this Paper.

MAN, Unqualified (26), seeks change with prospects; 11 years' Retail and Wholesale experience, Drug, Pricing, etc. 29/9, Office of this Paper.

PROFESSIONAL/TRADE PROPAGANDA, SALES. — Doctors, Chemists, Licensed Traders; car; long experience; salary and expenses. "Boaz," General Gordon Hotel, Weymouth.

REPRESENTATIVE of famous Perfumery House calling Chemists, Hairdressers, Stores, Wholesale and Retail, Hants, Dorset, Somerset, Devon, Cornwall, desires carry other proprietary lines; half expenses and commission. 24/9, Office of this Paper.

REPRESENTATIVE; resident Edinburgh; highest credentials; most successful Propagandist and Salesman, Medical, Dental, Hospitals, Pharmacists; disengaged. "Energy," 4 N. St. David Street, Edinburgh.

SALESMAN-PROPAGANDIST requires re-engagement shortly; over 20 years' experience calling on leading Physicians, Surgeons, Chemists and Institutions; energetic; can think originally; practical Organiser. M.P.S., 12 Cunningham Place, N.W.8.

TABLET-MAKER; 25 years' practical experience all branches, Sugar and Chocolate Coating, etc.; capable of taking charge. "F. W. B.," 39 Chaucer Road, E.17.

THE advertiser is a gentleman very well known and connected with Chemists, Doctors and a few Veterinary Surgeons in London and Southern Counties; he has had exceptionally good experience in Propaganda work with the Medical Profession; should any house of repute be interested the advertiser would be pleased to get into touch with them. Write 24/31, Office of this Paper.

UNQUALIFIED seeks Wholesale or Laboratory work; Part I; start small salary. W. Price, 318 Kennington Park Road, S.E.11.

FOR SALE.

6s. for 50 words or less ; 6d. for every additional 10 words or less, prepaid. (Box No., 1s. extra.)

(Articles to the value of £5-£50.)

"NATIONAL" Cash Register; medium size; prints and adds total; perfect condition; reasonable price. Write P. Tubbs, 1 Guildford Road, E.17.

MISCELLANEOUS.

10s. for 60 words or less ; 1s. for every additional 10 words or less, prepaid. (Box No., 1s. extra.)

A. BERNARD SLACK has written for benefit of Chemists and their friends a short article headed "*Why you should convert your business into a private limited company,*" and cost. Write for a free copy, study it and be wise and act on free advice given. 721 Princess Road, West Didsbury, Manchester.

CHEMISTS.—When you are wanting Shopfittings send your requirements to GEORGE COOK, The Working Shop Fitter, over 40 years' experience, 37 Macclesfield Street, City Road, London, E.C.1. 'Phone: Clerkenwell 5371. Sketches and Estimates free. Shop Fronts, Drug Fittings, Wall Cases, Dispensing Screens, Silent Salesmen, Counter Drawers.

CHEMISTS' FITTINGS.—New and Second-hand Drug Runs, Dispensing Screens, Glass-fronted Counters, Perfumery Cases, Nests of Drawers, Wall Cases, Silent Salesmen, Upright and Flat Counter Cases, Plate-glass Counters, Cash Tills, Display Stands and Glass Shelves, etc., at competitive prices. F. MAUND & E. BERG (SHOWCASES), LTD., Shopfitters and Shop Front Builders, 175/9 Old Street, London, E.C.1.

£78.—BARGAIN in Shop-soiled Mahogany Fittings, comprising 10-ft. Drug Fitting, 6-ft. Wall Case, 10-ft. Glass-fronted Counter, 6-ft. Dispensing Screen, Counter Drawers. PHILIP JOSEPHS & SONS, LTD., 90/92 St. John Street, Clerkenwell, E.C.1. Telephone: Clerk. 4111/2. "Pharmacy Fitters for over a Century."

£?—COMPLETE CHEMIST FITTINGS at any price you wish to pay. We have erected in our showrooms a Complete Chemist's Shop with Metal Shop Front, Window Backs, Correct Window Lighting, Signs and Modern Interior Fittings. Apply for Lists, D. MATTHEWS & SON, LTD., "The Liverpool Shop Fitters," 14 and 16 Manchester Street, Liverpool. Est. 1848.

Printed in Great Britain for the Proprietors by EYRE AND SPOTTISWOODE LIMITED, His Majesty's Printers, East Harding Street, London, E.C.4, and Published by the Proprietors, MORGAN BROTHERS (Publishers), Limited, at 28 Essex Street, Strand, London, W.C.2.—*July* 4, 1936. [50/44]

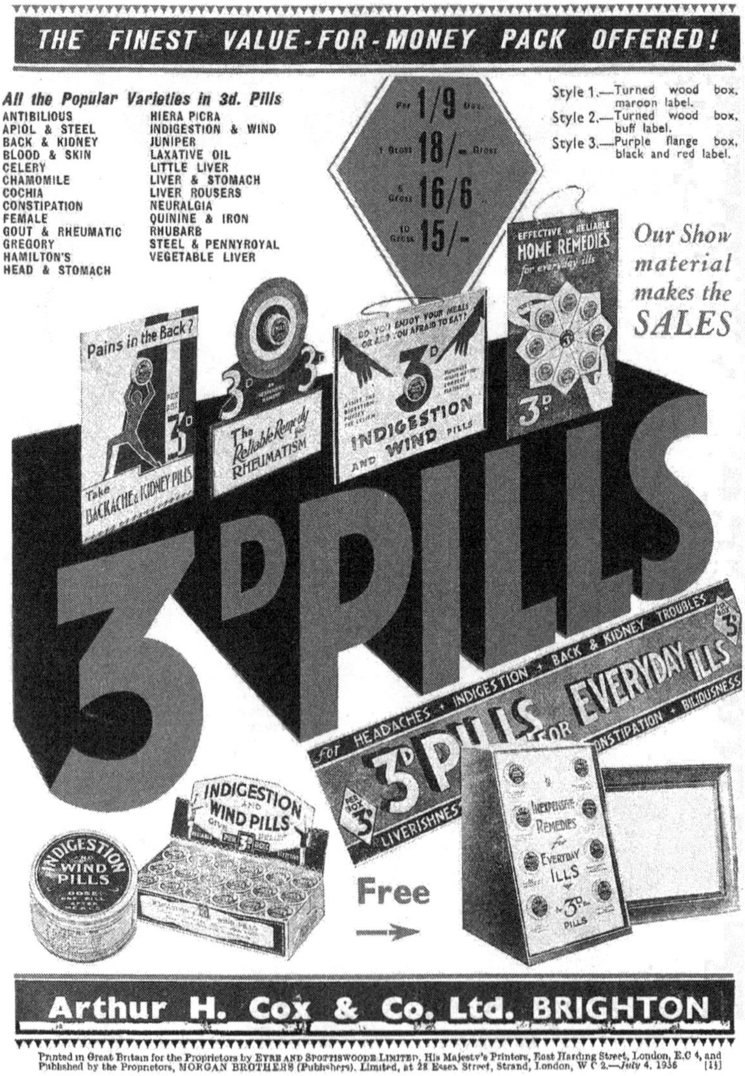

Printed in Great Britain for the Proprietors by EYRE AND SPOTTISWOODE LIMITED, His Majesty's Printers, East Harding Street, London, E.C 4, and Published by the Proprietors, MORGAN BROTHERS (Publishers), Limited, at 28 Essex Street, Strand, London, W C 2.—*July* 4, 1936 [1½]

THE CHEMIST AND DRUGGIST

RETAIL and DISPENSING PRICE LIST

ISSUED QUARTERLY · FIFTEENTH YEAR OF PUBLICATION

Use in conjunction with the "C. & D. Price List Formulary" and "C. & D. Poisons Guide"

THE SELLING PRICES in this List are based on the given cost and calculated for the quantities specified, the total oncost for that turnover being then added, together with the net profit, to the nearest figure. In case of fractions the prices are rounded up or down to the most suitable figure. As in arriving at the prices allowance has been made for variations in specific gravity, *liquids should be sold by fluid measure and solids by weight.*

INTERMEDIATE QUANTITIES should be calculated on the lower figure until midway is passed, then on the *higher figure.* The range of the quantities quoted in the List may be increased as follows: For **one pint** add one-fourth to the 16 oz. selling price. The **gallon price** for oils is obtained by dividing the cwt. price by 6; for **7-lb.** sales multiply the lb. cost by 10; for **14-lb.** by 20; and for **28-lb.** by 38. For *intermediate drachm prices* divide 1-oz. quotations by **7** and multiply by the number of drachms required. To obtain the *grain prices* divide the drachm selling price by 50.

PRICE ADJUSTMENT.—While standard wholesale prices are used as the starting point for calculating the retail prices, it may be desired to adjust the selling price for variations in cost. This may be effected by the following simplified method: To obtain the **lb. selling price** add half to the cost price (yielding 33⅓ per cent. on return); for the **4-oz. selling price** divide the lb. cost by 10 and multiply by 4 (yielding 37.5 per cent.); for the **1-oz. selling price** divide the lb. cost by 9 (yielding 43.75 per cent.). This method also applies to lozenges and pastilles which remain at a firm cost price.

DISPENSING CHARGES.—The two systems given (p. 2) are based on a special investigation and should be used for all dispensing other than contract work. When the Rapid Method is employed the Edinburgh private mark MELBORACIS should be used. In the case of a prescription containing one or more ingredients of an expensive nature the Costing Method is used and the mark "C. & D." only ought then to be indicated beneath the chemist's stamp.

MONTHLY CHANGES.—Important changes in prices occurring between the quarterly issues of this List are notified in THE CHEMIST AND DRUGGIST. Subscribers are recommended to carry out these alterations in ink as they are published, and so keep the quarterly List up to date.

"C. & D." DRUG INDEX

DRUGS (1913=100)		
—	1935	1936
Jan.	144·3	147·0
Feb.	144·4	147·0
Mar.	144·6	147·4
April	144·6	147·4
May	144·7	147·4
June	144·7	147·0
July	145·0	
Aug.	144·6	
Sept.	146·0	
Oct.	146·8	
Nov.	146·9	
Dec.	147·0	

DRESSINGS (1913=100)		
—	1935	1936
Jan.	136·3	136·2
Feb.	136·3	136·2
Mar.	136·2	136·5
April	136·2	136·5
May	136·2	136·5
June	136·2	136·6
July	136·2	
Aug.	136·2	
Sept.	136·2	
Oct.	136·2	
Nov.	136·2	
Dec.	136·2	

ABBREVIATIONS.—The references to standards or formulas in the List are: B.P. (British Pharmacopœia); U.S.P. (United States Pharmacopœia); B.P.C. (British Pharmaceutical Codex); M.O.H. (Ministry of Health); P.L.F. (Price List Formulary); N.I.F. (National Insurance Formulary).

SALES RESTRICTIONS.—The small capital letters and figures on the left-hand side of the retail price indicate restrictions on sale in Great Britain under the Pharmacy and Poisons Act, 1933, and the Poisons Rules and relate to the classification in *The Chemist and Druggist* "Poisons Guide," in which an extended list of poisons is given. In Northern Ireland and the Irish Free State different restrictions apply, although in many instances the letters may be taken as an indication that restrictions exist in these two countries. Dangerous drugs ("D.D." in Price List), are the same in Great Britain, Northern Ireland and the Irish Free State. Irish readers should refer to *The Chemist and Druggist* Poisons Cards.

PRICE LIST FORMULARY ("P.L.F.")—For the many unofficial preparations in active sale for which no standard formulas exist a special formulary has been compiled from "Pharmaceutical Formulas," "Veterinary Counter Practice" and other *C. & D.* publications. The cost and retail prices are given in this List and alterations made each month where changes in cost of ingredients render this necessary. The Price List Formulary is published at 2*s.* 6*d.* post free.

DRUG INDEX.—This *C. & D.* feature furnishes a comparative figure of the cost of drugs and appliances in 1913 and the present time. It is an important factor in accounting for the differences in retail charges now and before the war, and in the valuation of retail businesses.

STOCKTAKING SHEETS.—These sheets are used in conjunction with this List, in the annual stocktaking of drugs and chemicals, and form the simplest and quickest system of stock-taking for the drug-trade. The sheets, fastened into a pad, consist of the names of the articles printed on ruled paper in the same order as these occur in the List, which much facilitates the subsequent stage of pricing the stock from the cost figures. The sheets are sold in pads (2*s.* 6*d.* post free) with blank pages at the end.

Published as a Supplement to THE CHEMIST AND DRUGGIST, at 28 Essex Street, Strand, London, W.C.2

CONTENTS

PRICING PRESCRIPTIONS

DISPENSED MEDICINES

There are two systems of charging for medicines dispensed on prescription, as follows :—

1. RAPID METHOD.—The cost represents a definite proportion of the charge and refers to ordinary drugs and chemicals with infusions or decoctions. Tinctures, syrups, extracts, if prescribed in any quantity, require the price adjusting by the list according to Method 2. The prices quoted are exclusive of containers. (See below.)

Mixtures of simple medicaments :—

Size	Dose ʒj.	Dose ʒij.	Dose ʒiv.	Dose ℥j.
	s. d.	s. d.	s. d.	s. d.
℥j.	1 0	0 10	0 9	0 8
℥ij.	1 6	1 2	1 0	0 10
℥iij.	—	1 6	1 3	1 0
℥iv.	—	1 10	1 6	1 2
℥vj.	—	—	2 0	1 6
℥viij.	—	—	2 6	1 10

		s. d.
Gargles, lotions, injections	8 oz.	1 6
Pills and powders	12	1 6
Cachets and dry-filled capsules	12	2 6
Ointments, mixed .. .. 1 oz., 1s. 3d.;	2 oz.	1 6
Suppositories, bougies, pessaries	12	2 0
Small shaped blisters	each	1 0
Plasters, 6 in. × 6 in.	each	2 6

An extra fee of 6d. per prescription is made for night attendance.

When this method of pricing is employed, the first dispenser of the prescriptions should mark the price charged by private mark. The Edinburgh private mark

M	e	l	b	o	r	a	c	i	s
1	2	3	4	5	6	7	8	9	0

which has been in use for many years, should be adopted.

Larger quantities, or those containing appreciable amounts of tinctures, etc., should be priced by Method 2.

2. COSTING METHOD.—This method is calculated on the average time taken for the various operations involved in dispensing, and is based on the recommendations in 1915 of the Departmental Committee on the National Insurance Act Drug Tariff and the results obtained by numerous correspondents. The three components of the price of a prescription to be added together are as follows :—

A. The **selling prices** in this list are calculated upon costing principles and form a correct basis for obtaining the cost of the ingredients of a prescription. For finding the price of drachm quantities other than those quoted in the list, the rule that should be adopted is to divide the ounce quantity by seven and multiply the figures obtained by the number of drachms required.

B. Prices of **containers** are given in the list. (See below.)

C. Special **"oncost"** included in the terms "time" and "labour" to perform the work, and the special **establishment charges** of the dispensary above and beyond that already included in the distribution "oncost."

Modern medical treatment sometimes requires forms of medication needing long periods of time in their preparation. No standard fee can be laid down since time, the guiding factor, is unknown until the prescription is completed. A basic figure covering time with its essential oncost and actual labour may be calculated on a rate of 60d. per hour or portions thereof in making up the final professional charge.

The accountant's figures for "oncost" are as follows :—

		s. d.
Uncompounded medicines of whatever nature		0 6
Mixtures, lotions, liniments, drops, rectal injections		0 8
Emulsions		0 10
Pills and weighed powders	doz.	0 10
Ointments, confections, etc.		0 9
Blisters		0 8
Cachets	doz.	1 3
Capsules, hard (cachet fitting) (each extra doz. 6d.) ..	doz.	1 0
Bougies, suppositories, pessaries	doz.	1 4
Plasters		1 8
Granules, pastilles, lozenges, soft capsules	doz.	2 0
Silvering, varnishing, and otherwise coating pills ..	doz. 3d.	extra
Ampoules (filling and sterilising)	doz.	3 0
Solutions and oils in bulk (sterilising)	to 500 mils.	3 6
Oculenta (sterilised)	to 1 oz.	2 6
Powders, mixed, in bulk	to 4 oz.	0 10
Injections and hypodermic sterilising	to 1 oz.	2 6
Injections, intravenous and diagnostic sterilising ..	to 100 mils.	3 6
Hire of appliances	per week	2 6
Special registration fee of medicaments		0 3
Tuberculin and protein dilutions	per dose	2 6
	per 6 doses	3 0

As these charges cover average time, the oncost for larger quantities can be calculated according to the length of time required on the above basis.

When the Costing Method is used, mark "C. & D." under the name stamp on the prescription.

CONTAINERS

Retail charge

Medicine and Poison Bottles

	Sell s. d.		Sell s. d.		Sell s. d.
2 dr., 4 dr., 1 oz.	0 2	10 oz. ..	0 3	20 oz. ..	0 4
2 oz., 3 oz. ..	0 2	12 oz. ..	0 3	32 oz. ..	0 6
4 oz.	0 2	16 oz. ..	0 4	40 oz. ..	0 7
6 oz., 8 oz. ..	0 2				

Iodine bottles add price of rubber stopper (3d.) to poison bottles.

Ointment Pots	Sell s. d.	Stoppered Bottles	Sell s. d.	Powder Bottles	Sell s. d.
1 dr., 2 dr., ½ oz.	0 6	1 oz. ..	0 7	½ oz., 1 oz. ..	0 4
1 oz., 1½ oz. ..	0 7	2 oz. ..	0 8	2 oz.	0 5
2 oz.	0 8	4 oz. ..	0 9	4 oz.	0 7
3 oz.	0 10	6 oz. ..	0 10	6 oz.	0 8
4 oz ..	0 11	8 oz. ..	0 11		

Cost d.	per	Drugs and Chemicals	Selling Price 16 oz. s. d.	4 oz. s. d.	1 oz. s. d.	1 dr. s. d.
33·5	25	Abidon Caps	4 0	each	—	—
12	lb.	Absinthium	1 6	0 6	0 2	—
72	lb.	"A.C.E." anæsthet. P.I. (10)	7 6	2 6	—	—
60	lb.	Acaciæ gummi alb. elect. ..	7 6	2 2	0 7	—
51	lb.	Acaciæ gummi alb. parv. opt. ..	6 3	1 11	0 7	—
42	lb.	Acaciæ gummi alb. parv. sec. ..	5 3	1 6	0 5	—
48	lb.	Acaciæ gummi alb. pulv. opt. ..	6 0	1 9	0 6	—
39	lb.	Acaciæ gummi alb. pulv. sec. ..	4 10	1 5	0 5	—
30	lb.	Acaciæ gummi var. opt. ..	3 9	1 2	0 4	—
27	oz.	Acetamidosalol	—	—	4 0	0 7
4	oz.	Acetanilidum .. ..P.I. (8)	—	—	0 7	0 2
22	oz.	Acetannin	—	—	3 3	0 6
18	lb.	Acetonum	2 6	0 9	0 3	—
17	lb.	Acetonum coml.	2 2	0 8	0 3	—
228	lb.	Acetum aromaticum P.L.F. ..	—	—	—	0 4
41	lb.	Acet. arom. P.L.F. (synth. ol.)	—	—	—	0 3
30	lb.	Acet. cantharidini ..S.I. (5)	—	1 1	0 4	0 1
33	lb.	Acet. cantharidis . S.I. (5)	—	1 4	0 5	0 1
20	lb.	Acet. colchici .. P.I. (10)	—	0 9	0 3	—
8	lb.	Acet. destillatum album ..	1 0	0 4	0 1½	—
36	gal.	Acet. fuscum	gal.	4 6	pint	0 7
6	lb.	Acet. fuscum (Beaufoy) ..	—	0 3	0 1	—
27	lb.	Acet. ipecacuanhæ	—	1 0	0 4	—
27	lb.	Acet. odoratum meth. B.P.C. ..	—	1 0	0 4	—
16	lb.	Acet. rubi idæi	2 4	0 10	0 3	—
8	lb.	Acet. scillæ	1 2	0 5	0 2	—
78	gal.	Acet. vini Gallici	pint	1 3	0 2	—
13	tube	Acidol tablets	per	tube	1 6	—
49	50	Acidol pepsin (50 tabs.) ..	each	5 6	—	—
		Acida				
7	lb.	Acidum aceticum	1 0	0 4	0 1½	—
6	lb.	Acid. aceticum dilutum ..	0 9	0 3	0 1	—
16	lb.	Acid. aceticum glaciale ..	—	0 8	0 3	—
45	lb.	Acid. acetylsalicylicum	—	1 8	0 6	0 1
30	gm.	Acid. ascorbic synth.	—	0 3	grain	—
33	oz.	Acid. benzoicum nat.	—	—	4 10	0 8
5	lb.	Acid. benzoicum synth. ..	—	—	0 9	0 2
8	lb.	Acid. boricum cryst.	0 11	0 4	0 1½	—
9	lb.	Acid. borici pulv. subtil. ..	1 2	0 5	0 2	—
1.5	oz.	Acid. borici pulv. pkd. ..	—	0 7	0 2½	—
10	cwt.	Acid. borici coml. pulvis ..	7 lb.	4 0	—	—
7	lb.	Acid. borici coml. pulvis ..	1 0	0 4	0 1½	—
28	oz.	Acid. camphoricum	—	—	4 1	0 7
39	gal.	Acid. carbol. "misc." P.I. (8)	pint	0 8	—	—
60	gal.	Acid. carbol. "straw" P.I. (8)	1 0	0 4	0 2	—
5	lb.	Acid. carbol. (disinf. powder) ..	0 9	—	—	—
16	oz.	Acid. cinnamicum	—	—	2 4	0 4
21	lb.	Acid. citricum	2 7	0 9	0 3	—
22	lb.	Acid. citrici pulvis	2 9	0 10	0 3	—
28	lb.	Acid. cresyl. pur. (vap.)—P.I. (8)	—	1 2	0 4	—
30	lb.	Acid. formicum 50%	2 9	0 11	0 4	0 1
8	oz.	Acid. gallicum	—	—	1 2	0 3
7	oz.	Acid. glycerophosphoric. 20% ..	—	—	1 10	0 4
6	oz.	Acid. hippuricum	—	—	5 3	0 9
7	oz.	Acid. hydriodicum dilutum ..	—	—	1 1	0 2
6	lb.	Acid. hydrobrom. conc. 30% ..	—	1 8	0 7	—
5	lb.	Acid. hydrobrom. dilutum ..	—	0 9	0 3	0 1
0	lb.	Acid. hydrochlor. .. P.II. (8)	1 7	0 6	0 2	0 1
8	lb.	Acid. hydrochlor. dilutum P.II. (9)	—	0 5	0 2	—
6.5	lb.	Acid. hydrochlori. coml. P.II. (8)	1 0	0 4	0 2	—
7	oz.	Acid. hydrocyan. (fort) S.I. (5)	—	—	1 2	0 2
6	oz.	Acid. hydrocyan. dil. S.I. (5)	—	—	1 0	0 2
0	lb.	Acid. hydrofluor. coml. (by wt.) P.II. (8)	2 6	0 10	0 3	—
2	lb.	Ac. hydrofluor. dil. B.P.C 1923 P.II. (10)	1 8	0 6	0 2	—
0	lb.	Acid. hypophosphorosum dil. ..	—	1 2	0 7	0 1
6	oz.	Acid. lacticum	—	—	0 11	0 2

Ac—Al

Cost d.	per	Acida—(cont.)	Selling Price 16 oz. s. d.	4 oz. s. d.	1 oz. s. d.	1 dr. s. d.
18	lb.	Acid. lacticum dilutum ..	2 8	0 8	0 3	0 1
29	oz.	Acid. mandelic	—	—	4 3	0 8
12	oz.	Acid. molybdicum	—	—	2 0	0 4
17	lb.	Acid. nitricum .. P.II. (8)	3 2	0 11	0 3	—
8	lb.	Acid. nitricum dil. P.II. (9)	—	0 5	0 2	—
12	lb.	Acid. nitricum coml. P.II. (8)	2 3	0 8	0 3	—
8	lb.	Acid. nitro-hydrochlor. dil. P.II. (9)	—	0 5	0 2	—
12	lb.	Acid. oleicum	1 6	0 6	0 2	—
84	oz.	Acid. osmic. 1 per cent. sol. ..	—	—	12 0	1 9
21	lb.	Acid. oxalic. recryst. ..P.I. (8)	—	0 10	0 3	0 1
13	lb.	Acid. oxalic. coml. ..P.I. (8)	1 8	0 7	0 2	—
20	lb.	Acid. phosphoricum B.P. ..	—	1 4	0 5	—
8	lb.	Acid. phosphoricum dilutum ..	1 0	0 5	0 2	0 1
14	oz.	Acid. pyrogallicum sublim. ..	—	—	2 0	0 4
11	oz.	Acid. pyrogallicum cryst. ..	—	—	1 7	0 3
8	lb.	Acid. pyrolignosum	1 0	0 4	—	—
32	oz.	Acid. salicylicum nat.	—	—	4 8	0 10
30	lb.	Acid. salicylici pulvis	—	1 1	0 4	0 1
12	oz.	Acid. salicylsulphonicum ..	—	—	2 0	0 4
14	lb.	Acid. stearicum coml.	1 9	0 7	0 2	—
9	oz.	Acid. sulphanilic. recryst. ..	—	—	1 4	0 3
11	lb.	Acid. sulph. .. P.II. (8)	2 6	0 10½	0 3	—
8	lb.	Acid. sulph. dil. .. P.II. (9)	—	0 5	0 2	—
7.5	lb.	Acid. sulph. coml. P.II. (8)	1 9	0 6	0 2	—
8	oz.	Acid. sulph. aromat. P.II. (9)	—	—	1 2	0 2
8	lb.	Acid. sulphurosum	1 0	0 4	0 1	—
26	lb.	Acid. sulphuros. (in spirit) ..	—	1 0	0 4	—
7	oz.	Acid. tannicum	—	—	1 1	0 2
20	lb.	Acid. tartaricum cryst. mag. ..	2 6	0 9	0 3	—
21	lb.	Acid. tartaricum cryst. parv. ..	2 7	0 9	0 3	—
20	lb.	Acid. tartarici pulvis	2 6	0 9	0 3	—
15	oz.	Acid. trichloraceticum	—	—	2 3	0 4
15	oz.	Acid. valerianicum	—	—	2 3	0 4
21	lb.	Aconitum .. ..S.I. (4)	—	1 1	0 4	0 1
32	lb.	Aconitum pulverat. ..S.I. (4)	—	1 2	0 4	—
9	gr.	Aconitina .. ..S.I. (4)	per	gr.	1 6	—
13	gm.	Acriflavinum	per	gr.	0 2	7 7
113	oz.	Adalin	—	—	—	2 4
34	25	Adalin tablets gr. 5	doz.	2 6	—	—
22	lb.	Adeps benzoinatus	2 9	0 10	0 3	—
17	lb.	Adeps	2 1	0 8	0 3	—
18	lb.	Adeps lanæ	2 2	0 8	0 3	—
15	lb.	Adeps lanæ hydrosus	2 0	0 7	0 3	—
9	gr.	Adrenalinum .. ..P.I. (8)	per	gr.	1 4	—
41	oz.	Adrenalin.chlor.sol.1-1,000(P.D.) P.I. (8)	—	—	5 0	0 9
27	oz.	Adrephine (P.D.) ..P.I. (8)	—	—	3 0	—
39	lb.	Æther anæsthet. by wgt. ..	5 0	1 5	—	—
24	lb.	Æther methylicus 0.730 ..	3 0	1 0	0 4	—
9	oz.	Æther aceticus	—	—	1 4	0 3
72	lb.	Æther chloricus	—	2 6	0 9	—
8	oz.	Æther ozonicus	—	—	1 1	0 3
28	ea.	Æthylis chloride (30 c.c.) ..	ea.	3 6	—	—
40	ea.	Æthylis chloride (50 c.c.) ..	ea.	5 0	—	—
84	lb.	Agar (shredded)	—	3 2	0 11	—
90	lb.	Agar pulvis	—	3 3	1 0	—
51	oz.	Agotan .. .. ..℞ only	—	—	—	1 3
48	50	Agotan tablets .. ..℞ only	doz.	1 6	—	—
21	lb.	Agropyrum Ang.	—	0 10	0 3	—
50	oz.	Airol	—	—	—	1 1
90	oz.	Albargin	—	—	—	2 0
8	oz.	Albumen (egg) pulv.	—	—	1 2	0 2
6	oz.	Albumin. (blood) pulv. ..	—	—	0 11	—
12	oz.	Albumin. tannic.	—	—	1 9	0 3
262	pt.	Alcohol 90% sine rebate ..	24 0	7 0	1 9	0 4
108	pt.	Alcohol 90% c̄ rebate	11 0	3 3	1 0	0 2
274	pt.	Alcohol 95% s. r.	—	—	1 9	0 3

Cost d.	Cost per	Al—Am	16 oz. s. d.	4 oz. s. d.	1 oz. s. d.	1 dr. s. d.
315	lb.	Alcohol dehydrat.	—	10 3	2 8	0 5
144	lb.	Alcoholammon.fort.B.P.C.P.I.I.(9)	—	—	1 6	0 3
36	lb.	Alcohol amylicum	4 6	1 4	0 5	0 1
27	lb.	Alcohol amylicum coml.	3 4	1 0	0 4	—
36	pt.	Alcohol isopropylicum	4 0	1 1	0 4	—
360	lb.	Alcohol methylicum pur.	—	11 8	3 0	0 6
24	oz.	Aldehydum alcoh. 20%	—	—	3 6	—
42	dr.	Allantoinum	—	—	—	6 2
32	lb.	All Fours P.L.F. P.I. (13)	—	1 2	0 4	0 1
18	lb.	Allium sativum	2 3	0 8	0 3	—
120	oz.	Allobarbitonum ℞ only	—	—	—	2 6
162	100	Allonal tablets ℞ only	doz.	2 7	—	—
55	oz.	Allosan	—	—	7 0	1 4
40	lb.	Aloe Barbadensis	5 0	1 5	0 5	—
40	lb.	Aloe Barbadensis pulvis opt.	5 0	1 5	0 5	0 1
16	lb.	Aloe Capensis	2 0	0 7	0 2	—
21	lb.	Aloe Capensis pulvis	2 8	0 9	0 3	—
66	lb.	Aloe Socot. pulvis	8 3	2 5	0 9	0 2
15	oz.	Aloinum	—	—	2 3	0 4
28	gm.	Alopon (A. & H.) D.D.	per	gr.	0 4	—
60	lb.	Althææ flores	—	2 2	0 8	—
18	lb.	Althææ folia	2 3	0 8	0 3	—
24	lb.	Althææ rad. decort.	3 0	0 11	0 4	—
30	lb.	Althææ rad. dec. pulvis	3 9	1 1	0 4	—
13	lb.	Alumen	1 8	0 6	0 2	—
15	lb.	Alumen pulv.	2 0	0 7	0 2	—
4	lb.	Alumen coml.	0 7	0 2	0 1	—
252	cwt.	Alumen coml.	7 lb.	2 0	—	—
4.5	lb.	Alumen coml. pulv.	0 8	0 3	—	—
276	cwt.	Alumen coml. pulv.	14 lb.	4 0	7 lb.	2 2
21	lb.	Alumen chromicum recryst.	—	0 10	0 3	—
9	lb.	Alumen chromicum coml.	1 3	0 6	0 2	—
17	lb.	Alumen exsiccatum	2 2	0 8	0 3	—
18	lb.	Alumen exsiccatum pulv.	2 3	0 8	0 3	—
13	lb.	Alumen rupel	1 8	0 7	0 2	—
6	oz.	Aluminii acetas	—	—	0 11	0 2
8	oz.	Aluminii aceto-tartras	—	—	1 2	0 2
45	lb.	Aluminii chloridum (hydrated)	—	1 8	0 6	0 1
42	lb.	Aluminii hydroxidum	5 3	1 6	0 5	0 1
12	oz.	Aluminii salicylas	—	—	1 9	0 3
21	lb.	Aluminii sulphas	—	0 10	0 3	—
9	lb.	Aluminii sulphas coml.	1 2	0 4	—	—
16	oz.	Aluminii tannas	—	—	2 0	0 4
14	oz.	Amidol	—	—	1 9	0 3½
26	oz.	Amidopyrina ℞ only	—	—	3 9	0 7
42	oz.	Amidopyrin. camph. ℞ only	—	—	6 2	1 0
38	oz.	Amidopyrin. salicyl. ℞ only	—	—	5 7	0 10
51	lb.	Ammoniaci pulvis	—	—	0 6	0 1
45	lb.	Ammoniacum opt. (gtt.)	—	—	0 6	0 1
		Ammonium				
4	oz.	Ammon. acetas pur.	—	—	0 7	0 1
30	oz.	Ammon. benzoas nat.	—	—	4 5	0 8
78	lb.	Ammon. benzoas synth.	—	2 10	0 10	0 2
18	lb.	Ammon. bicarb.	—	0 8	0 3	0 1
36	lb.	Ammon. bichromas cryst.	—	1 4	0 5	—
37	lb.	Ammon. bromidum	—	1 4	0 5	—
19	lb.	Ammon. carb. resub.	2 5	0 9	0 3	—
16	lb.	Ammon. carb. resub. pulv.	2 0	0 7	0 2	—
13	lb.	Ammon. carb. coml.	1 8	0 7	0 2	—
10	lb.	Ammon. carb coml. (qty.)	1 3	—	7 lb.	7 0
11	lb.	Ammon. carb. coml. pulv.	1 4	0 5	0 2	—
11.5	lb.	Ammon. carb. coml. pulv. (qty.)	1 6	—	7 lb.	9 8
15	lb.	Ammon. chloridum pur.	1 10	0 7	0 2	—
11	lb.	Ammon. chloridum coml.	1 5	0 5	0 2	—
11	lb.	Ammon. chloridum "lumps"	1 5	—	7 lb.	8 3
7	oz.	Ammon. citras	—	—	1 1	0 2
60	lb.	Ammon. formas	—	2 3	0 8	0 2
36	oz.	Ammon. hippuras	—	—	5 3	1 9

Cost d.	Cost per	Am—An Ammonium—(cont.)	16 oz. s. d.	4 oz. s. d.	1 oz. s. d.	1 dr. s. d.
12	lb.	Ammon. hydrosulph. sol.	1 6	0 7	0 3	—
13	oz.	Ammon. hypophosphis	—	—	1 11	0 4
18	oz.	Ammon. iodidum	—	—	2 8	0 5
48	lb.	Ammon. monocarb. arom.	—	—	0 6	0 2
18	lb.	Ammon. nitras pur.	2 3	0 8	0 3	—
9	lb.	Ammon. nitras, coml.	1 2	0 4	0 2	—
27	lb.	Ammon. oxalas pur.	—	1 0	0 4	0 1
36	lb.	Ammon. persulphas	—	1 4	0 5	0 1
36	lb.	Ammon. phosphas	4 6	1 4	0 5	0 1
15	lb.	Ammon. phosphas coml.	1 10	0 7	0 2	—
42	lb.	Ammon. phosphas acid.	—	1 7	0 6	0 1
8	oz.	Ammon. salicylas	—	—	1 2	0 3
21	oz.	Ammon. succinas	—	—	3 1	0 6
12	lb.	Ammon. sulphas pur.	—	0 6	0 2	—
5	lb.	Ammon. sulphas coml.	0 8	0 3	—	—
210	cwt.	Ammon. sulphas coml.	7 lb.	1 8	—	—
42	lb.	Ammon. sulphocyanidum	—	—	0 6	0 1
6	oz.	Ammon. tartras	—	—	0 11	0 2
21	oz.	Ammon. valerianas cryst.	—	—	3 1	0 6
75	oz.	Ammona unstd.	—	—	—	1 10
67	5 amp	Amphotropin sol.	1 9	single	amp.	—
32	lb.	Amygdala amara	4 0	1 2	0 4	—
48	lb.	Amygdala dulcis Jordan	6 0	1 9	0 6	—
36	lb.	Amygdala dulcis Valent.	5 3	1 6	0 6	—
60	lb.	Amygd. dulc. pulv. alb.	7 6	2 2	0 7	0 1
24	lb.	Amygd. cont. (Almond meal)	3 0	0 11	0 3	—
27	lb.	Amyl acetas pur.	—	1 0	0 4	—
24	lb.	Amyl acetas coml.	3 1	0 11	0 4	—
9	oz.	Amyl nitris P.I. (8)	—	—	—	0 3
20	doz.	Amyl nitrite caps. ♏3 P.I. (13)	doz.	2 6	—	—
36	oz.	Amyleni hydras	—	—	5 3	0 9
360	cwt.	Amyli pulvis (maize)	7 lb.	2 9	—	—
7	lb.	Amyli pulvis (maize)	0 11	0 3	0 1	—
6	lb.	Amyli pulvis (potato)	0 9	0 3	0 1	—
7	lb.	Amyli pulvis (rice)	0 11	0 4	0 1	—
8	lb.	Amyli pulvis (wheat)	1 0	0 4	0 1	—
36	dr.	Amylocain hyd. S.I. (4)	—	—	—	0 3 (grain)
54	oz.	Anæsthesin P.I. (8)	—	—	—	1 2
14	lb.	Anchusæ radix	1 9	0 7	0 2	—
9	lb.	Anethi fructus E.I.	1 2	0 5	0 2	—
16	lb.	Anethi fructus pulvis	2 0	0 7	0 2	—
60	lb.	Angelicæ radix	7 6	2 2	0 8	—
72	lb.	Angelicæ radicis pulvis	9 0	2 7	0 9	—
4	oz.	Anilini hydrochlor.	—	—	0 7	0 1
16	lb.	Anilinum coml. opt.	2 0	0 7	0 2	—
12	lb.	Anisi fructus	1 6	0 6	0 2	—
15	lb.	Anisi fructus pulvis	2 0	0 7	0 3	—
14	lb.	Anisi fructus pulvis (crs.)	1 9	0 7	0 3	—
14	oz.	Anisole	—	—	2 0	0 4
54	lb.	Annatto (roll)	—	2 0	0 7	—
36	lb.	Annatto (liquid)	—	1 7	0 6	—
42	lb.	Anthemidis flores Ang.	—	1 6	0 5	—
30	lb.	Anthemidis flores exot.	3 9	1 2	0 4	0 1
33	lb.	Anthemidis florum exot. pulv.	—	1 3	0 4	0 1
26	lb.	Anthemidis flores exot. sec.	3 3	1 0	0 4	—
12	lb.	Antiformin substitute	1 6	0 6	0 2	—
60	oz.	Antikamnia, unstd.	—	—	—	1 6
60	oz.	Antikamnia tablets, unstd.	doz.	1 6	—	—
18	lb.	Antim. croc. pulv. S.I. (4)	2 3	0 8	0 3	—
7	oz.	Antim. et sod. tart. S.I. (4)	—	—	1 1	0 2
648	doz.	Antim. et sodii tart. sterules (M'dale) gr. ½ (box of 10) S.I.(4)	box	6 0	—	—
864	doz.	Antim. sod. tart. sterules (M'dale) gr.ij. (box of 10) S.I.(4)	box	8 0	—	—
12	lb.	Antim. nig. pulv. S.I. (4)	1 3	0 6	0 2	—
6	oz.	Antim. oxidum S.I. (4)	—	—	1 0	0 2

Cost d.	per	An—Ar	Selling Price 16 oz. s. d.	4 oz. s. d.	1 oz. s. d.	1 dr. s. d.
42	lb.	Antim. sulph. S.1. (4)	5 3	1 6	0 5	0 1
42	lb.	Antim. tartar. pv. S.1. (4)	5 3	1 6	0 6	0 1
6	oz.	Antim. et pot. tart. "intraven." S.1. (4)	—	—	1 0	0 2
43	oz.	Antitoxine tabs., unstd. ..	doz.	0 9	—	—
		Antitoxins (v. Serological Products, page 31)				
162	10c.c.	Antuitrin 'S' P.D. & Co. P.I. (13)	—	18 0	each	—
24	lb.	Apii grav. sem.	3 0	0 11	0 4	—
30	oz.	Apiol	—	—	—	0 8
10	gr.	Apomorph. hydroch. S.1. (4)	per	gr.	1 6	—
		Aquæ				
8	lb.	Aqua anethi	1 0	0 4	0 2	—
198	lb.	Aqua anethi conc.	—	7 0	2 0	0 4
8	lb.	Aqua anisi dest.	1 0	0 4	0 2	—
162	lb.	Aqua anisi conc. 1-40	—	5 9	1 7	0 4
19	lb.	Aqua aurantii flor. trip. ..	2 6	0 9	0 3	—
8	lb.	Aqua camphoræ	1 0	0 4	0 1½	—
54	lb.	Aqua camphoræ conc.	—	2 0	0 7	0 1
8	lb.	Aqua cari dest.	1 0	0 4	0 1½	—
174	lb.	Aqua cari conc. 1-40	—	6 2	1 10	0 4
8	lb.	Aqua caryophylli dest.	1 0	0 4	0 1½	—
192	lb.	Aqua caryophylli conc. ..	—	6 10	2 0	0 4
8	lb.	Aqua chloroformi	1 0	0 4	0 1½	—
60	lb.	Aq. chlorof. conc. B.P.C. P.I. (9)	—	2 2	0 8	0 2
9	lb.	Aqua cinnamomi	1 3	0 5	0 2	—
198	lb.	Aqua cinnamomi conc. ..	—	7 0	2 0	0 4
13	gal.	Aqua destillata	0 4	0 2	—	—
102	lb.	Aqua Florid. (isoprop.)	—	3 6	1 0	—
8	lb.	Aqua fœniculi	1 0	0 4	0 1	—
186	lb.	Aqua fœniculi conc.	—	6 7	1 10	0 4
18	lb.	Aqua laurocerasi S.1. (5)	2 3	0 8	0 3	—
294	lb.	Aqua lavand.opt.(isoprop.) P.L.F.	—	10 4	2 9	0 5
142	lb.	Aqua lavand.sec.(isoprop.) P.L.F.	—	5 0	1 4	0 3
81	lb.	Aqua mellis (isoprop.) P.L.F. ..	—	2 10	0 9	—
13	lb.	Aqua menthæ pip. dest. ..	1 8	0 7	0 2	—
216	lb.	Aqua menthæ pip. conc. Ang.1-40	—	7 6	2 0	0 4
198	lb.	Aqua menthæ pip. conc. exot.1-40	—	7 0	2 0	0 4
14	lb.	Aqua menthæ viridis dest. ..	1 9	0 7	0 2	—
14	lb.	Aqua picis P.L.F.	1 9	0 7	0 2	—
9	lb.	Aqua pimentæ dest.	1 2	0 5	0 2	—
198	lb.	Aqua pimentæ conc. 1-40 ..	—	7 6	2 1	0 4
8	lb.	Aqua pulegii dest.	1 0	0 4	0 1	—
13	lb.	Aqua rosæ dest.	1 8	0 7	0 2	—
18	lb.	Aqua rosæ trip. opt.	2 3	0 8	0 3	—
216	lb.	Aqua rosæ conc. 1-40	—	7 9	2 4	0 4
10	lb.	Aqua rosmarini	1 3	0 5	0 2	—
168	lb.	Aqua rosmarini conc. 1-40 ..	—	6 0	1 8	0 3
11	lb.	Aqua sambuci	1 5	0 6	0 2	—
24	lb.	Aqua sambuci trip.	3 0	0 11	0 3	—
228	lb.	Aqua sambuci conc. 1-40 ..	—	—	2 3	0 4
10	oz.	Araroba	—	—	1 6	0 2
24	dr.	Arbutin	—	—	—	3 6
18	lb.	Archil	2 4	0 9	0 3	—
17	lb.	Arctii radix	2 2	0 8	0 3	—
26	lb.	Arctii radicis pulvis	3 3	1 0	0 4	—
12	lb.	Areca	—	—	0 2	—
15	lb.	Arecæ pulvis	1 10	0 7	0 2	—
3	gr.	Arecolinæ hydrobromidum ..	per	gr.	0 6	—
72	oz.	Argenti bromidum	—	—	—	1 6
63	oz.	Argenti chloridum	—	—	—	1 4
72	oz.	Argenti iodidum	—	—	—	1 6
32	oz.	Argenti nitras cryst.	—	—	4 8	0 8
96	doz.	Argenti nit. (points in glass) ..	ea.	1 2	—	—
39	doz.	Argenti nit. ind. (in wood) ..	ea.	0 6	—	—
37	oz.	Argenti nit. mitigat. (sticks) ..	ea.	0 10	—	—
36	oz.	Argenti nucleinas	—	—	5 3	0 9

Cost d.	per	Ar—Be	Selling Price 16 oz. s. d.	4 oz. s. d.	1 oz. s. d.	1 dr. s. d.
63	oz.	Argenti oxidum	—	—	—	1 4
18	oz.	Argenti proteinatum	—	—	2 8	0 5
46	oz.	Argenti vitellin	—	—	6 9	1 0
60	oz.	Argentum colloidale	—	—	—	1 3
9	25	Argentum (fol.)	per	leaf	0 1	—
90	oz.	Argyrol	—	—	—	1 9
31	40	Arheol capsules	doz.	1 2	—	—
360	oz.	Aristochin	—	—	—	8 7
40	10gr.	Aristol	—	—	—	2 0
27	lb.	Aristolochiæ radix	3 6	1 0	0 4	—
36	lb.	Aristolochiæ radicis pulvis ..	4 6	1 4	0 5	—
24	lb.	Arnicæ flores	—	0 11	0 4	—
36	lb.	Arnicæ rhizoma	—	1 4	0 5	—
48	lb.	Arnicæ rhizomæ pulvis ..	—	—	0 6	0 1
15	lb.	Arsenic. alb. coml. S.1. P.II. (4)	2 0	0 7	0 3	—
11	lb.	Arsenic.alb.coml.plv. S.1.P.II.(4)	1 6	0 5	—	—
648	cwt.	Arsenic.alb.coml.plv. S.1.P.II.(4)	7 lb.	5 3	—	—
12	oz.	Arsenii bromidum S.1. P.I. (4)	—	—	—	0 4
36	oz.	Arsenii tri-iodidum S.1. P.I. (4)	—	—	—	0 9
20	lb.	Arsenii trioxid. S.1. P.II. (4)	—	—	0 3	—
21	lb.	Arsenii sulphid. flav. pulv. S.1. P.II. (4)	2 9	1 0	0 4	—
18	lb.	Arsenii sulphid. rub. pulv. S.1. P.II. (4)	2 3	0 10	0 4	—
42	oz.	Arseno-triferrin S.1. (5)	—	—	—	1 0
18	30	Arseno-trifer. tabs. gr. 5 S.1. (5)	doz.	1 3	—	—
66	lb.	Asafetida opt. (gtt.)	—	2 6	0 9	0 2
30	lb.	Asafetida coml.	—	1 2	0 5	—
63	lb.	Asafetidæ pulv.	—	—	0 8	0 2
72	lb.	Asbestos opt.	—	2 7	0 9	—
12	lb.	Asbestos coml.	1 6	0 6	0 2	—
78	oz.	Asparagin	—	—	11 4	1 9
9	lb.	Asphaltum	1 3	0 4	0 2	—
27	lb.	Asthma powder B.P.C.	—	1 0	0 4	—
72	oz.	Atophan .. .. ..℞ only	—	—	—	1 9
132	100	Atophan tablets gr. 7½ ..℞ only	doz.	2 1	—	—
132	100	Atoquinol tablets ..℞ only	doz.	2 1	—	—
48	dr.	Atropina S.1. (4)	per	gr.	0 3	—
42	dr.	Atropinæ sulphas ..S.1. (4)	per	gr.	0 3	—
78	lb.	Aurantii cortex Ang.	—	2 9	0 9	0 2
42	lb.	Aurantii cortex exot.	5 3	1 6	0 5	—
6	gr.	Auri bromidum	per	gr.	1 0	—
66	each	Auri chloridum (15 gr. tubes) ..	ea.	8 3	—	—
48	oz.	Auri chloridum sol. (2%) ..	—	—	6 6	—
		B				
26	lb.	Balsamum anisi P.L.F. ..	—	1 2	0 4	—
11	oz.	Balsamum Peruvianum ..	—	—	2 0	0 4
21	lb.	Balsamum sulphuris	3 6	1 0	0 4	—
6	oz.	Balsamum tolutanum	—	—	1 0	0 2
		Bandages—see page 30				
22	oz.	Barbitonum .. ..℞ only	—	—	3 3	0 6
23	oz.	Barbitonum solubile ..℞ only	—	—	3 5	0 7
21	lb.	Barii carb.pur.præc. S.1. P.II.(4)	2 9	0 10	0 3	—
10	lb.	Barii carb. coml. .. S.1. P.II. (4)	1 3	0 5	0 2	—
12	lb.	Barii chlori.pur. S.1. P.I. (4)	1 6	0 6	0 2	—
20	lb.	Barii hydrox. pur. ..S.1. P.I. (4)	2 6	0 9	0 3	—
20	lb.	Barii nit. pur. cryst. S.1. P.I. (4)	2 6	0 9	0 3	—
10	lb.	Barii nit. coml. S.1. P.I. (4)	1 3	0 5	0 2	—
24	lb.	Barii peroxid. anhyd. S.1. P.I. (4)	3 0	0 11	0 3	—
18	lb.	Barii sulphas B.P.	2 3	0 8	—	—
108	doz.	Barii sulphas puriss. pkd. ..	—	1 4	—	—
4	oz.	Barii sulphidum S.1 P.I. (4)	—	—	0 7	0 2
8	lb.	Bath powder P.L.F.	1 0	—	—	—
8	lb.	Battery solution P.L.F.	1 9	—	—	—
17	lb.	Bay rum (industrial) P.L.F. ..	2 0	0 7	0 3	—
81	doz.	Bay rum (indust.) pkd. ..	℥iij.	1 0	—	—
4.5	lb.	Bay salt	0 7	0 3	—	—
360	cwt.	Bay salt	7 lb.	2 9	14 lb.	5 0

Cost d.	per	Be—Bo	Selling Price 16 oz. s. d.	4 oz. s. d.	1 oz. s. d.	1 dr. s. d.
21	dr.	Beberinæ sulphas	—	—	—	3 1
51	lb.	Bellad. fol. Ang. S.I. (4)	—	—	0 7	—
69	lb.	Belladonna pulverata S.I. (5)	—	2 6	0 9	0 2
24	lb.	Belladonnæ rad. pulv. S.I. (4)	—	—	0 4	—
30	lb.	Benedict's reagent (qualit.)	4 3	1 4	—	—
5	oz.	Benzaldehydum pur.	—	—	0 9	0 2
33	dr.	Benzaminæ hydrochloridum	—	0 3	} per	4 10
33	dr.	Benzaminæ lactas	—	0 3	} gr.	4 10
42	dr.	Benzamin. base	—	—	—	6 4
15	lb.	Benzenum	1 9	0 6	0 2	—
30	oz.	Benzocaina P.I. (8)	—	—	—	0 8
51	lb.	Benzoinum Sumat.	—	2 0	0 7	0 1
54	lb.	Benzoini pulv.	6 9	2 0	0 7	0 1
4	pt.	Benzol coml.	—	0 8	0 3	—
7	oz.	Benzonaphthol	—	—	1 1	0 2
54	oz.	Benzosol	—	—	7 11	1 2
6	oz.	Benzyl benzoas	—	—	0 11	0 2
28	lb.	Berberidis pulvis	3 6	1 0	0 4	0 1
27	dr.	Berberinæ sulphas	—	—	—	4 0
33	oz.	Betainæ hydrochloridum	—	—	5 0	0 9
21	oz.	Betanaphthylis Sal	—	—	3 1	0 6
40	oz.	Betol	—	—	5 10	1 0
		"Bipp" (v. Past. bis. et iod.)				
30	lb.	Bird-lime	3 9	1 2	0 4	—
21	lb.	Bird-lime qty.	—	7-lb.	tins	18 3
126	lb.	Bisedia (Schacht) P.I. (13) *(Verify composition)*	—	4 0	1 0	0 2
		Bismuthum				
20	oz.	Bismuthi benzoas	—	—	3 0	0 6
26	oz.	Bismuthi betanaphthol.	—	—	3 9	0 7
114	lb.	Bismuthi carbonas	—	4 1	1 2	0 2
14	oz.	Bismuthi citras	—	—	2 0	0 4
21	oz.	Bismuthi et ammon. citras	—	—	3 1	0 6
18	oz.	Bismuthi hydroxidum	—	—	2 8	0 5
30	oz.	Bismuthi iodidum (oxy.)	—	—	4 5	0 8
26	oz.	Bismuthi lactas	—	—	3 9	0 7
10	oz.	Bismuthi nitras cryst.	—	—	1 6	0 3
10	oz.	Bismuthi oleas	—	—	1 6	0 3
22	oz.	Bismuthi oxidum	—	—	3 3	0 6
20	oz.	Bismuthi oxychloridum	—	—	2 11	0 5
21	oz.	Bismuthi oxychlor. puriss.	—	—	3 1	0 6
45	oz.	Bismuthi oxyiodogallas	—	—	6 9	1 0
66	oz.	Bismuthum precip.	—	—	—	1 5
12	oz.	Bismuthi salicylas	—	—	1 9	0 3
13	oz.	Bismuthi subgallas	—	—	1 11	0 4
102	lb.	Bismuthi subnitras	—	3 8	1 0	0 2
15	oz.	Bismuthi tannas	—	—	2 3	0 4
18	oz.	Bismuthi tartras solub.	—	—	2 8	0 5
25	oz.	Bismuthi tribromophen.	—	—	3 8	0 7
45	oz.	Bismuthi valerianas	—	—	6 9	1 0
80	lb.	Blue, Chin., pulv.	10 0	2 10	0 9	0 2
60	lb.	Blue, Pruss., pulv.	7 6	2 2	0 8	0 2
15	lb.	Boldo folia	2 0	0 7	0 2	—
8	lb.	Bole Armen.	1 0	0 4	0 1	—
32	lb.	Boraldehyde (D.F.)	1 6	bot.	2 6	bot.
16	lb.	Borax calcinatus	2 0	0 7	0 2	—
6.5	lb.	Borax cryst. (Howards)	1 0	0 4	0 1½	—
4.5	lb.	Borax coml. cryst.	0 7	0 2	0 1	—
6	lb.	Borax purificatus cryst.	0 9	0 3	0 1	—
6	lb.	Boracis purificati pulvis	0 9	0 3	0 1	—
—	—	Boracis purificati pulvis (pkd.)	—	0 6½	0 1½	—
5	lb.	Boracis coml. pulvis	0 8	0 3	0 1	—
360	cwt.	Boracis coml. pulvis	7 lb.	2 10	14 lb.	5 0
12	lb.	Bordeaux mixture P.L.F.	1 6	—	—	—
		Boric lint (see p. 31)				
		Boric wool (see p. 30)				
84	oz.	Bornyl valerianas	—	—	—	1 10

Cost d.	per	Bo—Ca	Selling Price 16 oz. s. d.	4 oz. s. d.	1 oz. s. d.	1 dr. s. d.
9	gm.	Borocaina S.I. (4)	grm.	1 0	—	—
12	tube	Borocain c̄ adren. tabs. S.I. (4)	tube	1 6	—	—
30	lb.	Borothymol	—	1 2	0 4	—
30	lb.	Boroglycerinum B.P.C.	3 9	1 1	0 4	0
16	10 gm	Brilliant green	—	—	—	1
174	lb.	Brilliantine, separable, P.L.F.	—	6 3	1 8	—
126	lb.	Brilliantine, separ. (isoprop.)	—	4 6	1 4	—
180	lb.	Brilliantine, inseparable, P.L.F.	—	6 5	1 9	—
90	lb.	Brilliantine, insepar. (isoprop.)	—	3 3	1 0	—
55	4 oz.	Bromidis unstd.	—	6 11	1 9	0
13	oz.	Bromoformum	—	—	—	0 1
6	oz.	Bromum	—	—	3 0	0
42	doz.	Bromum (2 c.c. tubes)	ea.	0 7	—	—
95	oz.	Bromural	—	—	—	2
39.5	20	Bromural tablets gr. 5	doz.	3 0	—	—
27	oz.	Brucina S.I. (4)	—	—	4 0	0
24	oz.	Brucinæ sulphas S.I. (4)	—	—	3 6	0
18	lb.	Bryoniæ albæ radix	2 3	0 8	0 3	—
45	lb.	Buchu	—	1 8	0 6	0
9	lb.	Burgundy mixture P.L.F.	1 2	—	—	—
15	oz.	Butyl-chloral hydras P.I. (8)	—	—	2 3	0
45	℥xx.	Bynin (A. & H.)	—	1 2	0 4	—
29	20	Butolan. tabs.	—	2 6	per	doz
		C				
12	oz.	Cadmii bromidum	—	—	1 9	0
21	oz.	Cadmii iodidum	—	—	3 1	0
11	oz.	Cadmii sulphide	—	—	1 8	0
17	oz.	Caffeina	—	—	2 6	0
12	oz.	Caffeinæ benzoas	—	—	1 9	0
12	oz.	Caffeinæ citras	—	—	1 9	0
46	lb.	Caffeinæ citras effervescens	—	1 8	0 6	—
27	oz.	Caffeinæ hydrobromidum	—	—	4 0	0
40	oz.	Caffeinæ iodidum	—	—	6 4	0 1
21	oz.	Caffeinæ salicylas	—	—	3 1	0
16	oz.	Caffeinæ sodio-benzoas	—	—	2 4	0
33	oz.	Caffeinæ sodio-iodidum	—	—	4 10	0
15	oz.	Caffeinæ sodio-salicylas	—	—	2 3	0
44	oz.	Caffeinæ valerianas	—	—	6 5	1
12	lb.	Calami aromatici radix	—	0 6	0 2	—
18	lb.	Calami aromatici rad. pulvis	2 3	0 9	0 3	—
30	lb.	Calamina artif. P.L.F.	3 9	1 2	0 4	0
26	lb.	Calamina præparata	3 3	1 0	0 4	—
		Calcium				
27	lb.	Calcii acetas	—	1 0	0 4	0
18	oz.	Calcii acetylsalicylas	—	—	2 8	0
7	oz.	Calcii bromidum exic.	—	—	1 1	0
6	lb.	Calcii carbonas	0 8	0 3	0 1	—
15	lb.	Calcii chloridum fusum	2 0	0 7	0 2	—
6	lb.	Calcii chloridum coml.	0 10	0 4	—	—
11	lb.	Calcii chloridum cryst.	1 5	0 6	0 2	—
13	lb.	Calcii chloridum gran.	1 9	0 7	0 2	—
9	oz.	Calcii citras	—	—	1 4	0
6	oz.	Calcii formas	—	—	0 9	0
7	oz.	Calcii gluconas	—	—	0 11	0
7	oz.	Calcii glycerophos.	—	—	1 1	0
96	oz.	Calcii guaiacol-sulphonas	—	—	14 0	2
11	lb.	Calcii hydroxid	1 5	0 6	0 2	—
6	oz.	Calcii hypophosphis	—	—	0 11	0
24	oz.	Calcii iodidum	—	—	3 6	0
26	lb.	Calcii lactas	3 3	0 11	0 3½	0
8	oz.	Calcii lactophosphas	—	—	1 2	0
3	oz.	Calcii oxalas	—	—	0 6	0
16	oz.	Calcii peroxidum	—	—	2 3	0
15	lb.	Calcii phosphas	3 9	1 1	0 4	—
8	lb.	Calcii phosphas coml.	1 0	0 4	0 2	—
12	lb.	Calcii phosphatis acidi pulvis	1 6	0 6	0 2	—

Cost d.	Cost per	Ca Calcium—(cont.)	Selling Price 16 oz. s. d.	4 oz. s. d.	1 oz. s. d.	1 dr. s. d.
54	lb.	Calcii phosphas di-acidus ..	—	1 10	0 7	0 1
36	lb.	Calcii phosph. mono-acid. ..	—	1 4	0 5	0 1
24	lb.	Calcii saccharas	3 0	0 11	0 3	—
5	lb.	Calcii sulphas	0 7	0 3	—	—
6	oz.	Calcii sulphocarbolas	—	—	0 9	0 2
4	lb.	Calcii superphosphas coml. ..	0 6	0 2	—	—
10	cwt.	Calcii superphosphas coml. ..	7 lb.	1 9	14 lb.	3 4
3	lb.	Calx	1 8	0 6	0 2	—
4	lb.	Calx chlorinata	0 10	0 3	0 1	—
4	oz.	Calx sulphurata	—	—	0 7	0 1
8	lb.	Calendulæ flores	—	1 9	0 6	0 1
		Calf lymph (v. Lymph) ..				
3	lb.	Calumbæ radix	1 8	0 7	0 2	—
5	lb.	Calumbæ radicis pulvis ..	1 11	0 8	0 3	—
8	oz.	Cambogia	—	—	1 2	0 2
9	oz.	Cambogiæ pulvis	—	—	1 4	0 3
7	lb.	Camphora (flores)	7 6	2 2	0 7	0 1
4	lb.	Camphora (1-oz. tab.)	—	—	0 8	—
6	lb.	Camphora (½-oz. tab.)	—	—	0 9	—
6	oz.	Camphora monobromata ..	—	—	2 4	0 5
5	lb.	Camphoræ synthet. pulv. ..	—	1 8	0 6	0 1
8	5	Campolon, 2 c.c.	each	1 9	—	—
0	lb.	Canary seed	1 3	0 5	—	—
0	lb.	Canellæ cortex	—	1 1	0 4	—
6	lb.	Canellæ corticis pulvis	—	1 4	0 5	0 1
8	oz.	Cannabinæ tannas ..S.I. (4)	—	—	11 4	1 8
.5	gr.	Cantharidinum .. ..S.I. (4)	—	—	—	1 0
4	lb.	Cantharis Chinensis ..S.I. (4)	—	2 0	0 7	—
2	lb.	Cantharis Chin. pulv. ..S.I. (4)	9 0	2 7	0 9	0 2
6	lb.	Cantharis Russ. .. ..S.I. (4)	—	5 7	1 7	—
4	lb.	Caoutchouc	—	3 0	1 0	—
6	box	Caprokol caps.	per	box	7 0	—
0	lb.	Capsici fructus	2 6	0 9	0 3	—
2	lb.	Capsici fructus pulvis sec. ..	2 9	0 10	0 3	—
1	oz.	Capsicin.	—	—	—	0 6
4	lb.	Carbo animalis gran.	1 9	0 6	0 2	—
1	lb.	Carbonis animalis pulvis ..	1 4	0 5	0 2	—
6	lb.	Carbo ligni	0 9	0 2½	0 1	—
.5	lb.	Carbonis ligni pulvis levigatus..	1 3	0 4½	0 1½	—
5	lb.	Carbonis ligni salicis pulvis ..	1 10	0 6	0 2	—
7	lb.	Carbon disulphidum	5 3	1 7	0 5	0 1
5	lb.	Carbon disulphidum coml. ..	3 0	1 0	0 4	—
8	lb.	Carbon tetrachloridum ..	6 0	1 10	0 7	0 1
1	oz.	Carbromalum	—	—	7 5	1 1
0	lb.	Cardamomi sem. pulv. dec. ..	—	4 3	1 2	0 2
2	oz.	Carminum opt.	—	—	6 4	0 11
3	oz.	Carminum sec.	—	—	4 10	0 9
	lb.	Carron oil P.L.F.	1 10	0 7	0 2	—
	lb.	Carum	1 7	0 7	0 2	—
	lb.	Carum pulvis	2 0	0 7	0 2	—
	lb.	Carum pulvis (coarse)	1 9	0 6	—	—
	lb.	Caryophyllum opt.	—	1 2	0 4	—
	lb.	Caryophyllum sec.	3 0	0 11	0 3	—
	lb.	Caryophylli pulvis sec.	3 0	0 11	0 3	—
	16 oz.	Cascara evacuant (P.D.) ..	15 9	4 6	1 4	0 3
	lb.	Cascarilla	—	3 8	1 0	0 2
	lb.	Caseinum (solub.)	3 0	1 0	0 4	0 1
	lb.	Caseinum album lev.	5 3	1 7	0 5	0 1
	lb.	Caseinum glycerophos. B.P.C...	4 6	1 4	0 5	—
	lb.	Cassiæ corticis pulvis	2 0	0 7	0 2	—
	lb.	Cassiæ fructus	—	0 7	0 2	—
	lb.	Cassiæ pulpa	—	1 6	0 6	—
	lb.	Cataplasma kaolini	1 3	0 6	—	—
	lb.	Catechu	2 7	0 10	0 3	—
	lb.	Catechu pulvis	3 3	1 0	0 4	—
	lb.	Catechu nigrum	1 9	0 7	0 2	—

Cost d.	Cost per	Ca—Co	Selling Price 16 oz. s. d.	4 oz. s. d.	1 oz. s. d.	1 dr. s. d.
20	lb.	Catechu nigri pulvis	2 6	0 9	0 3	—
28	oz.	Caulophyllinum	—	—	3 6	0 8
32	lb.	Cera alba in massa	4 0	1 2	0 4	—
34	lb.	Cera alba in placentis	4 3	1 3	0 4	—
42	lb.	Cera carnauba (grey)	5 3	1 6	0 5	—
54	lb.	Cera flava Ang.	6 9	2 0	0 7	—
32	lb.	Cera flava exot.	4 0	1 1	0 4	—
36	lb.	Cera flava exot. .. (1-oz. tab.)	4 6	1 3	0 4	—
12	lb.	Cera Japonica	1 6	0 6	0 2	—
33	lb.	Ceratum calaminæ	4 2	1 3	0 5	—
16	lb.	Ceresina coml. alba	2 0	0 7	0 2	—
15	lb.	Ceresina coml. flava	1 11	0 7	0 2	—
4	oz.	Cerii oxalas	—	—	0 7	0 1
28	lb.	Cetaceum	3 3	1 0	0 4	—
36	lb.	Cetacei pulvis	4 3	1 3	0 4	—
16	lb.	Cetraria Islandica	2 0	0 7	0 2	—
		Charta epispast. (11 in. × 8 in.)	each	1 3	—	—
48	lb.	Chilblain lotion P.L.F. ..	—	—	0 8	—
63	lb.	Chilblain paint P.L.F.	—	—	0 9	—
42	oz.	Chinosol	—	—	—	1 0
19	lb.	Chirata incisa	2 6	0 9	0 3	—
10	oz.	Chloral camph. B.P.C. ..P.I. (9)	—	—	—	0 3
20	oz.	Chloral formamidum ..P.I. (8)	—	—	2 11	0 5
7	oz.	Chloral hydras .. . P.I. (8)	—	—	1 1	0 2
7	oz.	Chloramina	—	—	1 1	0 2
126	oz.	Chloralose	—	—	—	2 8
24	oz.	Chlorbutol	—	—	—	0 6
66	oz.	Chloretone (P.D.)	—	—	—	1 5
123	doz.	Chloretone Inhalant, 10 c.c. ..	each	1 3	—	—
		Chlorodynum (v. Tinct. chlor. et morph. 1885)				
45	lb.	Chloroformum .. ..P.I. (8)	—	2 5	0 9	—
120	lb.	Chlorof. aconiti B.P.C. S.I. (5)	—	6 5	1 10	0 4
120	lb.	Chlorof. bellad. B.P.C. S.I. (5)	—	7 0	2 0	0 4
102	lb.	Chlorof. camph. B.P.C. P.I. (9)	—	—	1 9	0 4
24	oz.	Chlorophyllum (oil-sol.) ..	—	—	3 6	0 6
24	oz.	Chlorophyllum (spirit-sol.) ..	—	—	4 1	0 7
60	oz.	Cholesterol	—	—	8 9	1 3
27	lb.	Chondrus crispus elect. ..	3 5	1 0	0 4	—
6	oz.	Chromii trioxid	—	—	0 11	0 2
9	oz.	Chromii trioxid pur.	—	—	1 4	0 3
19	oz.	Chrysarobinum	—	—	2 10	0 5
10	oz.	Chrysoidin	—	—	1 6	0 3
13	gm.	Cignolin	—	0 3	per	grain
16	lb.	Cimicifugæ rhizoma	—	0 8	0 3	0 1
24	lb.	Cimicifug. rhizomæ pulvis ..	—	0 11	0 4	0 1
54	lb.	Cinchonæ calisayæ cort. pulvis	—	2 0	0 7	0 1
51	lb.	Cinchonæ pallid. cort. pulvis ..	—	2 0	0 7	0 1
45	lb.	Cinchonæ succirub. cortex ..	—	1 8	0 6	0 1
30	lb.	Cinchonæ succirub. cort. parv.	—	1 1	0 4	0 1
32	lb.	Cinchonæ succirub. cort. pulvis	—	1 2	0 4	0 1
87	oz.	Cinchonidina	—	—	—	1 10
54	oz.	Cinchonidinæ hydrochloridum	—	—	—	1 2
57	oz.	Cinchonidinæ sulphas	—	—	—	1 3
54	oz.	Cinchonina	—	—	—	1 2
48	oz.	Cinchoninæ hydrochloridum ..	—	—	—	1 0
42	oz.	Cinchoninæ sulphas	—	—	—	0 11
27	oz.	Cinchophenum	—	—	4 0	0 7
10	oz.	Cinnamic aldehyde	—	—	1 6	0 3
42	lb.	Cinnamomi cortex opt. ..	5 3	1 6	0 6	—
33	lb.	Cinnamomi cortex sec. ..	4 2	1 3	0 5	—
24	lb.	Cinnamomi cortex parv. ..	3 0	0 11	0 4	—
30	lb.	Cinnamomi cort. pulvis opt. ..	3 9	1 1	0 4	0 1
67	oz.	Citrarin	—	—	—	1 8
9	oz.	Cobalti chloridum	—	—	1 4	0 3
7	oz.	Cobalti nitras	—	—	1 1	0 2
96	dr.	Cocaina .. .. .. D.D.	per	gr.	0 5	14 0
90	dr.	Cocainæ hydrochlor. .. D.D.	per	gr.	0 5	13 0

Cost d.	Cost per	Co	Selling Price 16 oz. s. d.	4 oz. s. d.	1 oz. s. d.	1 dr. s. d.
90	dr.	Cocainæ nitras .. .. D.D.	per	gr.	0 5	13 0
90	dr.	Cocainæ salicylas .. D.D.	per	gr.	0 5	13 0
44	100cc	Cocaine eye-drops (factory) D.D.	℥ss.	1 8	—	—
36	lb.	Coccus (silver grain)	4 6	1 4	0 4	0 1
39	lb.	Cocci pulvis	5 0	1 5	0 5	0 1
28	lb.	Cocculi indici pulvis S.I. (4)	3 0	1 0	0 4	—
26	lb.	Coconut stearin	3 3	1 0	0 4	—
72	dr.	Codeina .. .. S.I. (4)	per	gr.	0 3	10 9
66	dr.	Codeinæ phosphas S.I. (4)	per	gr.	0 3	9 0
60	dr.	Codeinæ sulphas S.I. (4)	per	gr.	0 3	10 0
255	oz.	Codeonal .. .. .. ℞ only	—	—	—	6 0
29	10	Codeonal tablets, 2½ gr. ℞ only	doz.	4 4	—	—
22	lb.	Colch.corm. exot. pv.(20) P.I.(8)	—	0 10	0 3	—
36	lb.	Colch. sem. pulvis P.I. (8)	—	1 4	0 5	0 1
15	gr.	Colchicina .. S.I. (4)	per	gr.	2 3	—
15	gr.	Colchicinæ salicylas S.I. (4)	per	gr.	2 3	—
		Collodia				
33	lb.	Collodium flexile	—	1 3	0 5	0 1
42	lb.	Collodium acetonum B.P.C. ..	—	1 6	0 6	0 1
14	oz.	Collod. anodyn. B.P.C. .. S.I. (5)	—	—	2 0	0 4
10	oz.	Collod. bellad. B.P.C. .. S.I. (5)	—	—	1 6	0 3
50	lb.	Collod. salicyl. B.P.C. ..	—	1 10	0 7	0 1
120	lb.	Collod. sal. co. B.P.C. .. P.I. (9)	—	—	1 3	0 3
102	lb.	Collodium stypticum B.P.C. ..	—	—	1 0	0 2
18	oz.	Collodium vesicans .. S.I. (5)	—	—	2 8	0 6
36	℥iv.	Collosol argent. (Crookes) ..	—	4 0	1 6	0 3
54	℥iv.	Collosolarsen. (Crookes) S.I.P.I.(4)	—	6 0	1 9	0 3
54	℥iv.	Collosol bism. (Crookes) ..	—	6 0	1 9	0 3
41	℥iv.	Collosol hydr. (Crookes) ..	—	4 6	1 4	0 3
50	℥iij.	Collosol hydrarg. et sulphur. (Crookes)	—	5 6	1 6	0 3
22.5	℥iv.	Collosol iodine (Crookes) ..	—	2 6	0 9	0 2
45	℥iv.	Collosol iodine in oil	—	5 0	1 6	0 3
45	℥j.	Collosol manganese (inj.) ..	—	—	5 0	0 9
36	℥iv.	Collosol quinine	—	4 0	1 2	0 2
31.5	℥viij.	Collosol sulphur	—	2 0	0 6	0 1
78	lb.	Colocynthidis pulpa	—	2 9	0 9	0 2
78	lb.	Colocynthidis pulpæ pulvis ..	—	2 9	0 9	0 2
35	4 oz.	Colofine (Oppenheimer) ..	—	4 4	1 2	0 3
11	lb.	Colophonii pulv.	1 6	0 6	0 2	—
8	lb.	Colophonium	1 0	0 4	0 2	—
27	lb.	Composition essence	—	1 0	0 4	—
24	lb.	Composition powder P.L.F. ..	—	0 11	0 3	—
61	50	Compral tablets .. ℞ only	doz.	2 0	—	—
30	lb.	Confectio guaiaci co. B.P.C. ..	4 0	1 2	0 4	0 1
30	lb.	Confectio paraffini B.P.C. ..	3 9	1 2	0 4	—
30	lb.	Confectio petrolei	3 9	1 2	0 4	—
33	lb.	Confectio piperis	—	1 3	0 4	0 1
39	lb.	Confectio rosæ gallic.	—	1 3	0 5	—
18	lb.	Confectio sennæ	2 4	0 9	0 3	—
33	lb.	Confectio sennæ et sulph. B.P.C.	4 2	1 3	0 4	—
38	lb.	Confectio sulphuris	5 0	1 6	0 5	0 1
54	oz.	Congo Red	—	—	—	1 2
14	gr.	Coniina .. .. .. S.I. (4)	per	gr.	1 2	—
8	gr.	Coniinæ hydrobrom. .. S.I. (4)	per	gr.	1 2	—
39	lb.	Copaiba	5 0	1 5	0 6	0 1
9	oz.	Copaibæ resina	—	—	1 4	0 3
32	lb.	Copal elect.	4 3	1 3	0 5	—
30	lb.	Copal pulv.	3 9	1 4	0 5	—
36	each	Coramine 1·7c.c., 5 amps. ..	—	4 0	per	box
10	lb.	Coriandrum	1 3	0 5	0 2	—
13	lb.	Coriand. pulvis	1 7	0 6	0 2	—
11	lb.	Coriand. pulvis (crs.)	1 4	0 5	0 2	—
		Corn solvent (v. Collod. callos.)				
110	lb.	Coster's paste	—	—	0 8	0 2
54	dr.	Cotarninæ hydrochlor. .. S.I. (4)	per	gr.	2 2	8 4
54	dr.	Cotarninæ phthalas .. S.I. (4)	per	gr.	2 2	8 4

Cost d.	Cost per	Co—De	Selling Price 16 oz. s. d.	4 oz. s. d.	1 oz. s. d.	1 dr. s.
96	dr.	Cotoinum	per	gr.	0 3	—
15	oz.	Coumarinum	—	—	2 4	0
66	lb.	Creme d'amandes, scented ..	8 6	2 5	0 8	—
54	lb.	Creme d'amandes, unscented ..	6 9	2 0	0 7	—
54	lb.	Cremor bismuthi	8 6	2 10	0 9	—
44	lb.	Cremor frigidum P.L.F. ..	—	1 7	0 6	—
24	lb.	Cremor frigidum P.L.F. ..	—	1 0	0 4	—
24	lb.	Crem. frig. "American" P.L.F.	—	1 0	0 4	—
22	lb.	Crem. frigid. "theatrical" P.L.F.	2 9	0 10	—	—
39	lb.	Crem. zinci B.P.C.	4 9	1 5	0 5	—
15	oz.	Creosoti carbonas	—	—	2 2	0
42	lb.	Creosotum .. .. P.I. (8)	—	1 7	0 6	0
18	lb.	Cresol .. .. .. P.I. (8)	2 3	0 8	0 3	—
21	lb.	Creta cum camphora 12½% ..	2 8	0 10	0 3	—
15	lb.	Creta c. camph. 10%	2 0	0 7	0 3	—
18	lb.	Creta Gallica (tab.)	2 3	0 8	0 3	—
360	cwt	Cretæ Gall. pulvis	7 lb.	2 9	14 lb.	5
6	lb.	Cretæ Gall. pulvis	0 9	0 3	0 1	—
7	lb.	Cretæ Gall. pulvis subtil. ..	0 10	0 3	0 1	—
6	lb.	Creta præparata	0 9	0 3	0 1	—
8	lb.	Creta præparata rubra	1 0	0 4	0 2	—
72	oz.	Crocus Valent.	—	—	—	1
78	oz.	Crocus Valent. pulv.	—	—	—	1
54	lb.	Croup embrocation P.L.F. ..	6 9	2 0	0 7	—
36	10 gm	Cryogenine	—	—	—	2
18	10	Cryogenine tablets gr. 4 ..	doz.	2 9	—	—
20	oz.	Crystal violet (medicinal) ..	—	—	3 0	0
42	lb.	Cubebæ fructus	—	1 6	0 6	—
51	lb.	Cubebæ fructus pulvis	—	2 0	0 7	0
26	lb.	Cucumber cream	—	1 0	0 4	—
54	lb.	Cucumber paste	6 0	1 9	0 6	—
192	lb.	Cucumber pomade	—	6 10	2 0	—
22	lb.	Cudbear	—	0 10	0 3	—
15	lb.	Cumini fructus	2 0	0 7	0 2	—
21	lb.	Cumini fructus pulvis	2 9	0 10	0 3	—
18	lb.	Cumini fructus pulvis (crs.) ..	2 4	0 8	0 3	—
22	lb.	Cupri ammon. sulph.	2 9	0 10	0 3	—
54	lb.	Cupri carbonas pur.	—	2 0	0 7	—
36	lb.	Cupri chloridum pur.	4 6	1 4	0 5	—
39	lb.	Cupri nitras	5 0	1 5	0 5	—
46	lb.	Cupri oleas	5 9	1 8	0 6	0
5	oz.	Cupri oxidum pur.	—	—	0 10	0
24	lb.	Cupri oxidum coml.	2 8	0 9	0 3	—
48	lb.	Cupri oxyacet. pulv. (ærugo) ..	6 0	1 9	0 6	—
15	lb.	Cupri sulphas	2 0	0 7	0 2	—
6	lb.	Cupri sulphas coml. opt. ..	0 9	0 3	0 1	—
609	cwt.	Cupri sulphas coml.	7 lb.	4 8	14 lb.	8
9	lb.	Cupri sulphas coml. pulvis ..	1 2	0 4	—	—
30	lb.	Cupri sulphas exsiccatus ..	3 9	1 1	0 4	—
60	lb.	Cuprum (filings)	—	2 2	0 8	—
54	lb.	Cuprum (foil)	—	2 0	0 7	—
42	lb.	Cuprum (turnings)	5 3	1 6	0 5	0
10	lb.	Curcumæ rhizoma	1 3	0 5	0 2	—
12	lb.	Curcumæ rhizomæ pulvis ..	1 6	0 6	0 2	—
10	lb.	Curcumæ rhizomæ pulvis (crs.)	1 3	0 5	0 2	—
36	lb.	Currie powder opt. P.L.F. ..	4 6	1 4	0 5	—
22	lb.	Currie powder sec. P.L.F. ..	2 9	0 10	0 3	—
60	lb.	Cydoniæ semina	—	2 2	0 8	—
		D				
30	lb.	Dale's plaster P.L.F. .. S.I. (6)	—	1 1	0 4	—
42	lb.	Damar gummi	5 3	1 7	0 5	—
36	lb.	Daturæ tatulæ pulvis .. S.I. (5)	—	1 4	0 5	0 1
24	gr.	Daturina .. .. S.I. (4)	per	gr.	3 6	—
24	gr.	Daturinæ sulphas .. S.I. (4)	per	gr.	3 6	—
36	lb.	Dec. agropyri conc. 1 to 7 ..	—	1 4	0 6	0 1
12	lb.	Dec. agropyri recens	1 6	0 6	0 2	—
24	lb.	Dec. aloes co.	—	0 11	0 3	—

Cost d.	per	De—Ea	16 oz. s. d.	4 oz. s. d.	1 oz. s. d.	1 dr. s. d.
33	lb.	Dec. aloes co. conc. 1 to 3 ..	—	1 3	0 4	0 1
30	lb.	Dec. aloes co. recens	3 9	1 2	0 4	—
39	lb.	Dec. cinch. conc. 1 to 7 ..	—	1 6	0 6	0 1
36	lb.	Dec. cinchonæ flav. c. 1 to 7 ..	—	1 4	0 5	0 1
54	lb.	Dec. cuspariæ conc. 1 to 7 ..	—	2 0	0 7	0 1
44	lb.	Dec. dulcamar. conc. 1 to 7 ..	—	1 7	0 6	0 1
24	lb.	Dec. gossypii rad. cort. rec. ..	3 0	1 0	0 3	—
51	lb.	Dec. granati cort. conc. 1 to 7..	—	2 0	0 7	0 1
30	lb.	Dec. hæmat. conc. 1 to 7 ..	—	1 2	0 4	0 1
14	lb.	Dec. hæmatoxyli recens ..	1 9	0 7	0 2	—
54	lb.	Dec. hemidesmi conc. 1 to 7 ..	—	2 1	0 8	0 2
42	lb.	Dec. mezerei conc. 1 to 7 ..	—	1 7	0 6	0 1
30	lb.	Dec. papaveris conc. 1 to 7 P.I. (10)	—	1 2	0 5	0 1
45	lb.	Dec. papav. et anth. conc. P.I. (10)	—	1 8	0 6	0 1
48	lb.	Dec. pareiræ conc. 1 to 7 ..	—	1 9	0 6	0 1
36	lb.	Dec. quercus conc. 1 to 7 ..	—	1 4	0 5	0 1
66	lb.	Dec. sarsæ Jam. (simp.) conc. 1 to 7	—	2 5	0 9	0 2
60	lb.	Dec. sarsæ co. conc. 1 to 7 ..	—	2 4	0 8	0 2
30	lb.	Dec. scoparii conc. 1 to 7 ..	—	1 1	0 4	0 1
38	lb.	Dec. senegæ conc. 1 to 7 ..	—	1 5	0 5	0 1
42	lb.	Dec. taraxaci conc. 1 to 7 ..	—	1 8	0 6	0 1
57	lb.	Dec. ulmi conc. B.P.C. 1 to 7 ..	—	2 1	0 7	0 1
32	lb.	Dec. uvæ ursi conc. 1 to 7 ..	—	1 2	0 4	0 1
31	oz.	Dermatol	—	—	4 7	0 8
39	lb.	Derris pulv.	5 0	1 5	0 5	—
40	30	Devegan tabs. .. .. S.I. (6)	doz.	1 6	—	—
10	lb.	Devonshire oils P.L.F. ..	—	0 5	0 2	—
7	lb.	Dextrin. alb.	0 11	0 4	0 2	—
7	lb.	Dextrin. flav.	0 11	0 4	0 2	—
14	lb.	Dextrosum	1 9	0 7	0 2	—
	12	Dial tablets, orig. tube ℞ only	tube	2 0	—	—
96	100	Dial tablets .. .. ℞ only	doz.	1 6	—	—
14	oz.	Diamidophenol. hydrochloridum	—	—	1 9	0 3
93	dr.	Diamorphinæ hydrochl. D.D.	per	gr.	0 4	—
15	lb.	Diapente P.L.F.	2 0	0 7	0 2	—
24	oz.	Diastasum	—	—	3 0	0 7
48	lb.	Dicalcium phosphate (P.D.) ..	6 0	2 0	—	—
36	oz.	Dichloramin.—T.	—	—	5 3	0 9
24	lb.	Dichlorobenzene ortho. ..	—	1 4	0 5	—
24	lb.	Dichlorobenzene para	—	1 4	0 5	—
38	15c.c.	Digalen .. .. S.I. (6)	—	—	8 6	1 4
24	25	Digifoline tablets S.I. (6)	doz.	1 6	—	—
23	oz.	Digifortis (P.D.) S.I. (6)	—	—	—	0 7
15	gr. 15	Digipuratum .. S.I. (6)	per	gr.	0 2	—
21	10c.c.	Digipuratum liq. S.I. (6)	—	—	—	1 4
24	12	Digipuratum tablets S.I. (6)	doz.	3 0	—	—
7	gr.	Digitalinum amorph. S.I. (6)	per	gr.	1 1	—
8	gr.	Digitalinum cryst. S.I. (4)	per	gr.	15 10	—
24	40	Digitaline gran. (Nativ.) S.I. (6)	doz.	0 11	—	—
2	lb.	Digitalis folia Ang. S.I. (4)	—	1 6	0 6	0 1
7	lb.	Digitalis pulverata S.I. (5)	—	—	0 8	0 2
9	gr.	Digitonin .. P.I. (10)	—	—	—	—
4	100	Dimol pulverettes	doz.	1 0	—	—
1	4 oz.	Dimol syrup	—	—	1 4	0 3
0	gm.	Dioninum .. S.I. (4)	per	gr.	0 4	—
3	oz.	Diuretin	—	—	—	1 0
2	20	Diuretin tablets gr. 7½	doz.	1 8	—	—
8	oz.	Dolichos pubes	—	—	7 6	1 2
4	oz.	Dormigene pulv. (A. & H.) ..	—	—	—	2 7
2	gr.	Duboisinæ sulphas S.I. (4)	per	gr.	1 10	—
1	lb.	Dulcamara	—	0 9	0 3	—
8	lb.	Dusting powder P.L.F. ..	—	1 3	0 4	—
		E				
0	lb.	Eau de Cologne opt. P.L.F. ..	34 6	10 0	2 10	0 6
2	lb.	Eau de Cologne opt. (isoprop.)	—	5 9	1 9	0 4

Cost d.	per	Ea—El	16 oz. s. d.	4 oz. s. d.	1 oz. s. d.	1 dr. s. d.
216	lb.	Eau de Cologne sec.	23 0	6 0	1 9	0 5
		Eau de Cologne sec. pkd. ..	—	8 6	℥ij.	2 6
126	lb.	Eau de Cologne sec. (isoprop.)	—	4 6	1 4	0 3
14	oz.	Eikonogen	—	—	1 9	0 4
6	gr.	Elaterinum .. P.I. (8)	per	gr.	1 0	—
72	dr.	Elaterium Ang. .. P.I. (8)	per	gr.	0 3	—
24	lb.	Elemi	—	1 0	0 4	—
		Elixir				
54	lb.	Elixir aletridis B.P.C.	—	2 0	0 7	0 1
90	lb.	Elixir aromaticum B.P.C. ..	—	3 6	1 0	0 2
96	lb.	Elixir aurantii B.P.C.	—	3 6	1 0	0 2
99	lb.	*Elixir aurantii comp.* B.P.C. ..	—	3 6	1 0	0 2
54	lb.	Elixir benzyl benzoatis	—	2 2	0 7	—
54	lb.	Elixir bismuthi B.P.C.	—	2 3	0 8	—
48	lb.	Elixir bismuth sal. B.D.H. ..	—	2 2	0 8	—
48	lb.	Elixir bromoformi B.P.C. ..	—	2 0	0 7	—
72	lb.	Elixir camphoræ monobromatæ	—	2 10	0 9	—
123	lb.	Elixir cascaræ et euonymi B.P.C.	—	5 6	1 5	—
80	lb.	Elixir cascaræ sag. P.L.F. ..	10 0	2 10	0 10	—
32	lb.	Elixir cascaræ sag.	—	1 7	0 6	—
75	lb.	Elixir cinchonæ B.P.C. ..	—	2 10	0 9	0 2
54	lb.	Elixir cocæ B.P.C. P.I. (13)	—	2 0	0 7	—
57	lb.	Elixir codein. co. P.I. (13)	—	2 8	0 8	—
57	lb.	Elixir codein. co. B.D.H. P.I. (13)	—	2 2	0 8	—
48	lb.	Elixir diamorph. et pini co. D.D.	—	2 0	0 8	—
45	lb.	Elixir diamor. et ter. B.P.C. D.D.	—	1 9	0 6	0 1
72	lb.	Elixir diamorph. et terp. c. apomorph. B.P.C. S.I. (5)	—	2 9	0 10	—
68	16 oz.	Elixir enzymes (Armour) ..	—	2 2	0 7	0 1
54	lb.	Elixir ephedrin	—	2 0	0 7	—
54	lb.	Elix. ethylmorph. et terp. P.I. (3)	—	2 3	0 9	—
102	lb.	Elixir ferri, quin. et strych. phos. B.P.C. .. P.I. (13)	—	4 6	1 4	—
45	lb.	Elixir formatum B.P.C. ..	—	1 9	0 6	0 1
56	lb.	Elixir formatum co. P.I. (13)	—	2 2	0 8	0 2
66	lb.	Elixir glusidi B.P.C.	—	2 6	0 9	—
92	lb.	Elixir guaiacol. co.	—	3 3	0 11	—
32	lb.	Elixir idæi co.	—	1 10	0 6	—
30	lb.	Elixir ipecacuanhæ B.P.C. ..	—	1 2	0 4	0 1
30	lb.	Elixir kolæ B.P.C.	—	1 2	0 4	0 1
19	4 oz.	Elixir lactated pepsin (Armour)	—	2 9	0 9	0 2
70	16 oz.	Elixir lactopeptin.	—	2 3	0 8	0 2
63	lb.	Elixir lecithin B.P.C.	—	2 4	0 8	—
72	lb.	Elixir lecithini compositum ..	—	2 8	0 10	0 2
66	lb.	Elixir luminal .. ℞ only	—	2 6	0 10	—
93	lb.	Elixir papaini B.P.C.	—	3 5	1 0	—
72	lb.	Elixir pepsini B.P.C.	—	2 7	0 9	0 2
68	lb.	Elixir pepsini co. P.L.F. ..	—	2 5	0 8	—
57	lb.	Elixir pepsini et bism. co. B.P.C.	—	2 2	0 8	—
54	lb.	Elixir peptolacticum	—	2 3	0 8	—
66	lb.	Elixir phosphori B.P.C. ..	—	2 5	0 8	0 2
90	lb.	Elixir phosphori co. B.P.C. ..	—	3 3	1 0	—
54	lb.	Elixir pini compositum D.D.	—	2 3	0 9	—
30	lb.	Elixir pruni virg.	—	1 4	0 6	—
90	lb.	Elixir quininæ ammon. B.P.C.	—	3 3	0 11	0 2
78	lb.	Elixir quininæ amm. co. B.P.C.	—	2 10	0 10	—
52	lb.	Elixir rhei B.P.C.	—	2 2	0 7	0 2
32	lb.	Elixir rubi idæi	—	1 9	0 6	—
33	lb.	Elixir sennæ fructus B.P.C. ..	—	1 3	0 5	—
30	lb.	Elixir simplex B.P.C.	—	1 6	0 5	0 1
72	16 oz.	Elixir terpheroini co. (D.F.) D.D.	—	3 0	0 10	—
108	16 oz.	Elixir terpheroini (Squire) D.D.	—	3 6	1 0	0 2
78	lb.	Elixir terpheroini co. .. D.D.	—	3 6	1 0	—
96	lb.	Elixir viburn. prunif. B.P.C. ..	—	3 5	1 0	0 2
105	lb.	Elixir viburn. prun. co. B.P.C.	—	3 11	1 1	0 2

Cost d.	Cost per	Em—Et	Selling Price 16 oz. s. d.	4 oz. s. d.	1 oz. s. d.	1 dr. s. d.
7	gr.	Emetina S.1. (4)	per	gr.	1 2	—
7	gr.	Emetin. period S.1. (4)	per	gr.	1 1	—
6	gr.	Emetin. bismuthi iod. ..S.1. (4)	per	gr.	0 11	—
6	gr.	Emetinæ hydrochlor. ..S.1. (4)	per	gr.	0 11	—
36	lb.	Emuls. acriflavinæ	4 6	1 4	—	—
84	lb.	Emulsio benzyl benzoate ..	—	3 4	1 0	—
48	lb.	Emulsio bismuth et magnesiæ	—	2 2	0 8	—
15	lb.	Emulsio chloroformi B.P.C. ..	—	—	0 3	0 1
60	lb.	Emuls. iodoformi 10 per cent.	—	3 0	0 10	—
48	lb.	Emuls. menth. pip. B.P.C. ..	—	1 9	0 6	—
18	lb.	Emuls. olei morrhuæ B.P.C. ..	2 3	0 8	0 3	—
		Emuls. ol. morrh. 50% pkd. ..	℥ vj.	1 9	℥ xij.	3 0
27	lb.	Emuls. ol. morrh.c.hypoph.B.P.C.	3 6	1 0	—	—
51	lb.	Emuls. ol. morrh. pancr. B P.C.	6 6	2 0	0 7	—
56	lb.	Emuls. ol. morrh. pancr. et malti B.P.C.	7 2	2 3	0 7	—
28	lb.	Emuls. ol. olivæ B.P.C. ..	3 10	1 2	—	—
66	lb.	Emuls. ol. olivæ co. B.P.C. ..	9 0	2 7	—	—
21	lb.	Emuls. petrolei (agar)	2 6	0 9	—	—
18	lb.	Emuls. petrolei c. agar N.I.F.	2 4	0 9	0 3	—
18	lb.	Emuls. petr. agar phenolphthal. N.I.F...	2 4	0 9	0 3	—
21	lb.	Emuls. petr. phenolphthal.(agar)	2 6	0 9	—	—
18	lb.	Emuls. petr. c. hypoph. B.P.C.	2 0	0 7	0 2	—
144	doz.	Emuls. petrolei .. .. pkd.	—	1 6	℥ viij.	1 9
24	dr.	Ephedrina alk. .. ..P.I. (8)	per	gr.	0 2	3 6
16	dr.	Ephedrinæ hydrochlor...P.I. (8)	per	gr.	0 2	2 4
18	dr.	Ephedrine sulphas ..P.I. (8)	per	gr.	0 2	2 8
15	oz.	Ergota preparata ..S.1. (6)	—	—	2 3	0 4
108	.1gm.	Ergotoxin ethanesulph. S.1. (4)	0 4	for	0.1	gm.
60	.1gm.	Ergotoxin phosph. ..S.1. (4)	0 3	for	0.1	gm.
90	4 oz.	Emutin S.1. (6)	—	—	2 10	0 6
51	dr.	Erythrityl tet. dil. ..P.I (9)	per	gr.	0 3	—
102	dr.	Erythrol tetranitras ..P.I. (8)	per	gr.	0 5	—
21	lb.	Esbachs solution	—	0 10	0 3	—
42	oz.	Ess. ambræ grisem	—	—	6 2	1 0
24	oz.	Ess. amygdalæ 1 in 16	—	—	3 6	0 6
24	oz.	Ess. anisi 1 in 5	—	—	3 6	0 6
28	oz.	Ess. apricot	—	—	3 10	0 8
114	lb.	Ess. camphoræ B.P.C.	—	3 9	1 0	—
13	oz.	Ess. cherry, fruit	—	—	2 0	0 4
30	oz.	Ess. cinnamomi	—	—	4 5	0 9
78	lb.	Ess. cinnam. et quin. P.L.F. ..	—	2 9	0 9	—
27	oz.	Ess. Iridis	—	4 0	—	0 7
246	lb.	Ess. limonis (soluble)	—	9 0	2 6	0 4
456	lb.	Ess. menth. pip. (Ang.) 1 in 5 ..	—	—	3 6	0 7
336	lb.	Ess. menth. pip. (Ang.) 1 in 10	—	—	3 1	0 6
252	lb.	Ess. menth. pip. (exot.) 1 in 10	—	8 6	2 4	0 4
51	oz.	Ess. moschi	—	—	7 5	1 2
75	oz.	Ess. moschi fort.	—	—	10 2	1 6
16	oz.	Ess. pear (jargonelle)	—	—	2 9	0 6
22	oz.	Ess. pineapple	—	—	2 4	0 4
96	lb.	Ess. pulegii 1 in 10	—	3 5	1 0	0 2
14	oz.	Ess. raspberry (fruit)	—	—	2 0	0 4
14	lb.	Ess. rennet	1 9	0 7	0 3	—
17	oz.	Ess. strawberry	—	—	2 6	0 5
24	oz.	Ess. vanillæ P.L.F.	—	—	3 6	0 6
36	oz.	Ess. vanillæ fort.	—	—	5 3	0 9
14	oz.	Ess. vanillæ (isoprop.)	—	—	2 0	0 4
16	oz.	Ess. vanillin P.L.F.	—	—	2 8	0 5
87	lb.	Ess. zingiberis	9 10	2 10	0 9	0 2
42	oz.	Estoral	—	—	5 3	1 0
10	oz.	Ethyl bromidum	—	—	—	0 6
74	50 cc.	Ethyl chaulmoogras	per cc.	0 3	—	—
31	ea.	Ethyl chloridum (30 c.c.) ..	ea.	4 0	—	—
42	ea.	Ethyl chloridum (50 c.c.) ..	ea.	5 3	—	—
74	50 cc.	Ethyl hydnocarpas	per c.c.	0 3	—	—
31	oz.	Ethyl iodidum	—	—	—	1 4

Cost d.	Cost per	Et—Ex	Selling Price 16 oz. s. d.	4 oz. s. d.	1 oz. s. d.	1 s.
72	dr.	Ethyl morphinæ hydrochl.S.1. (4)	per	gr.	0 4	-
74	50 cc.	Ethyl morrhuas	per	c.c.	0 3	-
5	oz.	Ethyl phthalate	—	—	0 9	0
96	oz.	Eucainæ hyd. (beta)	—	—	—	2
96	oz.	Eucainæ lact. (beta)	—	—	—	2
20	lb.	Eucalypti folia Ang.	2 6	0 9	0 3	-
24	lb.	Eucalypti fol. pulv.	3 0	0 11	0 3	-
7	oz.	Eucalyptol	—	—	1 1	0
50	oz.	Eugallol	—	—	6 0	1
12	oz.	Eugenol	—	—	1 9	0
36	oz.	Euonyminum virid.	—	—	5 3	0
16	lb.	Eupad	2 0	0 8	0 3	-
42	lb.	Euphorb. gum. pulv.	—	1 6	0 6	-
192	oz.	Euquinine	—	—	—	4
45	oz.	Euresol	—	—	—	1
22.4	amp.	Evipan sodium .. ..℞ only	—	2 6	per	am
		Extracta				
21	oz.	Ext. aconiti radicis alc. S.1. (6)	—	—	3 2	0
10	oz.	Ext. adonis vernalis liq. ..	—	—	1 8	0
51	lb.	Ext. agropyri liquidum ..	—	2 0	0 8	0
108	lb.	Ext. aletridis liquidum B.P.C.	—	4 0	1 1	0
54	lb.	Ext. aloes pulvis	—	2 0	0 7	0
36	oz.	Ext. aloes Barbadensis glac. ..	—	—	4 6	0
9	oz.	Ext. aloes Socotrinæ pulvis ..	—	—	1 9	0
24	oz.	Ext. anthemidis pulvis '98 ..	—	—	3 1	0
14	oz.	Ext. apocyni liquidum	—	—	2 0	0
150	lb.	Ext. arnica liq.	—	5 5	1 7	0
60	lb.	Ext. belæ liquidum	—	2 2	0 8	0
12	oz.	Ext. bellad. siccum ..S.1. (5)	—	—	1 9	0
108	lb.	Ext. bellad. liquidum ..S.1. (5)	—	4 6	1 4	0
102	lb.	Ext. bellad. viride '98 ..S.1. (5)	—	3 9	1 0	0
13	oz.	Ext. bellad. viridis pulv. '98 S.1. (5)	—	—	1 11	0
13	oz.	Ext. boldo liquidum	—	—	1 10	0
36	oz.	Ext. bone marrow	—	—	4 6	0 1
24	oz.	Ext. buchu	—	—	3 6	0
138	lb.	Ext. buchu liquidum B.P.C. ..	—	5 0	1 6	0
15	oz.	Ext. cacti grandiflori liquidum..	—	—	2 3	0
39	oz.	Ext. calendulæ	—	—	5 9	0 1
14	oz.	Ext. calendula liq.	—	—	2 2	0
15	oz.	Ext. calumbæ	—	—	2 3	0
52	dr.	Ext. cannabis indicæ .. D.D.	—	—	—	7
108	lb.	Ext. cascaræ sag. sicci pulvis ..	—	3 10	1 1	0
32	lb.	Ext. cascaræ sag. liquidum ..	4 2	1 3	0 4	0
51	lb.	Ext. cascaræ sag. liquidum insip.	6 4	1 11	0 7	0
126	lb.	Ext. caulophylli liquidum ..	—	4 2	1 2	0
8	oz.	Ext. cinchonæ	—	—	1 2	0
60	lb.	Ext. cinchonæ liquidum ..	—	2 4	0 8	0
144	lb.	Ext. cocæ liquidum .. D.D.	—	5 6	1 7	0
24	oz.	Ext. colchici acet. ..S.1. (5)	—	—	3 6	0
9	oz.	Ext. colchici liq. ..S.1. (5)	—	—	1 4	0
30	oz.	Ext. colchici sicc. ..S.1. (5)	—	—	4 5	0
30	oz.	Ext. colch. sem. acet. ..S.1. (5)	—	—	4 5	0
10	oz.	Ext. collinsonia liq.	—	—	1 6	0
23	oz.	Ext. colocynthidis pulvis ..	—	—	3 5	0
6	oz.	Ext. colocynthidis co.	—	—	1 0	0
99	lb.	Ext. condurango liquidum ..	—	3 7	1 0	0
8	oz.	Ext. conii S.1. (5)	—	—	1 2	0
11	oz.	Ext. conii liquidum ..S.1. (6)	—	—	1 8	0
18	oz.	Ext. convallariæ liquidum ..	—	—	2 8	0
14	oz.	Ext. coto liquidum	—	—	2 0	0
22	oz.	Ext. damianæ pulvis	—	—	3 3	0
108	lb.	Ext. damianæ liquidum ..	—	4 0	1 1	0
18	oz.	Ext. droseræ rotund. liquidum	—	—	2 8	0
57	oz.	Ext. ergotæ S.1. (5)	—	—	8 4	1
60	oz.	Ext. ergotæ pulvis ..S.1. (5)	—	—	8 9	1
156	lb.	Ext. ergot. liq. S.1. (5)	—	5 9	1 8	0

Ex

Cost d.	per	Extracta—(cont.)	16 oz. s. d.	4 oz. s. d.	1 oz. s. d.	1 dr. s. d.
168	lb.	Ext. ergotæ liq. '14 S.I. (5)	—	6 1	1 9	0 3
192	lb.	Ext. ergot. ammon. liq. S.I. (6)	—	7 1	2 2	0 4
30	oz.	Ext. euonymi	—	—	4 5	0 8
76	lb.	Ext. euphorbiæ liquidum ..	—	2 10	0 10	0 2
14	oz.	Ext. fellis bovinum	—	—	2 0	0 4
16	oz.	Ext. fellis bovinum pulv. ..	—	—	2 4	0 4
10	oz.	Ext. filicis	—	—	1 6	0 3
9	oz.	Ext. fuci B.P.C. pulv.	—	—	1 4	0 3
60	lb.	Ext. fuci liquidum	7 6	2 2	0 8	0 2
12	oz.	Ext. fuci pulvis	—	—	1 9	0 3
30	oz.	Ext. gelsemii alcoh. S.I. (5)	—	—	4 5	0 8
38	lb.	Ext. gentianæ	—	1 4	0 5	0 1
66	lb.	Ext. gentianæ pulvis	—	2 5	0 9	0 2
54	lb.	Ext. glycyrrhizæ	—	2 0	0 7	0 1
26	lb.	Ext. glycyrrhizæ liquidum ..	—	1 0	0 4	0 1
02	lb.	Ext. gossypii rad. cort. liquidum	—	3 7	1 2	0 2
93	lb.	Ext. granati rad. cort. liquidum	—	3 4	0 11	0 2
72	lb.	Ext. grindeliæ liquidum ..	—	2 9	0 10	0 2
18	lb.	Ext. hæmatox. exot.	—	0 8	0 3	0 1
30	lb.	Ext. hæmatox. pulvis	—	1 2	0 4	0 1
16	oz.	Ext. hamamelidis (fol.) ..	—	—	2 4	0 4
72	lb.	Ext. hamamelidis liquidum ..	9 0	2 7	0 9	0 2
12	oz.	Ext. hellebor. nig.	—	—	1 9	0 3
79	—	Ext. hepatis siccum	9s.	for	3	tubes
50	lb.	Ext. hepat. liq.	—	5 4	—	—
84	oz.	Ext. hydrastis siccum	—	—	—	1 9
30	oz.	Ext. hydrastis liquidum ..	—	—	4 5	0 8
10	oz.	Ext. hyoscyam. liq. P.I. (9)	—	—	1 6	0 3
18	oz.	Ext. hyoscyami siccum S.I. (5)	—	—	2 8	0 5
20	oz.	Ext. hyoscy. vir. pul. S.I. (5)	—	—	2 11	0 5
21	oz.	Ext. ipecacuanhæ liquidum ..	—	—	3 2	0 6
15	oz.	Ext. iridis sicc. B.P.C.	—	—	2 3	0 4
84	lb.	Ext. jaborandi liq. P.I. (9)	—	3 0	0 10	0 2
22	oz.	Ext. jalapæ pulvis	—	—	3 3	0 6
26	lb.	Ext. kavæ liquidum	—	4 8	1 4	0 3
81	lb.	Ext. kolæ liquidum	—	2 11	0 11	0 2
22	oz.	Ext. krameriæ pulvis	—	—	3 3	0 6
17	oz.	Ext. lactucæ pulvis	—	—	2 2	0 5
18	oz.	Ext. lupuli pulvis	—	—	2 8	0 5
10	lb.	Ext. malti	1 4	—	—	—
14	lb.	Ext. malti ferratum	1 10	0 7	—	—
26	lb.	Ext. malti c. cascar. sag. wgt. ..	3 3	1 0	—	—
21	lb.	Ext. malti c. glycerophos. wgt. P.I. (13)	2 8	0 11	—	—
24	lb.	Ext. malti c. hæmoglobin. wgt.	3 0	1 0	—	—
22	lb.	Ext. malti c. hypophosph. wgt.	2 9	1 0	—	—
12	lb.	Ext. malti c. ol. morrh. B.P.C.	1 6	—	—	—
44	doz.	Ext. malti c. oleo morrh. pkd.	1 6		2-lb.	2 6
14	lb.	Ext. malti c. syr. fer. phos. co. wgt.	1 10	0 7	—	—
16	lb.	Ext. malti liquidum	2 8	1 0	0 3	—
27	lb.	Ext. malti liq. c. casc. sag. ..	—	1 3	0 5	—
33	lb.	Ext. malti liq. c. glyceroph. ..	4 3	1 4	0 5	—
30	lb.	Ext. malti liq. c. hæmoglob. ..	4 0	1 3	0 4	—
30	lb.	Ext. malti liq. c. hypophos. ..	3 9	1 2	0 4	—
26	lb.	Ext. malti liq. c. syr. East. P.I. (13)	3 6	1 1	0 4	—
20	lb.	Ext. malti liq. c.syr. ferri phos. co.	2 9	0 11	0 3	—
59	lb.	Ext. marubii liquidum	—	2 7	0 9	0 2
3	oz.	Ext. maticæ liq.	—	—	2 0	0 4
60	lb.	Ext. medullæ rubræ liquidum ..	—	2 3	0 8	0 2
0	oz.	Ext. nuc. vom. sicc. S.I. (5)	—	—	1 6	0 3
63	lb.	Ext. nuc. vom. liq. S.I. (5)	—	2 4	0 8	0 2
60	lb.	Ext. opii liquidum .. D.D.	—	2 2	0 8	0 2
63	oz.	Ext. opii siccum .. D.D.	—	—	—	1 4
64	lb.	Ext. papaveris liq. P.I. (9)	—	2 0	0 7	0 1
72	lb.	Ext. pareiræ liquidum	—	2 7	0 9	0 2
61	oz.	Ext. physostigmatis S.I. (6)	—	—	7 5	1 1
3	oz.	Ext. picrorhizæ liquidum ..	—	—	2 0	0 4

Ex—Fe

Cost d.	per	Extracta—(cont.)	16 oz. s. d.	4 oz. s. d.	1 oz. s. d.	1 dr. s. d.
8	oz.	Ext. pini canadensis liquidum ..	—	—	1 4	0 3
22	lb.	Ext. pini (for baths)	2 9	0 10	0 3	—
11	oz.	Ext. pulsatillæ liquidum ..	—	—	1 8	0 3
126	lb.	Ext. pyrethri rad liq.	—	4 7	1 4	0 3
20	oz.	Ext. quassiæ pulvis	—	—	2 11	0 6
44	lb.	Ext. quassiæ liq.	—	1 7	0 6	0 1
66	lb.	Ext. quillaiæ liquidum	—	2 6	0 9	0 2
12	oz.	Ext. rhamni frang. liquidum ..	—	—	1 9	0 3
15	oz.	Ext. rhei pulvis	—	—	2 2	0 4
11	oz.	Ext. rhus. arom. liquidum ..	—	—	1 8	0 3
14	oz.	Ext. rhus. toxicod. liquidum ..	—	—	2 0	0 4
27	oz.	Ext. rutæ	—	—	4 0	0 9
13	oz.	Ext. sabal liq.	—	—	2 0	0 4
102	lb.	Ext. salicis nigræ liquidum ..	—	3 9	1 1	0 2
15	oz.	Ext. sarsæ Jam. simp.	—	—	2 3	0 4
13	oz.	Ext. sarsæ Jam. co.	—	—	1 11	0 4
7	oz.	Ext. scillæ liquidum	—	—	1 1	0 2
99	lb.	Ext. senegæ liquidum	—	—	1 1	0 2
36	lb.	Ext. sennæ liquidum	—	1 6	0 6	0 1
16	oz.	Ext. serpentariæ liq.	—	—	2 4	0 4
20	oz.	Ext. stramonii foliæ S.I. (5)	—	—	2 11	0 6
33	oz.	Ext. stramonii sem. S.I. (5)	—	—	4 10	0 8
24	oz.	Ext. strophanthi S.I. (5)	—	—	3 6	0 6
30	oz.	Ext. sumbul	—	—	—	0 8
54	lb.	Ext. taraxaci	—	2 0	0 7	0 1
66	lb.	Ext. taraxaci pulvis	—	2 5	0 10	0 2
6	oz.	Ext. uvæ ursi liq.	—	—	0 11	0 2
18	oz.	Ext. valerianæ pulvis	—	—	2 8	0 5
39	oz.	Ext. viburni prunifolii	—	—	5 9	1 10
102	lb.	Ext. viburni liquidum	—	3 8	1 0	0 2
		F				
30	lb.	Fehling's solution No. 1 ..	—	1 6	0 5	—
30	lb.	Fehling's solution No. 2 ..	—	1 6	0 5	—
		Ferrum				
21	oz.	Ferri albuminas	—	—	3 1	0 6
26	lb.	Ferri alum. pur.	3 3	1 0	0 4	—
8	oz.	Ferri arsenas .. S.I. (4)	—	—	1 2	0 2
56	oz.	Ferri cacodylas .. S.I. (4)	—	—	—	1 4
18	lb.	Ferri carbonas saccharatus ..	2 3	0 8	0 3	—
8	oz.	Ferri citras	—	—	1 2	0 2
37	lb.	Ferri et ammonii citras ..	—	1 5	0 5	0 1
56	lb.	Ferri et ammonii citras vir. ..	—	2 0	0 7	0 1
6	oz.	Ferri et ammonii tartras ..	—	—	0 11	0 2
16	oz.	Ferri et bismuthi citras ..	—	—	2 4	0 4
11	oz.	Ferri et mangan. citras ..	—	—	1 8	0 3
10	oz.	Ferri et mang. phosphas ..	—	—	1 6	0 3
6	oz.	Ferri et potassii tartras ..	—	—	0 11	0 2
19	oz.	Ferri et quininæ citras	—	—	2 10	0 5
30	oz.	Ferri et quin. cit. c. strych. S.I. (6)	—	—	4 1	0 7
14	oz.	Ferri et strych. citras S.I. (5)	—	—	1 9	0 3
12	oz.	Ferri glycerophosphatis pulvis ..	—	—	1 9	0 3
13	oz.	Ferri hypophosphis	—	—	1 11	0 4
15	oz.	Ferri iodidum	—	—	2 3	0 4
10	oz.	Ferri lactas	—	—	1 6	0 3
18	oz.	Ferri lactophosphas	—	—	3 0	0 6
11	lb.	Ferri limat.	1 5	0 6	0 2	—
30	lb.	Ferri nitras	—	1 2	0 4	—
48	lb.	Ferri oleas	—	2 0	0 7	0 1
4	oz.	Ferri oxalas (ferric) P.I. (8)	—	—	0 7	0 1
12	lb.	Ferri oxidum præcipitatum rubrum	1 6	0 6	0 2	—
30	lb.	Ferri oxidum sacch. B.P.C. ..	—	1 2	0 4	—
12	lb.	Ferri perchloridum cryst. ..	1 9	0 5	0 2	—

Fe—Gl

Cost d.	per	Ferrum—(cont.)	Selling Price 16 oz. s. d.	4 oz. s. d.	1 oz. s. d.	1 dr. s. d.
33	lb.	Ferri phosphas saccharatus ..	—	1 3	0 5	—
5	oz.	Ferri phosphas solubilis ..	—	—	0 11	0 2
7	oz.	Ferri pyrophosphas	—	—	1 1	0 2
14	oz.	Ferri salicylas	—	—	2 0	0 4
15	oz.	Ferri succinas	—	—	2 3	0 4
7	lb.	Ferri sulphas pur.	0 11	0 3	0 1	—
7	lb.	Ferri sulphas pur. granulatus ..	0 11	0 3	0 1	—
14	lb.	Ferri sulphas exsiccatus ..	1 9	0 7	0 2	—
4	lb.	Ferri sulphas coml.	0 6	0 2	—	—
8	lb.	Ferri sulphidum (cake) ..	1 0	0 4	0 2	—
16	oz.	Ferri valerianas	—	—	2 4	0 4
16	oz.	Ferrier's snuff P.L.F. .. D.D.	—	—	2 6	0 6
31.5	8 oz.	Ferro-malt (Crookes)	—	2 0	0 6	—
36	8 oz.	Ferro-malt glycerophos. ..	—	2 3	0 7	0 1
43	oz.	Ferropyrin	—	—	—	1 0
6	oz.	Ferrum redactum	—	—	0 11	0 2
21	oz.	Fluorescein technical	—	—	3 1	0 6
36	oz.	Fluorescein solubile	—	—	5 3	0 9
17	lb.	Fœniculi pulvis	2 2	0 7	0 2	—
15	lb.	Fœniculi pulvis (coarse) ..	1 10	0 7	0 2	—
8	lb.	Fœnugreci sem. pulvis	1 0	0 3	—	—
7	lb.	Fœnugreci sem. pulvis (crs.) ..	0 11	0 3	—	—
570	cwt.	Fœnugreci sem. pulvis (crs.) ..	0 9	—	7 lb.	4 6
13	oz.	Formamol	—	—	2 0	0 4
10	3 oz.	Formolyptol, unstd.	—	—	0 5	—
22	lb.	Foot powder, antisep. P.L.F. ..	2 9	1 0	0 4	—
8	lb.	Foot-rot paste P.L.F.	1 0	0 4	—	—
74	lb.	Foot-rot powder P.L.F. ..	9 3	2 6	—	—
54	lb.	Frosting	6 9	2 0	0 7	—
26	oz.	Fuchsinum pur.	—	—	3 9	0 7
5	lb.	Fuller's earth	0 8	0 3	—	—
6	lb.	Fuller's earth pulvis	0 9	0 3	—	—
7	lb.	Fuller's earth levig.	0 11	0 4	—	—
7	lb.	Fuller's earth levig. alb. ..	0 11	0 4	—	—
		G				
32	oz.	Galactosum	—	—	4 8	0 8
12	lb.	Galangalæ rhizoma	1 8	0 6	0 2	—
8	oz.	Galbani pulvis	—	—	1 2	0 2
27	lb.	Gallæ cærul.	3 6	1 0	0 4	—
36	lb.	Gallæ cærul. pulvis	4 6	1 4	0 5	—
18	25	Gardan tablets .. ℞ only	per	bot.	2 6	—
72	lb.	Gelatinum sheet No. 1 ..	8 6	2 5	0 8	—
84	lb.	Gelatinum incisum	10 6	3 0	0 10	—
102	lb.	Gel.codein.etglyc. P.L.F. P.I. (13)	—	3 9	1 0	—
20	lb.	Gelatum zinci	2 6	0 9	—	—
30	lb.	Gelat. zinci dur. P.L.F. ..	3 9	1 2	—	—
18	gr.	Gelseminæ hydrochlor. S.I. (4)	per	gr.	2 8	—
15	lb.	Gentianæ rad. incis.	2 0	0 7	0 2	—
17	lb.	Gentianæ rad. pulvis	2 3	0 8	0 3	—
598	cwt.	Gentianæ rad. pulvis (crs.) ..	7 lb.	4 8	14 lb.	9 0
18	oz.	Geraniol	—	—	2 8	0 5
20	oz.	Geraniol acetas	—	—	3 0	0 6
22	oz.	Gingerin. (African)	—	—	3 3	0 6
54	oz.	Gingerin. (Jam.)	—	—	7 11	1 2
7	lb.	Glucosum (liq.) .. .. wgt.	1 0	0 4	0 2	—
8	lb.	Glucosum (solid)	1 0	0 4	0 2	—
2	lb.	Glucosum pulv.	1 6	0 6	0 2	—
36	lb.	Glue, surg. (Sinclair) P.L.F. ..	4 6	1 2	—	—
		Glycerina				
78	lb.	Glycerin bismuth carb. ..	—	4 0	1 1	0 2
50	lb.	Glycerin pepsin fort.	—	2 7	0 9	0 2
20	lb.	Glycerin phenolis P.II. (9)	—	1 2	0 4	0 1
12	lb.	Glycerinum	2 1	0 7	0 3	—
12	lb.	Glycerinum (wgt.)	1 6	0 6	—	—
22	lb.	Glyc. acidi borici	3 6	1 0	0 4	—

Gl—He

Cost d.	per	Glycerina—(cont.)	Selling Price 16 oz. s. d.	4 oz. s. d.	1 oz. s. d.	1 dr. s. d.
38	lb.	Glyc. acidi gallici	—	1 9	0 6	0 1
86	8 oz.	Glyc. ac. pepsin (Bullock) ..	—	6 0	1 7	0 4
28	lb.	Glyc. acidi tannici	—	1 5	0 5	0 1
24	lb.	Glyc. aluminis	—	1 2	0 4	—
33	lb.	Glyc. amyli	—	1 3	0 5	—
44	lb.	Glyc. atropinæ .. S.I. (5)	—	2 6	0 8	—
54	lb.	Glyc. bellad. 50% S.I. (5)	10 2	2 6	0 9	—
60	lb.	Glyc. bellad. .. S.I. (5)	—	2 8	0 9	—
16	lb.	Glyc. boracis	—	0 11	0 3	—
72	lb.	Glyc. carminini B.P.C. ..	—	3 11	1 2	—
28	lb.	Glyc. diamorph. B.P.C. D.D.	—	1 9	0 6	—
34	lb.	Glyc. Eastoni .. P.I. (13)	—	1 9	0 6	0 1
26	lb.	Glyc. et cucum.	—	1 0	0 4	—
14	lb.	Glyc. et aqua rosæ 1 in 3 ..	2 0	0 7	0 2	—
27	lb.	Glyc. glycerophosphatum co. ..	—	1 4	0 5	—
24	lb.	Glyc. ichthamol.	—	1 3	0 5	0 1
6	oz.	Glyc. iodi B.P.C.	—	—	1 9	—
51	lb.	Glyc. pancreatini	—	1 9	0 7	0 1
84	lb.	Glyc. papaini	—	3 6	1 0	0 2
32	lb.	Glyc. pepsini	—	1 6	0 5	0 1
26	lb.	Glyc. plumbi subacet. P.I. (9)	—	1 6	0 6	0 1
11	lb.	Glyc. thymolis co.	1 6	0 6	0 2	—
54	lb.	Glyc. tragacanthæ	—	1 10	0 7	0 1
30	oz.	Glycine	—	—	4 5	0 8
33	lb.	Glycothymoline, unstd. ..	—	1 3	0 4	—
24	lb.	Glycyrrhizæ radix decort. ..	3 0	1 0	0 4	—
12	lb.	Glycyrrhizæ radicis pulvis ..	1 6	0 6	0 2	—
28	lb.	Glycyrrhizæ radicis decort. pulv.	3 6	1 0	0 4	—
10	lb.	Glycyrrhizæ radicis pulvis (crs.)	1 3	0 5	0 2	—
560	cwt.	Glycyrrhizæ radicis pulvis (crs.)	7 lb.	4 2	14 lb.	7 9
16	oz.	Glycyrrhizinum ammoniatum ..	—	—	2 4	0 4
54	lb.	Gossypii radicis cort. pulvis ..	—	2 0	0 7	—
21	lb.	Gran. paradisi pulv.	2 8	0 9	0 3	—
17	lb.	Granati cortex	—	0 8	0 3	—
27	lb.	Granati radicis cortex	—	1 0	0 4	—
35	4 oz.	Grindeline (Oppenheimer) ..	—	4 4	1 2	0 3
7	lb.	Guaiaci ligni rass.	0 11	0 4	0 1	—
5	oz.	Guaiaci resinæ pulvis	—	—	0 9	0 2
20	oz.	Guaiacol (cryst.)	—	—	3 0	0 5
18	oz.	Guaiacol	—	—	2 8	0 5
30	oz.	Guaiacol. benzoas	—	—	4 5	0 8
16	oz.	Guaiacol. carbonas	—	—	2 4	0 4
42	oz.	Guaiacol. cinnamas	—	—	6 4	0 11
108	oz.	Guaiacol. salicylas	—	—	—	2 4
8	oz.	Guaranæ pulvis	—	—	1 2	0 2
9	oz.	Guttæ fluorescinæ B.P.C. ..	—	—	1 4	0 3
		H				
8	lb.	Hæmatox. lignum incis. ..	1 0	0 4	0 1	—
13	lb.	Hæmatox. ligni pulvis	1 8	0 7	0 2	—
19	dr.	Hæmatoxylinum	—	—	—	2 10
6	oz.	Hæmoglobini pulvis	—	—	0 11	0 2
90	lb.	Hæmorrhaline (Hewlett) ..	—	3 3	0 11	0 2
33.6	10c.c.	Halibut liver oil	4 0	each	—	—
33.5	box25	Haliverol capsules ♏3 P.D. ..	4 0	each	—	—
302	doz.	Haliverol (P.D. & Co.) ..	—	—	5 c.c.	3 0
21	oz.	Hamamelinum	—	—	3 1	0 6
30	10 v.	Hebaral sod. P.D. gr. 3 ℞ only	3 3	each	—	—
14	oz.	Heliotropin. cryst.	—	—	2 0	0 4
22	lb.	Hellebori nigri radicis pulvis ..	2 9	0 10	0 3	—
40	oz.	Helmitol	—	—	—	0 11
14	lb.	Hennæ folia	1 9	0 7	0 2	—
17	lb.	Hennæ fol. pulvis	2 3	0 8	0 3	—
18	oz.	Hexamin benzoas.	—	—	2 8	0 5
18	oz.	Hexamin salicylas	—	—	2 8	0 5
5	oz.	Hexamina	—	—	0 9	0 2

He—In

Cost d.	Cost per	He—In	Selling Price 16 oz. s. d.	4 oz. s. d.	1 oz. s. d.	1 dr. s. d.
24	oz.	Hexamina resorcin.	—	—	3 6	0 8
12	oz.	Hexamin. sodii acet.	—	—	1 9	0 3
90	doz.	Hirudines	ea.	1 2	—	—
5	gr.	Homatropina .. S.1. (4)	per	gr.	0 9	—
5	gr.	Homatrop. hydrobrom. S.1. (4)	per	gr.	0 9	—
22	lb.	Hoof ointment P.L.F. I. ..	2 9	—	—	—
21	lb.	Hoof ointment P.L.F. II. ..	2 8	—	—	—
5	lb.	Hordeum perlatum	0 8	0 3	0 1	—
70	100	Hormotone tablets	per	doz.	1 3	—
		Hydrargyrum				
168	lb.	Hyd. bisulphidum (cinnabar) ..	20 6	5 11	1 9	—
108	lb.	Hyd. bisulph. (vermilion) ..	13 6	4 0	1 1	—
14	oz.	Hyd. bromidum	—	—	2 0	0 4
24	oz.	Hyd. cyanidum .. S.1. (4)	—	—	3 6	0 6
19	oz.	Hyd. iodid. flav. S.1. P.II. (4)	—	—	2 10	0 5
15	oz.	Hyd. iodid. rub. S.1. P.II. (4)	—	—	2 3	0 4
18	oz.	Hyd. iodid. virid.	—	—	2 8	0 5
60	lb.	Hyd. oleas .. S.1. (4)	—	2 2	0 8	0 2
120	lb.	Hyd. oxid. flav. P.I. (8)	—	—	1 3	0 3
132	lb.	Hyd. oxid. rub. P.I. (8)	—	—	1 4	0 3
18	oz.	Hyd. oxycyanidum S.1. (4)	—	—	2 8	0 5
99	lb.	Hyd. perchloridum S.1. P.II. (4)	—	—	1 1	0 2
120	lb.	Hyd. persulphas (alb.) ..	—	4 3	1 2	0 2
22	oz.	Hyd. salicylas .. S.1. (4)	—	—	3 3	0 6
111	lb.	Hyd. subchloridum	—	—	1 1	0 2
11	oz.	Hyd. subchl. præc. subtil. ..	—	—	1 8	0 3
150	lb.	Hyd. subsulphas flavus ..	—	5 5	1 7	0 3
120	lb.	Hyd. sulphuretum c. sulphure ..	—	4 3	1 2	0 2
18	oz.	Hyd. sulphocyanid. P.I. (8)	—	—	2 8	0 5
23	oz.	Hyd. tannas .. S.1. (4)	—	—	3 5	0 7
78	lb.	Hydrargyrum	10 0	2 10	0 9	—
114	lb.	Hyd. ammoniatum P.I. (8)	—	4 1	1 2	0 2
38	lb.	Hyd. cum creta	—	1 5	0 5	0 1
8	gr.	Hydrastina	per	gr.	1 2	—
8	gr.	Hydrastininæ hydrochlor. ..	per	gr.	1 2	—
63	16 oz.	Hydrated bismuth (P.D.) ..	—	2 5	0 9	0 2
21	16 oz.	Hydrated magnesia (P.D.) ..	2 6	1 0	0 3	—
84	lb.	Hydroquinone	—	2 9	0 9	0 2
7	gr.	Hyoscin. hydrobrom. S.1. (4)	per	gr.	1 2	—
27	lb.	Hyoscyami semina S.1. (4)	—	1 0	0 4	—
5	gr.	Hyoscyamina cryst. S.1. (4)	per	gr.	0 10	—
5	gr.	Hyoscyamin. sulph. S.1. (4)	per	gr.	0 10	—
		I				
43	oz.	Ichthalbin	—	—	—	1 0
20	30	Ichthalbin tablets gr. 5 ..	doz.	1 2	—	—
40	lb.	Ichthammol	—	1 5	0 5	0 1
72	lb.	Ichthyocolla Brazil. incis. ..	9 0	2 7	0 9	0 2
114	lb.	Ichthyol	—	4 2	1 2	0 2
6.6	amp.	Icoral 0.5%	0 10	per	amp.	—
7.3	amp.	Icoral 5.0%	1 0	per	amp.	—
51	lb.	Incense P.L.F.	6 5	1 10	—	—
42	oz.	Indicarminum	—	—	6 4	1 0
22	oz.	Indigo synthetic	—	—	3 3	0 6
24	oz.	Indigo (carmine dry)	—	—	3 6	0 6
42	lb.	Indigo (carmine paste)	—	1 6	0 5	—
40	lb.	Indigo sulphatis sol.	—	1 5	0 5	—
12	lb.	Infusa recenta	1 6	0 6	0 2	—
		Infusa Concentrata 1—7				
37	lb.	Inf. agropyri conc.	—	1 5	0 5	0 1
46	lb.	Inf. anthemidis conc.	—	1 9	0 6	0 1

In—Ir

Cost d.	Cost per	In—Ir Infusa—(cont.)	Selling Price 16 oz. s. d.	4 oz. s. d.	1 oz. s. d.	1 dr. s. d.
21	lb.	Inf. amarum conc.	—	0 11	0 4	0 1
36	lb.	Infus. aromat co.	—	1 6	0 6	0 1
36	lb.	Inf. aurantii conc.	—	1 4	0 5	0 1
36	lb.	Inf. aurantii co. conc.	—	1 4	0 5	0 1
42	lb.	Inf. buchu conc.	—	1 6	0 6	0 1
24	lb.	Inf. calumbæ conc.	—	1 0	0 4	0 1
27	lb.	Inf. caryophylli conc.	—	1 0	0 4	0 1
60	lb.	Inf. cascarillæ conc.	—	2 2	0 7	0 1
45	lb.	Inf. catechu conc.	—	1 8	0 7	0 1
30	lb.	Inf. chiratæ conc.	—	1 5	0 5	0 1
42	lb.	Inf. cinchonæ acid. conc. ..	—	1 7	0 7	0 1
54	lb.	Inf. cinchonæ flav. conc. ..	—	2 0	0 7	0 1
60	lb.	Inf. cinchonæ pallid. conc. ..	—	2 2	0 7	0 1
45	lb.	Inf. cuspariæ conc.	—	1 8	0 6	0 1
43	lb.	Inf. dulcamaræ conc.	—	1 8	0 6	0 1
69	lb.	Inf. ergotæ conc. S.1. (5)	—	2 6	0 9	0 2
25	lb.	Inf. gentianæ (simp.) conc. ..	—	1 0	0 4	0 1
30	lb.	Inf. gentianæ co. conc. ..	—	1 1	0 4	0 1
39	lb.	Inf. jaborandi conc.	—	1 5	0 6	0 1
33	lb.	Inf. krameriæ conc.	—	1 4	0 5	0 1
56	lb.	Inf. lupuli conc.	—	2 0	0 7	0 1
44	lb.	Inf. marubii conc.	—	1 9	0 6	—
45	lb.	Inf. maticæ conc.	—	1 10	0 7	0 1
40	lb.	Inf. pruni serot. conc.	—	1 5	0 6	0 1
21	lb.	Inf. quassiæ conc.	—	0 10	0 3	0 1
40	lb.	Inf. rhei conc.	—	1 6	0 6	0 1
48	lb.	Inf. rosæ acidum conc. ..	—	1 9	0 5	0 1
30	lb.	Inf. scoparii conc.	—	1 1	0 5	0 1
38	lb.	Inf. senegæ conc.	—	1 5	0 5	0 1
36	lb.	Inf. sennæ conc.	—	1 4	0 5	0 1
54	lb.	Inf. serpentariæ conc.	—	2 0	0 7	0 1
45	lb.	Inf. simarubæ conc.	—	1 8	0 6	0 1
30	lb.	Inf. uvæ ursi conc.	—	1 2	0 4	0 1
32	lb.	Inf. valerianæ conc.	—	1 2	0 4	0 1
		Injectiones				
23	oz.	Inject. apomorph. hypod. S.1.(6)	—	—	3 10	0 7
32	oz.	Inject. cocainæ hypod. .. D.D.	—	—	4 8	0 8
48	oz.	Inject. coc. hyp. (10%) .. D.D.	—	—	7 0	1 0
28	oz.	Inject. morphinæ hypod. D.D.	—	—	5 0	0 9
6	oz.	Inject. strychnin. hypod. S.1. (5)	—	—	1 0	0 2
32	lb.	Insect powder (Dalm.)	4 0	1 2	0 4	—
22	lb.	Insect powder sec.	2 9	0 9	0 3	—
13.5	ea.	Insulin, 5 c.c. .. P.I. (13)	orig.	bot.	1 6	—
25.5	ea.	Insulin, 10 c.c. .. P.I. (13)	orig.	bot.	2 10	—
28	lb.	Inulæ radicis pulvis	3 9	1 2	0 4	—
24	lb.	Inulæ radicis pulvis (crs.) ..	3 5	1 0	0 4	—
27	oz.	Inulin	—	—	4 0	0 7
15	oz.	Iodatol 10%	—	—	2 0	0 5
30	oz.	Iodatol 25%	—	—	3 9	0 9
90	lb.	Iodine, alcoholic sol. (Factory)	—	2 10	0 9	—
117	100 gm.	Iodipin 10%	—	—	—	0 9
96	oz.	Iodival	—	—	—	2 4
13	oz.	Iodoformum	—	—	2 0	0 4
108	lb.	Iodoform varnish (Whitehead's)	—	4 0	1 3	—
54	20	Iodothyrine tablets gr. 3 ..	doz.	4 0	—	—
10	oz.	Iodum resubl.	—	—	1 6	0 3
38	oz.	Iononum 10%	—	—	5 7	0 10
15	oz.	Ipecac. pulverata	—	—	2 0	0 4
180	lb.	Ipecac. rad. (Rio) pulvis ..	—	5 4	1 6	—
19	lb.	Iridis rad. flor.	—	0 9	0 3	—
108	lb.	Iridis rad. flor. trimmed ..	—	4 0	1 1	—
23	lb.	Iridis rad. flor. pulv.	3 0	0 11	0 4	—
122	lb.	Iridis rad. flor. (fingers) ..	—	4 4	1 2	—

Cost d.	Cost per	Ja—Li	Selling Price 16 oz. s. d.	4 oz. s. d.	1 oz. s. d.	1 dr. s. d.
		J				
18	lb.	Jaborandi fol. .. ..P.I.(8)	—	0 8	0 3	—
30	lb.	Jalap. pulverata	—	1 3	0 5	0 1
38	oz.	Jalapæ resinæ pulvis	—	—	5 7	0 10
48	oz.	Jalapin	—	—	7 0	1 0
9	lb.	Juniperi fructus	1 2	0 4	0 2	—
19	lb.	Juniperi fructus contus. ..	2 5	0 9	0 3	—
		K				
5	lb.	Kainit	0 8	0 3	—	—
5	oz.	Kamala (sifted)	—	—	0 9	—
18	lb.	Kaolinum puriss.	2 3	0 8	0 3	—
11	lb.	Kaolinum pur. pulvis	1 5	0 5	1 1	—
6	lb.	Kaolinum coml. pulvis opt. ..	0 9	0 3	—	—
68	dr.	Kerocain .. ..S.I. (4)	per	gr.	0 3	8 6
25	50	Kerol caps. (intest.)	doz.	0 9	—	—
20.5	50	Kerol caps. (stom.)	doz.	0 8	—	—
8	lb.	Kieselguhr (alb.)	1 0	0 4	0 1½	—
7	lb.	Kieselguhr (grey)	0 11	0 4	0 1½	—
		L				
40	oz.	Lactopeptine, unstd.	—	—	5 3	1 0
70	lb.	Lactopept. elix., unstd. ..	8 9	2 3	0 7	0 1
40	oz.	Lactopept. tab. gr. 5, unstd. ..	doz.	0 10	—	—
17	lb.	Lactosum	2 2	0 8	0 3	—
9	dr.	Lactucarium	—	—	—	1 4
15	oz.	Lævulosum	—	—	2 3	0 4
28	lb.	Lambing oils P.L.F.	3 6	—	—	—
24	50	Lamellæ	3 6	per	tube	—
36	50	Lamellæ homatropin. . S.I. (5)	4 6	per	tube	—
6	lb.	Lapis cariosi pulvis	0 9	0 3	0 1	—
11	oz.	Lapis divinus (sticks)	—	—	1 8	0 3
7	lb.	Lapis Hibern. pulvis	0 10	0 4	0 2	—
8	lb.	Lapis pumicis elect.	1 0	0 4	0 2	—
5	lb.	Lapis pumicis pulvis	0 8	0 3	0 1	—
7	lb.	Lapis pumicis pulvis levig. ..	1 0	0 4	0 2	—
18	lb.	Laricis cortex	—	0 9	0 2	—
30	lb.	Laricis corticis pulvis	—	1 1	0 4	—
14	lb.	Lauri fructus	—	0 6	0 2	—
18	lb.	Lauri fructus pulvis	—	0 8	0 3	—
108	lb.	Lavandulæ flores Ang.	—	4 0	1 1	0 2
45	lb.	Lavandulæ flores Gall. opt. ..	5 9	1 7	0 6	—
42	lb.	Lavandulæ flores Gall. sec. ..	5 3	1 6	0 6	—
42	oz.	Lecithin (ovo)	—	—	6 2	1 8
36	lb.	Leeming's ess. P.L.F. S.I. (11)	4 6	1 4	—	—
48	oz.	Lenigallol	—	—	—	1 2
10	oz.	Leptandrinum	—	—	1 6	0 3
15	lb.	Ligroinum	—	0 6	0 2	—
72	lb.	Limonis cortex sicc. Ang. ..	—	2 7	0 9	0 2
36	lb.	Linctus diamorphinæ .. D.D.	—	1 6	0 6	—
24	lb.	Linctus diamorph. N.H.I. D.D.	—	1 0	0 4	—
36	lb.	Linctus diamorph. camph. B.P.C. S.I. (5)	—	1 5	0 6	—
42	lb.	Linctus diamorph. c. ipecac. B.P.C. S.I. (5)	—	1 9	0 7	—
36	lb.	Linctus diamorph. et scillæ B.P.C. S.I. (5)	—	1 5	0 6	—
60	lb.	Linctus diamorph. et thymi B.P.C. S.I. (5)	—	2 2	0 8	—
22	lb.	Linctus scillæ (Gee) P.I. (13)	3 0	0 11	0 3	—
28	lb.	Linctus simplex P.L.F. ..	—	1 4	0 5	—

Cost d.	Cost per	Li	Selling Price 16 oz. s. d.	4 oz. s. d.	1 oz. s. d.	1 dr. s. d.
30	lb.	Linctus tussi P.L.F. P.I. (13)	5 0	1 6	0 5	—
480	cwt.	Lini semina	7 lb.	3 6	14 lb.	7 0
6	lb.	Lini semina Ang. sifted ..	0 11	0 4	—	—
396	cwt.	Lini semina contusa E.I. ..	7 lb.	3 0	14 lb.	5 6
5.5	lb.	Lini semina contusa	0 9	0 3	—	—
5	lb.	Lini sem. farina (sine oleo) ..	0 9	0 3	—	—
		Linimenta				
96	lb.	Lin. A.B.C. .. . S.I. (5)	—	3 4	0 11	0 2
39	lb.	Lin. A.B.C. meth. . S.I. (5)	—	1 5	0 5	0 1
102	lb.	Lin. aconiti .. . S.I. (5)	—	3 3	0 9	0 2
42	lb.	Lin. acon. co. meth. N.I.F S.I. (5)	—	1 5	0 5	—
22	lb.	Lin. aconiti meth. . S.I. (5)	—	0 8	0 3	—
34	lb.	Lin. æruginis P.L.F.	—	1 3	0 4	—
16	lb.	Lin. album (acetic)	2 0	0 7	0 2	—
15	lb.	Lin. album (ammon.)	2 0	0 7	0 2	—
32	lb.	Lin. album conc.	4 0	1 2	0 4	—
21	lb.	Lin. anodyn. .. P.I. (12)	—	0 10	0 3	—
15	lb.	Lin. album (B.P.C.)	2 0	0 7	0 2	—
14	lb.	Lin. alb. N.H.I.	—	0 7	0 2	—
42	lb.	Lin. ammoniæ	—	1 5	0 5	—
96	lb.	Lin. belladonnæ . S.I. (5)	—	3 3	0 11	0 2
28	lb.	Lin. bellad. meth. S.I. (5)	—	0 11	0 4	0 1
126	lb.	Lin. betulæ co. (Hewlett) ..	—	4 6	1 3	—
		Lin. calaminæ B.P.C.	4 0	1 9	0 6	—
		Lin. calaminæ co. B.P.C. ..	4 0	1 9	0 6	—
15	lb.	Lin. calcis	1 10	0 7	0 2	—
22	lb.	Lin. camphoræ	2 3	0 8	0 3	—
78	lb.	Lin. camph. ammoniatum ..	—	2 9	0 9	—
21	lb.	Lin. camph. ammoniatum meth.	—	0 9	0 3	—
96	lb.	Lin. capsici B.P.C.	—	3 8	1 0	—
33	lb.	Lin. capsici co. meth.	—	1 3	0 5	—
42	lb.	Lin. capsici meth.	—	1 5	0 5	—
50	lb.	Lin. chloroformi P.I. (12)	—	2 3	0 9	0 2
132	lb.	Lin. crotonis .. P.I. (12)	—	4 9	1 4	0 3
51	lb.	Lin. hydrargyri	—	3 0	1 0	0 2
24	oz.	Lin. menthol	—	—	3 6	0 7
50	lb.	Lin. methyl salicylatis	—	1 10	0 6	0 1
57	lb.	Lin. methyl salicylatis co. ..	—	2 0	0 7	0 1
22	lb.	Lin. methyl sal. N.H.I. ..	—	0 11	0 4	—
87	lb.	Lin. opii .. .. S.I. (5)	—	3 1	0 10	0 2
95	lb.	Lin. opii ammon. S.I. (6)	—	3 5	1 0	0 2
39	lb.	Lin. opii ammon. meth. S.I. (6)	—	1 5	0 5	—
51	lb.	Lin. opii meth. .. S.I. (5)	—	1 10	0 7	0 1
72	lb.	Lin. potassii iodidi B.P.C. ..	—	2 7	0 9	0 2
30	lb.	Lin. potassii iodidi c. sapone ..	—	1 1	0 4	—
72	lb.	Lin. saponis	—	2 6	0 8	—
12	lb.	Lin. saponis meth.	1 8	0 6	0 2	—
102	lb.	Lin. sinapis	—	3 11	1 1	0 2
42	lb.	Lin. sinapis meth.	—	1 6	0 5	—
20	lb.	Lin. terebinthinæ	2 6	0 9	0 3	—
27	lb.	Lin. terebinthinæ aceticum ..	3 4	1 0	0 4	—
20	lb.	Lin. universale P.L.F.	3 0	0 11	0 3½	—
		Liquores				
132	lb.	Liq. actææ rac. conc. (Hewlett)	—	4 9	1 4	0 3
38	lb.	Liq. acidi chromici	—	1 5	0 5	0 1
24	lb.	Liq. acriflavini B.P.C.	3 0	1 0	0 4	—
20	oz.	Liq. adrenalin. hydrochlor. P.I.(13)	—	—	2 11	0 5
20	lb.	Liq. aluminii acetatis	2 6	0 9	0 3	—
21	lb.	Liq. alumin. aceto-tart. ..	2 8	0 9	0 3	—
8.5	lb.	Liq. ammoniæ dil. P.II. (9)	1 2	0 4	0 1	—
9	lb.	Liq. ammon. fort. 0.888 P.II. (9)	1 2	0 4	0 2	—
10	lb.	Liq. ammon. fort. 0.880 P.II. (9)	1 3	0 5	0 2	—
11	lb.	Liq. ammonii acetatis dil. ..	1 5	0 5	0 2	—
15	lb.	Liq. ammon. acet. fort. ..	—	0 10	0 3	—
18	lb.	Liq. ammon. citratis	2 3	0 9	0 3	—

Li

Cost d.	per	Liquores—(cont.)	Selling Price 16 oz. s. d.	4 oz. s. d.	1 oz. s. d.	1 dr. s. d.
33	lb.	Liq. ammon. citr. fort. (1 to 3)	—	1 6	0 6	—
12	lb.	Liq. antim. chlor. coml. S.1. (5)	2 0	0 8	0 3	—
12	lb.	Liq. arsenicalis .. S.1. (5)	—	0 7	0 3	—
28	lb.	Liq. arsenii bromidi S.1. (5)	—	1 2	0 4	—
14	lb.	Liq. arsenici hydrochlor. S.1. (5)	—	0 9	0 3	—
24	lb.	Liq. arsen. et hydr. iodid. S.1. (5)	—	0 11	0 4	—
10	oz.	Liq. atropinæ sulphatis S.1. (5)	—	—	1 9	0 4
17	oz.	Liq. auri et arsen. brom. S.1. (5)	—	—	2 2	0 5
15	lb.	Liq. azonubri	—	—	0 2	0 1
30	lb.	Liq. bismuthi conc. B.P.C. ..	—	—	0 5	0 2
19	lb.	Liq. bismuthi et am. cit. ..	—	0 10	0 3	—
54	lb.	Liq. bismuthi (Schacht) ..	—	1 10	0 6	0 1
78	lb.	Liq. bromidi co. B.P.C. S.1. (5)	—	2 10	0 10	0 2
57	lb.	Liq. bromochloral co. B.P.C. S.1. (5)	—	2 0	0 7	—
4	lb.	Liq. calcii bisulphitis	0 7	0 3	—	—
9	lb.	Liq. calcii chloridi	1 2	0 4	0 2	—
21	gal.	Liq. calcii hydroxid.	pint	0 5	—	—
9	lb.	Liq. calcis chlorinatæ	1 2	0 5	0 2	—
9	lb.	Liq. calcis chlor. c. ac. bor. B.P.C.	1 0	0 4	—	—
11	lb.	Liq. calcis saccharatus	1 5	0 5	0 2	—
12	lb.	Liq. calcis sulphuratæ	1 6	0 6	0 2	—
66	lb.	Liq. caoutchouc	—	3 7	1 0	—
56	pt.	Liq. carb. deter. (Wright) unstd.	—	—	0 5	0 1
48	lb.	Liq. carmini	6 0	1 9	0 6	0 1
01	lb.	Liq. cauloph. et puls. co. (Oppenheimer)	—	3 9	1 0	—
84	lb.	Liq. cauloph. et pulsat. B.P.C.	—	3 0	0 10	0 2
15	lb.	Liq. chlori	2 0	0 8	—	—
32	lb.	Liq. cocci cact.	—	1 2	0 4	—
96	lb.	Liq. cocci cact. B.P.C.	—	3 5	1 0	—
75	lb.	Liq. cop. et buc. et cub. B.P.C.	—	2 9	0 10	0 2
13	lb.	Liq. cresolis sapon. P.II. (12)	2 1	1 1	0 4	—
13	oz.	Liq. epispasticus S.1. (5)	—	—	1 10	0 4
26	25 gm	Liq. ergosterol irrad.	—	0 2	per	mil
15	oz.	Liq. ethyl nitritis	—	—	2 0	0 4
10	oz.	Liq. euonymi	—	—	1 6	1 3
96	lb.	Liq. euonymi et cascaræ ..	—	3 9	1 0	0 2
66	lb.	Liq. euonymi et iridini ..	—	2 5	0 8	0 2
75	lb.	Liq. euonymini et papaini ..	—	2 9	0 10	0 2
51	lb.	Liq. euonymini et pepsini ..	—	2 0	0 7	0 1
97	lb.	Liq. euonymini et pepsini c̄ bis. co. (Oppenheimer)	—	3 9	1 0	—
20	lb.	Liq. ferri acetatis	—	1 0	0 4	—
72	lb.	Liq. ferri albuminatis B.P.C. ..	—	2 10	0 10	—
20	lb.	Liq. ferri dialysatus '85	—	0 10	0 3	—
66	lb	Liq. ferri peptonatis	—	2 6	0 9	—
10	lb	Liq. ferri perchloridi fortis ..	—	0 8	0 3	—
9	lb.	Liq. ferri perchloridi	—	0 6	0 2	—
13	lb.	Liq. ferri pernitratis	—	0 7	0 2	—
16	lb.	Liq. ferri persulphatis	—	0 9	0 3	—
11	lb.	Liq. formaldehydi P.II. (12)	1 6	0 6	0 2	—
48	lb.	Liq. formald. sapon. P.II. (12)	6 0	1 9	0 6	—
10	oz.	Liq. gutta-perch. B.P.C. P.I. (9)	—	—	2 10	—
11	oz.	Liq. glyceryl trinitratis P.I. (13)	—	—	1 8	0 3
21	lb.	Liq. hamamelidis	2 9	0 10	0 3	—
5	oz.	Liq. hydrarg. nitr. acidus S.1. (5)	—	—	1 3	0 3
9	lb.	Liq. hydrarg. perchloridi P.II. (10)	—	0 5	0 2	—
7	lb.	Liq. hydrogenii perox. 10 vol. ..	1 0	0 4	0 2	—
11	lb.	Liq. hydrogenii perox. 20 vol. ..	1 6	0 6	0 2	—
78	lb.	Liq. iodi. fortis	—	2 9	0 9	0 2
60	lb.	Liq. iodi. mitis	7 6	2 2	0 7	0 1
02	lb.	Liq. iodi. simp.	—	3 9	1 0	—
0.5	lb.	Liq. magnesii bicarbonatis ..	1 6	0 5	0 2	—
		Liq. magnesii bicarbonatis pkd.	℥vj.	1 0	—	—
10	oz.	Liq. morphinæ acetatis D.D.	—	—	1 6	0 3
13	oz.	Liq. morphinæ bimeconatis D.D.	—	—	1 11	0 4
10	oz.	Liq. morphinæ hydrochloridi D.D.	—	—	1 6	0 3

Cost d.	per	Liquores—(cont.)	Selling Price 16 oz. s. d.	4 oz. s. d.	1 oz. s. d.	1 dr. s. d.
10	oz.	Liq. morphinæ sulphatis D.D.	—	—	1 11	0 4
13	oz.	Liq. morphinæ tartratis D.D.	—	—	1 9	0 4
78	lb.	Liq. opii sedativus B.P.C. D.D.	—	2 9	0 9	0 2
84	lb.	Liq. opii sedativus P.L.F. D.D.	—	3 0	0 10	0 2
258	lb.	Liq. opii sed. (Battley) .. D.D.	—	8 6	2 5	0 5
78	lb.	Liq. pancreaticus P.L.F. ..	—	2 10	0 9	—
101	lb.	Liq. pancreat. (Benger) .. fl.	—	3 6	1 0	0 2
60	lb.	Liq. pancreatis	—	2 2	0 8	0 2
48	lb.	Liq. papaini et iridini B.P.C. ..	—	1 9	0 6	0 1
84	lb.	Liq. pepsini P.L.F.	—	2 2	0 9	0 2
84	lb.	Liq. pepsini et papaini	—	3 0	0 10	0 2
24	lb.	Liq. pepticus B.P.C.	—	0 11	0 3	—
120	lb.	Liq. pepticus (Benger)	—	3 9	1 0	0 2
96	lb.	Liq. picis carbonis	—	3 5	1 0	0 2
18	lb.	Liq. picis carbonis meth. ..	2 0	0 7	0 2	—
11	lb.	Liq. plumbi subacet. f t. P.I. (9)	1 9	0 7	0 2	—
4	lb.	Liq. plumbi subacetatis ..	0 6	0 2	0 1	—
10	lb.	Liq. potassæ	1 3	0 5	0 2	—
8.5	lb.	Liq. potassii permanganatis ..	1 1	0 4	0 2	—
50	lb.	Liq. quin. ammon.	—	1 9	0 6	0 1
75	lb.	Liq. quin. ammon. c. cinnam. ..	—	2 8	0 9	0 2
42	lb.	Liq. rhei dulcis P.L.F. ..	—	1 7	0 6	0 1
28	lb.	Liq. rosæ dulcis B.P.C. ..	—	1 0	0 4	0 1
63	lb.	Liq. sabal. co.	—	—	0 8	0 2
12	lb.	Liq. sacch. ust. B.P.C.	—	—	0 2	0 1
144	lb.	Liq. santali co. B.P.C. ..	—	5 2	1 4	—
120	lb.	Liq. santali co. P.L.F.	—	5 4	1 6	0 3
150	lb.	Liq. santali flav. c. buchu et cubeb. (Hewlett)	—	4 10	1 3	0 3
39	lb.	Liq. saponis æther meth. ..	4 9	1 4	0 5	—
114	lb.	Liq. sedans (P.D.)	—	3 9	1 0	0 2
30	lb.	Liq. sennæ dulcis	—	1 3	0 5	0 1
11	oz.	Liq. senecio co.	—	—	1 8	0 3
11	lb.	Liq. sodæ	1 6	0 6	0 2	—
11	lb.	Liq. sodæ chlorinatæ	1 6	0 6	0 2	—
11	lb.	Liq. sodæ chlor. c. ac. bor. B.P.C. (conc. 1-9)	—	1 5	0 6	0 1
11	lb.	Liq. sod. chlor. c. sod. bic. B.P.C. (conc. 1-9)	—	1 5	0 6	0 1
11	lb.	Liq. sod. chlor. chir.	1 6	0 6	—	—
15	lb.	Liq. sodii arsenatis S.1. (5)	—	0 7	0 3	—
4.5	lb.	Liq. sodii bisulphitis	0 7	0 3	0 1	—
26	oz.	Liq. sodii ethylatis	—	—	3 9	0 7
20	lb.	Liq. sodii phenatis co. P.II. (12)	—	0 9	0 3	—
30	lb.	Liq. strychninæ hydrochl. S.1. (5)	—	1 1	0 6	0 1
45	lb.	Liq. taraxaci	—	1 9	0 6	0 1
16	lb.	Liq. tartrazin co.	—	—	0 2	0 1
30	lb.	Liq. thymol. co.	3 6	1 1	0 4	—
90	lb.	Liq. trinitrophenolis P.I. (12)	11 3	3 2	—	—
76	lb.	Liq. trypsin.	—	—	0 10	0 2
9	oz.	Liq. viburni prunif. co. ..	—	—	1 4	0 3
30	lb.	Liq. zinci chloridi pur. ..	—	1 4	0 5	—
12	lb.	Liq. zinci chloridi coml. ..	2 2	0 8	—	—
36	14 oz.	Listerine, unstd.	—	1 4	0 4	—
33	oz.	Lithii acetylsalicylas	—	—	4 10	0 9
14	oz.	Lithii benzoas	—	—	2 0	0 4
16	oz.	Lithii bromidum	—	—	2 4	0 4
15	oz.	Lithii carbonas	—	—	2 3	0 4
11	oz.	Lithii citras	—	—	1 8	0 3
45	lb.	Lithii citras effervescens ..	—	1 8	0 6	—
39	oz.	Lithii glycerophos.	—	—	5 9	0 10
40	oz.	Lithii guaiacas	—	—	5 10	0 10
45	oz.	Lithii hippuras	—	—	6 7	1 1
22	oz.	Lithii iodidum	—	—	3 3	0 6
24	oz.	Lithii lactas	—	—	3 9	0 7
14	oz.	Lithii salicylas	—	—	2 0	0 4
15	oz.	Lithii sulphas	—	—	2 3	0 4
240	24v.	Liver extract (P. D. & Co.) ..	each	26 8	—	—

Cost		Lo—Ma	Selling Price			
d.	per		16 oz. s. d.	4 oz. s. d.	1 oz. s. d.	1 dr. s. d.
39	lb.	Lobelia pkts. P.I. (8)	—	1 5	0 5	—
30	lb.	Lobeliæ pulvis P.I. (8)	—	1 1	0 4	—
8	lb.	Lotio acidi borici 1 in 32	1 0	0 6	0 2	—
12	lb.	Lotio ac. carbol. rub. 5p.c. P.II. (12)	1 8	0 7	0 3	—
16	lb.	Lotio calaminæ B.P.C.	2 0	0 7	0 2	—
222	lb.	Lotio crinalis B.P.C.	—	8 0	2 2	0 4
15	lb.	Lotio hydrarg. flav. P.I. (12)	2 3	0 10	0 3	—
15	lb.	Lotio hydrarg. nig. P.I. (12)	2 3	0 8	0 3	—
8.5	lb.	Lotio hyd. perch. 1 in 1,000 P.II. (12)	1 2	0 4	0 2	—
14	lb.	Lotio plumbi c. opio P.I. (12)	1 9	0 6	—	—
44	lb.	Lotio resorcin. composita	6 0	1 9	0 6	—
15	lb.	Lotio rubra	2 0	0 7	—	—
8	lb.	Lot. plumbi	1 0	0 4	—	—
115	oz.	Luminal ℞ only	—	—	—	2 6
72	100	Luminal tablets gr. 1½ ℞ only	doz.	1 2	—	—
126	oz.	Luminal, sodium ℞ only	—	—	—	3 0
18	oz.	Lupulinum	—	—	2 8	0 5
36	lb.	Lupulus	4 6	1 4	0 5	—
11	oz.	Lycopodium	—	—	1 8	0 3
5	ea.	Lymph. calf	ea.	0 8	—	—
13	lb.	Lysol P.II. (12)	1 10	1 1	0 4	—
		M				
60	lb.	Macis opt.	7 6	2 2	0 8	—
48	lb.	Macis opt. parv.	5 9	1 9	0 6	—
60	lb.	Macidis pulvis opt.	7 6	2 2	0 8	—
48	lb.	Madder	6 0	1 9	0 6	—
22	50	Magisal tab. (Martindale)	doz.	0 9	—	—
		Magnesium				
34	lb.	Magnesia levis	4 3	1 3	0 5	—
44	lb.	Magnesia ponderosa	5 8	1 8	0 6	—
84	lb.	Magnes. boro-citras	—	3 0	0 10	0 2
13	lb.	Magnes. carbonas levis	1 8	0 7	0 2	—
15	lb.	Magnes. carbonas ponderosus	1 10	0 7	0 2	—
84	lb.	Magnes. citras (ver.)	—	3 0	0 10	0 2
21	lb.	Magnes. cit. gran. efferv.	2 9	0 9	0 3	—
		Magnes. cit. eff. opt. pkd.	—	1 0	8 oz.	1 9
19	lb.	Magnes. cit. gran. eff. sec.	2 6	0 9	0 3	—
8	oz.	Magnes. formas	—	—	1 2	0 2
14	oz.	Magnes. glycerophosphas	—	—	2 0	0 4
33	lb.	Magnes. hydroxidum	—	1 3	0 5	0 1
13	oz.	Magnes. hypophosphis	—	—	2 0	0 4
11	oz.	Magnes. lactas	—	—	1 8	0 3
9	oz.	Magnes. peroxidum 15%	—	—	1 4	0 3
4	oz.	Magnes. phosph. acid	—	—	0 7	0 1
39	lb.	Magnes. phosphas	—	1 5	0 5	0 1
12	oz.	Magnes. salicylas	—	—	1 9	0 3
48	lb.	Magnes. silicas pur. precip.	—	1 9	0 6	0 1
4	lb.	Magnes. sulphas opt.	0 6	0 3	0 1	—
		Magnes. sulphas opt. pkd.	—	0 4	0 2	—
5	lb.	Magnes. sulphas (Howards)	0 8	0 4	0 2	—
7	lb.	Magnes. sulphatis pulvis	1 0	0 4	0 2	—
10	lb.	Magnes. sulphatis pulvis exsicc.	1 3	0 5	0 2	—
5	lb.	Magnes. sulphatis pulvis color.	0 9	0 3	—	—
8	lb.	Magnes. sulphatis pulvis exsicc.	1 0	0 4	0 2	—
5	lb.	Magnes. sulphatis pulvis color.	0 9	0 3	—	—
312	cwt.	Magnes. sulphas color.	7 lb.	2 5	14 lb.	4 4
3	lb.	Magnes. sulphas coml.	0 5	0 2	—	—
40	cwt.	Magnes. sulphas coml.	7 lb.	2 0	14 lb.	3 6
27	lb.	Magnes. sulphas efferv.	3 5	1 0	0 4	—
14	oz.	Magnesium (powder)	—	—	2 0	0 4
21	oz.	Magnesium (ribbon)	foot	0 3	2 9	—
24	16 oz.	Magneslait (D.F.)	bot.	1 3	0 4	—
15	oz.	Malachite green	—	—	2 3	0 4
30	oz.	Maltose	—	—	4 5	0 8
36	lb.	Mangan. carbonas	—	—	0 5	0 1

Cost		Ma—Mi	Selling Price			
d.	per		16 oz. s. d.	4 oz. s. d.	1 oz. s. d.	1 dr. s. d.
21	lb.	Mangani chloridum	—	0 8	0 3	—
22	oz.	Mangani glycerophosphas	—	—	3 3	0 6
11	oz.	Mangani hypophosphis	—	—	1 8	0 3
8	lb.	Mangani oxidum nig. coml.	1 0	0 4	0 2	—
9	lb.	Mangani oxidum nig. gran.	1 2	0 4	0 2	—
7	oz.	Mangani peroxidum pur. præcip.	—	—	1 1	0 2
24	lb.	Mangani sulphas	—	0 11	0 3	—
20	lb.	Mange dressing P.L.F.	2 6	0 9	—	—
144	lb.	Manna elect. nov.	—	5 0	1 5	0 3
15	oz.	Mannite	—	—	2 3	0 4
72	lb.	Maranta Bermuda ver.	9 0	2 7	0 9	0 2
39	lb.	Maranta Bermuda	4 11	1 5	0 5	—
24	lb.	Maranta St. Vincent opt.	3 0	0 11	0 3	—
18	lb.	Maranta St. Vincent sec.	2 3	0 9	0 3	—
180	lb.	Marking ink P.L.F.	—	—	1 9	0 4
12	lb.	Marrubium sicc.	1 6	0 6	0 2	—
14	lb.	Marylebone cream	1 9	0 7	—	—
66	lb.	Mastich. elect.	—	2 5	0 9	0 2
14	lb.	Maw seed	1 9	0 6	0 2	—
114	oz.	Medinal ℞ only	—	—	—	2 4
129	100	Medinal tablets gr. 5 ℞ only	doz.	2 4	—	—
192	100	Medinal tablets gr. 7½ ℞ only	doz.	3 6	—	—
18	lb.	Mel Ang.	2 3	0 8	0 3	—
14	lb.	Mel Calif.	1 9	0 7	0 2	—
12	lb.	Mel Jam.	1 6	0 6	0 2	—
14	lb.	Mel New Zealand	1 9	0 7	—	—
10	lb.	Mel W.I.	1 3	0 5	0 2	—
16	lb.	Mel boracis	2 0	0 7	0 3	—
15	lb.	Mel depuratum	2 0	0 7	0 3	—
24	lb.	Mel rosæ	—	0 11	0 4	—
16	lb.	Mentha pulegium	2 0	0 7	0 2	—
25	oz.	Menthol	—	—	3 8	0 7
14	oz.	Menthol, synthetic	—	—	2 0	0 4
42	oz.	Menthol cones (4 to oz.)	ea.	1 6	—	—
45	oz.	Menthol cones (8 to oz.)	ea.	0 10	—	—
18	oz.	Menthol snuff	—	—	2 8	0 5
126	oz.	Menthol camphoras	—	—	—	3 0
60	oz.	Menthol valerianas	—	—	—	1 3
12	lb.	Mercurial cream wgt.	—	—	1 6	0 4
60	10c.c.	Mercurochrome solut. S.1. (6)	per	c.c.	0 11	—
48	16 oz.	Metatone (P. D. Co.)	6 0	8 oz.	3 6	—
24	oz.	Methylacetanilidum P.I. (8)	—	—	3 6	0 6
18	oz.	Methyl orange	—	—	2 9	0 6
96	lb.	Methyl orange sol.	—	3 6	1 0	—
30	lb.	Methyl salicylas	—	1 2	0 5	0 1
36	oz.	Methylsulphonal ℞ only	—	—	5 3	0 9
26	oz.	Methylthionin chlor.	—	—	3 9	0 7
18	oz.	Metol	—	—	2 3	0 4
18	lb.	Mezerei cortex	—	0 8	0 3	—
18	20	Migranine tablets gr. 5½	doz.	1 8	—	—
		Misturæ				
8.5	lb.	Mistura alba	1 0	0 5	0 2	—
120	lb.	Mist. ammoniaci co. conc. (1 to 7)	—	4 3	1 2	0 2
15	lb.	Mist. amygdalæ	2 0	0 7	0 2	—
54	lb.	Mist. bism. c. morph. P.I. (13)	7 0	2 1	0 8	—
30	lb.	Mist. bism. co. B.P.C. P.I. (13)	4 0	1 2	0 4	—
42	lb.	Mist. bis. co. c.p. B.P.C. P.I. (13)	—	1 8	0 6	—
123	16 oz.	Mist. bismuthi (Seller) fl.	—	3 10	1 0	0 2
36	lb.	Mist. carminativa B.P.C., 1923	4 6	1 4	0 5	—
14	lb.	Mist. cascaræ co. B.P.C.	1 10	0 7	0 2	—
18	lb.	Mist. chlori B.P.C.	2 6	0 9	0 3	—
22	lb.	Mist. chlorof. co. B.P.C. P.I. (13)	2 10	0 10	0 3	—
26	lb.	Mist. creosoti conc.	—	—	1 1	0 2
20	lb.	Mist. cretæ co. B.P.C.	2 9	0 9	—	—
28	lb.	Mist. diarrhœa (B. of H.) P.L.F. P.I. (13)	3 6	1 0	0 4	—
38	lb.	Mist. ferri aromatica	5 0	1 7	0 5	—

Mi—Oc

Cost d.	per	Misturæ—(cont.)	Selling Price 16 oz. s. d.	4 oz. s. d.	1 oz. s. d.	1 dr. s. d.
26	lb.	Mist. ferri composita	3 3	1 0	0 4	—
18	lb.	Mist. (gripe) P.L.F.	—	℥ viij.	1 3	—
27	lb.	Mist. guaiaci	3 4	1 0	0 4	—
36	lb.	Mist. (influenza) P.L.F.	—	℥ viij.	2 6	—
16	lb.	Mist. magnesii hydroxidi	2 7	0 9	0 3	—
24	lb.	Mist. olei ricini	3 0	1 0	0 3	—
30	lb.	Mist. pepsini co. P.I. (13)	4 0	1 3	0 5	—
150	lb.	Mist. pepsini et bis. (Hewlett)	—	5 5	1 7	—
14	lb.	Mist. sennæ co.	2 1	0 7	0 2	—
150	lb.	Mist. senecio. co. (Hewlett)	—	5 5	1 7	—
42	lb.	Mist. tonic sedat. (Hewlett)	—	1 6	0 6	—
33	lb.	Mist. tussi rub. (Hewlett) P.I. (13)	—	1 3	0 4	—
126	lb.	Mist. veronigen co. (Hewlett) ℞ only	—	4 5	1 3	—
36	lb.	Mithridate (vet.) P.L.F.	4 6	1 4	—	—
18	75 g.	Mitigal liquid	—	each	2 0	—
87	dr.	Morphina pur. D.D.	per	gr.	0 4	12 7
69	dr.	Morphinæ acetas D.D.	per	gr.	0 4	10 1
69	dr.	Morphinæ hydrochloridum D.D.	per	gr.	0 4	10 1
69	dr.	Morphinæ sulphas D.D.	per	gr.	0 4	10 1
87	dr.	Morphinæ tartras D.D.	per	gr.	0 4	12 7
360	dr.	Moschus Chin. in gran.	per	gr.	1 2	—
27	oz.	Moschus artificial.	—	—	4 0	0 8
22	lb.	Mucilago acaciæ	2 9	0 10	0 3	—
18	lb.	Mucilago tragacanthæ	2 3	0 9	0 3	—
30	lb.	Mustard F	3 9	1 2	0 5	—
36	lb.	Mustard D.S.F.	4 6	1 3	0 5	—
7	lb.	Mustard bran	0 10½	0 4	—	—
40	lb.	Myristicæ 64's	—	1 5	0 5	—
32	lb.	Myristicæ 80's	—	1 2	0 4	—
26	lb.	Myristicæ pulvis	—	0 11	0 3	—
84	lb.	Myrrh. elect.	—	3 0	0 10	0 2
48	lb.	Myrrh. sorts	—	1 9	0 6	0 1
36	lb.	Myrrh. sorts, parv.	4 6	1 4	0 4	0 1
66	lb.	Myrrh. pulv. opt.	—	2 5	0 9	—
30	lb.	Myrrh. pulv. sec. (vet.)	3 9	1 2	—	—
		N				
14	pt.	Naphtha solvent	pint	1 9	—	—
48	lb.	Naphthalin. pur.	—	1 9	0 6	—
7	lb	Naphthalin. coml. flake	0 11	0 3	0 1	—
7	lb.	Naphthal. coml. glob.	0 11	0 3	0 1	—
30	oz.	Naphthalin tetrachlor.	—	—	4 5	0 8
6	oz.	Naphthol (beta)	—	—	0 11	0 2
24	oz.	Naphthol salicyl.	—	—	3 6	0 6
23	dr.	Narcotina	—	—	—	3 5
26	25	Neo-bornyval perles	doz.	1 9	ea.	3 6
99	oz.	Neo-protosil	—	—	—	1 7
39	4 oz.	Nepenthe D.D.	—	5 0	1 4	0 3
42	lb.	Nessler's solution	—	1 8	0 6	—
36	lb.	Nickel chloridum	—	1 4	0 5	—
12	lb.	Nickel sulphas coml.	1 3	0 5	0 2	—
21	oz.	Nicotina coml. S.1. P.II. (4)	—	—	3 1	0 6
162	lb.	Nicotine fumigant P.L.F. S.1. (6)	—	—	1 8	—
16	lb.	Nitrobenzenum P.II. (8)	—	0 7	0 2	—
58	oz.	Novalgin pulv.	—	—	8 6	1 3
18	25 t.	Novalgin tabs.	—	2 6	tube	—
18	gm.	Novocain S.1. (4)	per	gr.	0 3	—
22	lb.	Nucis vomicæ pulvis S.1. (5)	2 9	1 0	0 4	0 1
21	lb.	Nux vomic. pulverata S.1. (5)	—	—	0 4	0 1
		O				
4	oz.	Oculentum acidi borici	—	—	0 6	0 1
72	doz.	Oculenta in tubes	—	1 0	each	—
14	oz.	Oculent. atropinæ S.1. (5)	—	—	2 0	0 4
6	oz.	Oculent. flavum P.I. (9)	—	—	0 10	0 2
10	oz.	Oculent. flav. c. atrop. S.1. (5)	—	—	1 6	0 4

Oc—Ol

Cost d.	per		Selling Price 16 oz. s. d.	4 oz. s. d.	1 oz. s. d.	1 dr. s. d.
12	oz.	Oculent. physostigminæ S.1. (5)	—	—	1 6	0 4
30	oz.	Oleo-resin cubebæ	—	—	4 5	0 9
		Olea				
66	lb.	Oleum abietis	—	2 6	0 8	0 2
24	lb.	Ol. adipis	—	0 11	0 3	—
150	dr.	Ol. allii	per	min.	0 6	—
60	oz.	Ol. amygd. Ang. ess. s.a.p.	—	—	8 6	1 3
51	lb.	Ol. amygdalæ Ang.	—	1 10	0 7	—
48	lb.	Ol. amygdæ dulc. exot.	6 0	1 9	0 6	—
21	oz.	Ol. anethi Ang.	—	—	3 1	0 6
252	oz.	Ol. angelicæ rad.	—	—	—	5 2
84	gal.	Ol. animale	1 3	0 5	0 2	—
60	lb.	Ol. anisi	—	2 2	0 7	0 1
30	dr.	Ol. anthemidis	per	min.	0 1	4 5
57	oz.	Ol. apii	—	—	8 4	1 3
13	lb.	Ol. arachis	1 8	0 7	0 2	—
18	lb.	Ol. arachis pallid	2 3	0 8	0 3	—
20	oz.	Ol. aurantii amari	—	—	—	0 5
17	oz.	Ol. aurantii dulcis	—	—	—	0 5
36	oz.	Ol. aurantii tangierin	—	—	—	0 9
17	oz.	Ol. bergamottæ	—	—	2 6	0 5
30	lb.	Ol. cadinum	—	1 1	0 4	0 1
6	oz.	Ol. cajuputi	—	—	1 1	0 2
27	oz.	Ol. calam. arom.	—	—	4 0	0 7
24	lb.	Ol. camphoræ ess. alb.	—	0 11	0 3	—
36	lb.	Ol. camphoræ ess. fusc.	—	1 4	0 5	—
27	oz.	Ol. canangæ	—	—	4 0	0 7
19	lb.	Ol. carbolicum 5 % P.II. (9)	2 3	0 8	0 3	—
17	lb.	Ol. carbol. (vet.) 5% P.II. (9)	2 0	0 7	—	—
21	oz.	Ol. cari exot.	—	—	3 0	0 5
9	oz.	Ol. caryophylli	—	—	1 4	0 3
9	oz.	Ol. cassiæ	—	—	1 4	0 3
14	oz.	Ol. cedri ligni (micros.)	—	—	2 0	0 4
51	lb.	Ol. cedri ligni	—	1 11	0 7	0 1
54	gal.	Ol. cetacei	0 11	0 4	0 2	—
6	oz.	Ol. chaulmoogræ	—	—	1 0	0 2
16	oz.	Ol. chenopodii	—	—	2 4	0 4
8	oz.	Ol. cinereum	—	—	2 4	0 4
54	oz.	Ol. cinnamomi	—	—	—	1 2
10	oz.	Ol. cinnamomi fol.	—	—	1 6	0 3
4	oz.	Ol. citronellæ	—	—	0 7	0 1
12	lb.	Ol. cocois nuciferæ	1 6	0 6	0 3	—
52	gal.	Ol. colzæ (quantity)	gal.	6 6	pint	0 11
7	oz.	Ol. copaibæ	—	—	1 1	0 2
48	oz.	Ol. coriandri Ang.	—	—	—	1 0
27	oz.	Ol. coriandri exot.	—	—	—	0 7
14	oz.	Ol. crotonis P.I. (8)	—	—	2 0	0 4
24	oz.	Ol. cubebæ Ang.	—	—	3 6	0 6
26	lb.	Ol. eucalypti	3 3	1 0	0 4	—
24	lb.	Ol. eucalypti amygdalæ	—	0 11	0 4	—
11	oz.	Ol. eucalypti citriodoræ	—	—	1 8	0 3
54	lb.	Ol. eucalypti glob.	—	2 0	0 8	—
54	oz.	Ol. fœniculi Ang.	—	—	—	1 4
14	oz.	Ol. fœniculi exot.	—	—	2 0	0 4
14	oz.	Ol. gaultheriæ	—	—	2 0	0 4
36	oz.	Ol. geranii Afric.	—	—	5 3	0 9
18	oz.	Ol. geranii E.I.	—	—	2 8	0 5
54	oz.	Ol. geranii Gall.	—	—	8 0	1 2
66	gal.	Ol. gossypii sem.	1 0	0 4	0 2	—
27	lb.	Ol. gurgun.	—	1 0	0 4	—
30	oz.	Ol. hippoglossi	—	—	4 5	0 8
5	oz.	Ol. hydnocarp.	—	—	0 9	0 2
90	dr.	Ol. iridis concret.	—	—		13 2
13	oz.	Ol. jasmini	—	—	2 0	0 4
48	oz.	Ol. juniperi bacc. Ang.	—	—	7 0	1 0
8	oz.	Ol. juniperi bacc. exot.	—	—	1 2	0 2

Ol

Cost d.	per	Olea—(cont.)	Selling Price 16 oz. s. d.	4 oz. s. d.	1 oz. s. d.	1 dr. s. d.
60	lb.	Ol. juniperi ligni	—	2 2	0 7	0 1
114	oz.	Ol. lavandulæ Ang.	—	—	—	2 4
46	oz.	Ol. lavandulæ ab flor.	—	—	6 9	1 0
52	oz.	Ol. lavandulæ redist.	—	—	7 7	1 1
312	lb.	Ol. lavandulæ Gall.	—	—	3 2	0 6
144	lb.	Ol. lavandulæ spic. ver. ..	—	5 2	1 6	0 3
96	lb.	Ol. lavandulæ spic. coml. ..	—	3 2	1 0	0 2
36	oz.	Ol. limettæ dest.	—	—	5 3	0 9
120	oz.	Ol. limettæ (hand pressed) ..	—	—	—	2 6
16	oz.	Ol. limonis	—	—	2 4	0 4
15	oz.	Ol. limonis (Messina)	—	—	2 3	0 4
36	oz.	Ol. linaloes	—	—	4 6	0 10
51	gal.	Ol. lini opt.	pint	0 10	0 2	—
54	gal.	Ol. lini (boiled)	pint	0 11	0 2	—
36	gal.	Ol. lini (cattle)	pint	0 8	gal.	4 6
174	dr.	Ol. lupuli Ang.	per	min.	0 5	—
15	oz.	Ol. marjoram	—	—	2 3	0 4
144	lb.	Ol. menthæ Jap. (dementh.) ..	—	5 0	1 5	0 2
78	oz.	Ol. menthæ pip. (Mitcham) ..	—	—	—	1 8
240	lb.	Ol. menthæ pip. redest. ..	—	8 6	2 6	0 5
100	oz.	Ol. menthæ vir. Ang.	—	—	—	2 6
20	oz.	Ol. menthæ vir. exot.	—	—	2 10	0 6
96	gal.	Ol. morrhuæ (British)	1 4	0 6	0 2	—
102	gal.	Ol. morrhuæ (Newfl.)	1 6	0 7	0 2	—
108	gal.	Ol. morrhuæ (Nor.)	1 6	0 7	0 2	—
66	gal.	Ol. morrhuæ (vet.)	pint	1 0	gal.	8 6
13	oz.	Ol. myricæ acris ess.	—	—	2 0	0 4
17	oz.	Ol. myristicæ Ang.	—	—	2 6	0 5
12	oz.	Ol. myristicæ exot.	—	—	1 9	0 3
16	oz.	Ol. myristicæ express.	—	—	2 4	0 4
16	lb.	Ol. neatsfoot	2 0	0 7	0 2	—
63	dr.	Ol. neroli	per	min.	0 3	—
54	dr.	Ol. neroli Ital.	per	min.	0 2	—
60	oz.	Ol. neroli synth.	—	—	—	1 3
150	gal.	Ol. olivæ (cream)	2 1	0 7	0 2	—
132	gal.	Ol. olivæ (sublime)	1 10	0 7	0 2	—
114	gal.	Ol. olivæ (fine)	1 7	0 6	0 2	—
13	oz.	Ol. origani alb.	—	—	1 8	0 4
72	lb.	Ol. origani coml.	—	2 7	0 9	0 2
15	lb.	Ol. palmæ	2 0	0 7	0 2	—
22	oz.	Ol. palmarosæ	—	—	3 3	0 6
27	oz.	Ol. patchouli	—	—	—	0 7
30	lb.	Ol. persicæ Ang.	3 9	1 2	0 4	—
38	lb.	Ol. persicæ Ang. pall.	4 8	1 5	0 5	—
18	oz.	Ol. petitgrain	—	—	2 8	0 5
13	oz.	Ol. phosphoratum	—	—	1 11	0 4
12	lb.	Ol. picis	1 6	0 6	0 2	—
16	lb.	Ol. picis rectificatum	2 0	0 7	0 3	—
14	oz.	Ol. pimentæ exot.	—	—	—	0 4
13	oz.	Ol. pini pumilionis	—	—	2 0	0 4
90	lb.	Ol. pini sylvestris fact.	—	—	0 11	0 2
144	lb.	Ol. pini (spruce)	—	5 2	1 6	0 3
42	oz.	Ol. piperis	—	—	5 0	1 0
100	oz.	Ol. pulegii Ang.	—	—	14 0	2 5
108	lb.	Ol. pulegii exot.	—	4 0	1 1	0 2
66	gal.	Ol. rapii	1 0	0 4	0 2	—
36	oz.	Ol. rhodii (fact.)	—	—	5 3	0 9
20	lb.	Ol. ricini Ital. insip.	2 6	0 9	0 3	—
13	lb.	Ol. ricini (first)	1 8	0 7	0 4	—
10	lb.	Ol. ricini (cattle)	1 4	0 6	—	—
84	gal.	Ol. ricini (cattle)	pint	1 6	gal.	10 6
48	lb.	Ol. ricini aromaticum	—	1 9	0 6	—
60	lb.	Ol. rosæ color.	—	2 2	0 7	—
180	oz.	Ol. rosmarini Ang.	—	—	—	4 4
45	lb.	Ol. rosmarini exot.	—	1 7	0 6	0 1
66	lb.	Ol. rosmarini super.	—	2 5	0 9	0 2
90	lb.	Ol. rosmarini Gall.	—	3 2	0 11	0 2
27	lb.	Ol. rusci B.P.C.	—	1 0	0 4	—

Ol—Pa

Cost d.	per	Olea—(cont.)	Selling Price 16 oz. s. d.	4 oz. s. d.	1 oz. s. d.	1 dr. s. d.
84	lb.	Ol. rusci ver.	—	3 0	0 10	0 2
22	oz.	Ol. rutæ	—	—	3 3	0 6
16	oz.	Ol. sabinæ .. ..S.I. (4)	—	—	—	2 4
9	oz.	Ol. salviæ	—	—	1 4	0 3
18	lb.	Ol. sambuci viride	2 3	0 8	0 3	—
26	oz.	Ol. santal. Aust.	—	—	3 9	0 7
36	oz.	Ol. santali flav. Ang.	—	—	5 3	0 9
33	oz.	Ol. santali flav. E.I.	—	—	4 10	0 9
9	oz.	Ol. sassafras nat.	—	—	1 4	0 3
		Ol. sassaf. artif. (v. Safrol.) ..				
12	lb.	Ol. sesami	1 6	0 6	0 2	—
12	lb.	Ol. sinapis expressum	1 6	0 6	0 2	—
30	oz.	Ol. sinapis volatile	—	—	4 5	0 8
11	oz.	Ol. staphisagriæ S.I. (4)	—	—	1 8	0 3
22	oz.	Ol. staphisagriæ (æther.) ..	—	—	3 3	0 7
20	lb.	Ol. succini rectificatum ..	—	0 9	0 3	—
72	gal.	Ol. terebinthinæ	pint	1 2	0 2	—
21	lb.	Ol. terebinthinæ rectificatum ..	2 5	0 9	0 3	—
30	lb.	Ol. theobromatis opt.	3 9	1 1	0 4	0 1
12	oz.	Ol. thymi alb.	—	—	1 9	0 3
108	lb.	Ol. thymi	—	3 10	1 0	—
10	oz.	Ol. thymi rub.	—	—	1 6	0 3
66	gal.	Ol. "train" opt.	pint	1 0	—	—
6	oz.	Ol. verbenæ	—	—	0 11	0 2
42	oz.	Ol. vetivert	—	—	—	1 0
78	gal.	Ol. "whale" opt.	pint	1 3	—	—
72	oz.	Ol. ylang-ylang	—	—	—	1 7
28	lb.	Olibanum	—	1 1	0 4	0 1
43	gm.	Omnopon pdr. (Roche) D.D	per	gr.	0 6	—
27	20	Omnopon tabs. .. .. D.D.	doz.	2 0	—	—
28	oz.	Opium Turc. .. .. D.D.	—	—	4 1	0 7
30	oz.	Opii pulv. .. .. D.D.	—	—	4 5	0 8
60	5 gm.	Opoidine .. .. D.D.	per	gr.	0 5	—
50	100	Opoidine tablets gr. ⅛ .. D.D.	doz.	1 0	—	—
21	oz.	Optannin	—	—	—	0 6
11	20	Optannin tablets gr. 7½ ..	doz.	0 10	—	—
96	oz.	Orthocaina .. ..P.I. (8)	—	—	—	2 0
99	oz.	Orthoform. .. . P.I. (8)	—	—	—	2 2
24	lb.	Ossis sepiæ (medium)	3 0	0 11	0 3	—
27	lb.	Ossis sepiæ pulv. subtil. ..	3 4	1 0	0 4	—
150	dr.	Otto rosæ (virgin)	per	min.	0 5	—
30	dr.	Otto rosæ (synthetic)	per	min.	0 2	4 5
15	lb.	Oxymel	2 3	0 8	0 3	—
26	lb.	Oxymel ipecacuanhæ	3 10	1 2	0 4	—
12	lb.	Oxymel scillæ	2 3	0 8	0 3	—
24	oz.	Oxyquinolin. sulph. (ortho.) ..	—	—	3 9	0 7
		P				
67	10c.c.	Padutin	0 10	per	c.c.	—
18	oz.	Pancreatini	—	—	2 8	0 5
42	oz.	Papainum	—	—	6 4	0 10
69	dr.	Papaverina .. . S.I. (4)	per	gr.	0 4	—
69	dr.	Papaverin. sulph. ..S.I.(4)	per	gr.	0 4	—
132	100	Papaveris capsulæ Ang. P.I. (8)	ea.	0 3	—	—
12	lb.	Papaveris capsulæ cont. P.I. (8)	1 9	0 6	—	—
18	20	Paracodin tablets	doz.	1 7	—	—
8	lb.	Paraffinum durum	1 0	0 4	0 2	—
10	lb.	Paraffinum liquidum	1 4	0 6	0 2	—
		Paraffinum liquidum, pkd. ..	—	0 10	℥xij.	2 4
8	lb.	Paraffinum liquidum flavum ..	1 0	0 4	0 2	—
13	lb.	Paraffinum molle album ..	1 8	0 7	0 2	—
17	lb.	Paraffinum molle album ..	1-lb.	tins	2 2	—
8	lb.	Paraffinum molle flavum ..	1 0	0 4	0 2	—
11	lb.	Paraffinum molle flavum ..	1-lb.	tins	1 5	—
10	lb.	Paraffinum (toilet)	1 3	0 5	0 2	—
4	oz.	Paraformaldehydum	—	—	0 7	0 1
4	oz.	Paraldehydum	—	—	0 7	0 1

Cost d.	Cost per	Pa—Pi	Selling Price 16 oz. s. d.	4 oz. s. d.	1 oz. s. d.	1 dr. s. d.
18	oz.	Paramidophenol hyd.	—	—	2 3	0 6
34	lb.	Parenol (alb.) B.P.C.	4 0	1 2	0 4	—
44	lb.	Parenol liq. (alb.) B.P.C. ..	5 6	1 7	0 5	—
96	lb.	Parogenum B.P.C.	—	2 0	0 7	—
66	lb.	Parogenum iodi B.P.C. ..	—	2 5	0 8	0 2
41	lb.	Parolein (B.W.)	5 0	1 3	0 4	0 1
14	oz.	Pasta bismuthi et iodoformi ..	—	—	2 0	0 4
15	lb.	Pasta zinci ox. co.	2 0	0 7	0 2	—
22	lb.	Pasta zinci et gelat. B.P.C. ..	2 9	0 10	0 3	—
30	lb.	Pasta zinci et ichtham. B.P.C.	3 11	1 1	0 4	—
60	lb.	Pastilles, fumigating	—	2 2	0 8	—
95	100	Pavon tablets .. .. D.D.	doz.	1 6	—	—
6	gr.	Pelletierinæ tannas ..S.I. (4)	per	gr.	1 0	—
102	lb.	Pepsencia (Fairchild)	—	3 6	1 0	0 2
66	8 oz.	Pepsin. c. bism. co. (Schacht) ..	—	4 1	1 1	0 2
66	8 oz.	Pepsin. liquid. (Schacht) ..	—	4 1	1 1	0 2
16	oz.	Pepsinum porci	—	—	2 4	0 4
17	oz.	Pepsin. (scale)	—	—	2 6	0 5
64	8 oz.	Peptenzyme elixir unstd. ..	—	4 0	1 0	0 2
64	oz.	Peptenzyme pwdr., unstd. ..	—	—	7 4	1 1
17	oz.	Peptonum siccum	—	—	2 6	0 5
58	5.0	Percaine crystals, vials S.I. (4)	1 gm.	2 0	—	—
58	10	Percaine 1,200 amps. S.I. (6)	6 6	per	box	—
42	lb.	Perichthol	5 3	1 6	0 6	0 1
33	lb.	Petroleum leve.	3 9	1 0	0 4	—
6	oz.	Phenacetinum	—	—	0 11	0 2
57	oz.	Phenalgin unstd. P.I. (13)	—	—	—	1 5
51	oz.	Phenalgin tbs. gr. 5 unstd. P.I. (13)	doz.	1 0	—	—
13	oz.	Phenazonum	—	—	1 11	0 4
22	oz.	Phenazonum caff. cit.	—	—	3 3	0 6
20	oz.	Phenazoni salicylas	—	—	2 11	0 5
36	oz.	Phenobarbital .. ..℞ only	—	—	—	0 9
36	oz.	Phenobarbital, solubile ..℞ only	—	—	—	0 9
63	oz.	Phenocoli hydrochloridum ..	—	—	8 0	1 6
26	lb.	Phenol cryst. .. ..P.I. (8)	3 3	1 0	0 4	0 1
72	lb.	Phenol (iodised) P.II. (9)	—	—	0 9	0 2
19	lb.	Phenol. liquefact. . P.I. (9)	—	0 9	0 3	—
16	lb.	Phenol 2% alcoholic P.II. (10)	2 0	0 7	0 2	—
7	oz.	Phenolphthaleinum	—	—	1 1	0 2
26	oz.	Phenylenediaminæ hyd. ..	—	—	3 9	0 7
24	oz.	Phenylhydrazinæ hydroch. ..	—	—	3 6	0 8
10	gm.	Phloroglucin.	per	gr.	0 2	—
8	oz.	Phosphorus, amorph.	—	—	1 1	0 3
8	oz.	Phosphorus, yellow P.I. (8)	—	—	1 1	0 3
8	gr.	Physostigmin. sal. S.I. (4)	per	gr.	1 2	—
62	25 gm	Phytin	—	—	9 3	1 9
67.5	100	Phytin tablets	doz.	1 0	—	—
84	oz.	Phytolaccinum	—	—	12 4	2 0
60	dr.	Picrotoxinum .. . S.I. (4)	—	—	—	8 0
9	lb.	Pig powders P.L.F. I. S.I. (11)	—	½-oz.	3d. ea.	—
19	lb.	Pig powders P.L.F. II. S.I. (11)	2 6	0 9	0 3	—
48	lb.	Pigmentum aconiti co. meth. . S.I. (5)	—	—	0 7	0 1
60	lb.	Pig. caseini B.P.C.	—	2 3	0 7	—
11	oz.	Pig. chrysarobini B.P.C. ..	—	—	3 4	0 6
36	lb.	Pig. iodi (Mandl)	—	1 5	0 5	—
33	lb.	Pig. iodi N.I.F.	—	1 4	0 5	—
48	lb.	Pig. iodi fort. N.I.F.	—	1 10	0 7	—
25	lb.	Pigmentum iodi meth.	—	1 0	0 4	—
48	lb.	Pigmentum iodi meth. fort. ..	—	1 10	0 7	—
7	oz.	Pig. iodoformi	—	—	1 2	—
8	oz.	Pig. salol	—	—	1 4	—
3	gr.	Pilocarpin. hydrochlor. S.I. (4)	per	gr.	0 5	—
3	gr.	Pilocarpinæ nitras S.I. (4)	per	gr.	0 5	—
		Pilulæ				
63	lb.	Pil. aloes pulvis	—	2 4	0 8	0 2
66	lb.	Pil. aloes et asafetidæ pulvis ..	—	2 6	0 9	0 2
78	lb.	Pil. aloes et ferri pulvis ..	—	2 8	0 9	0 2

Cost d.	Cost per	Pi—Po Pilulæ—(cont.)	Selling Price 16 oz. s. d.	4 oz. s. d.	1 oz. s. d.	1 dr. s. d.
72	lb.	Pil. aloes et myrrhæ pulvis ..	—	2 7	0 9	0 2
75	lb.	Pil. aloes socot. pulvis	—	2 9	0 10	0 2
18	50	Pil. Alophen (P.D. & Co.) ..	ea.	2 0	—	—
84	lb.	Pil. cambogiæ co. pulvis ..	—	3 0	0 10	0 2
64	lb.	Pil. cochiæ	—	2 2	0 7	0 1
108	lb.	Pil. colocynthidis co. pulvis ..	—	4 0	1 1	0 2
162	lb.	Pil. colocynthidis et hyoscy. pulvis	—	5 10	1 7	0 3
52	lb.	Pil. conii co. .. P.I. (13)	—	2 0	0 7	0 1
24	lb.	Pil. ferri	—	1 0	0 4	0 1
15	oz.	Pil. ferri iodidi	—	—	2 3	0 4
114	lb.	Pil. galbani co. pulvis	—	5 0	1 3	0 3
78	lb.	Pil. hydrargyri pulvis	—	2 10	0 9	0 2
102	lb.	Pil. hyd. subchlor. co. pulvis S.I. (5)	—	3 9	1 0	0 2
126	lb.	Pil. ipecacuanhæ c. scilla S.I. (5)	—	4 3	1 2	0 2
10	oz.	Pil. phosphori	—	—	1 6	0 3
8	oz.	Pil plumbi c. opio S.I. (5)	—	—	1 2	0 2
48	oz.	Pil. quininæ sulphatis	—	—	7 0	1 0
60	lb.	Pil. rhei co. pulvis	—	2 2	0 8	0 2
12	oz.	Pil. saponis co. pulvis .. D.D.	—	—	1 9	0 3
21	oz.	Pil. scammonii co. pulvis ..	—	—	3 0	0 6
78	lb.	Pil. scillæ co. pulvis	—	2 9	0 10	0 2
57	gall.	Pine disinfecting fluid	1 0	per	pint	—
16	lb.	Pimentæ fructus	2 0	0 7	0 2	—
20	lb.	Pimentæ fructus pulvis ..	2 6	0 9	0 3	—
33	lb.	Piper album	4 2	1 2	0 4	—
33	lb.	Piperis albi pulvis	4 2	1 2	0 4	—
36	lb.	Piper longum	4 5	1 4	0 5	—
18	lb.	Piper nigrum extra	2 3	0 8	0 3	—
20	lb.	Piperis nigri pulvis	2 6	0 9	0 3	—
84	oz.	Piperazina	—	—	12 4	1 10
120	oz.	Piperina	—	—	—	2 6
54	6	Pitocin amps. .. P.I. (13)	ea.	6 0	—	—
54	6	Pitressin .. .. P.I. (13)	ea.	6 0	—	—
15	lb.	Pix Barbadense	2 0	0 9	—	—
21	lb.	Pix Burgundica ver.	2 8	0 9	0 3	—
15	lb.	Pix Burgundica fact.	1 9	0 6	0 2	—
16	lb.	Pix carbonis præp.	2 0	0 6	0 2	—
9	lb.	Pix liquida	1 3	0 5	0 2	—
·66	gm.	Platini chloridum	per	gr.	0 8	—
81	oz.	Platini chloridi sol. 5 per cent.	—	—	11 9	1 9
12	gr.	Platinum foil or wire	per	gr.	1 9	—
13	lb.	Plumbi acetas pur. P.I. (8)	1 8	0 7	0 2	—
11	lb.	Plumbi acetas coml. P.I. (8)	1 5	0 5	0 2	—
13	lb.	Plumbi arsen. wash P.L.F. S.I P.II. (6)	1 8	—	—	—
28	lb.	Plumbi carbonas pur.	3 6	1 0	0 4	0 1
22	oz.	Plumbi iodidum	—	—	3 3	0 6
48	lb.	Plumbi oleas (normal) S.I. (4)	6 0	1 9	0 7	—
10	lb.	Plumbi oxidum (litharge) ..	1 3	0 5	0 2	—
12	lb.	Plumbi oxidum rubrum ..	1 6	0 6	0 2	—
28	oz.	Podophylli resina	—	—	4 1	0 7
90	lb.	Pot-pourri P.L.F.	11 3	3 3	0 11	—
		Potassium				
39	lb.	Potassa caustica (st.) P.II. (15)	4 10	1 5	0 5	—
18	lb.	Potassa caustica (bl. ash) P.II. (15)	2 3	0 8	0 3	—
20	lb.	Potassa caustica (gran.) P.II. (15)	2 6	0 9	0 3	—
15	lb.	Pot. caust. lump coml. P.II. (15)	2 0	—	—	—
15	lb.	Potassa sulphurata	2 0	0 7	0 2	—
21	lb.	Potassii acetas gran.	2 8	0 10	0 3	—
5	oz.	Potassii arsenas .. S.I. (4)	—	—	0 10	—
27	oz.	Potassii benzoas nat.	—	—	4 0	0 7
8	oz.	Potassii benzoas synth. ..	—	—	1 2	0 3
11	lb.	Potassii bicarbonatis pulvis ..	1 5	0 5	0 2	—
28	lb.	Potassii bichromas	3 6	1 0	0 4	—
12	lb.	Potassii bichrom. coml.	1 9	0 6	0 2	—
51	lb.	Potassii borotartras	6 6	1 10	0 7	—
33	lb.	Potassii bromidum gran. ..	4 2	1 2	0 4	—

Po—Pu

Cost d.	per	Potassium—(cont.)	Selling Price 16 oz. s. d.	4 oz. s. d.	1 oz. s. d.	1 dr. s. d.
15	lb.	Potassii carbonas	2 0	0 7	0 2	—
8	lb.	Potassii carbonas coml. ..	1 0	0 4	0 2	—
14	lb.	Potassii chloras. pulvis pur. ..	—	0 7	0 2	—
9	lb.	Potassii chloratis pulvis coml. ..	—	0 4	0 2	—
12	lb.	Potassii chloridum pur. ..	1 6	0 6	0 2	—
8	lb.	Potassii chloridum coml. ..	1 0	0 4	—	—
114	gm.	Potassii chloroplatinis	per	gr.	1 0	—
34	lb.	Potassii chromas	—	1 3	0 5	—
34	lb.	Potassii citras	—	1 3	0 5	0 1
42	lb.	Potassii citras eff. B.P.C. ..	5 3	1 6	0 5	0 1
48	lb.	Potassii cyanidum 40% S.I. (4)	6 0	1 9	0 7	0 2
42	lb.	Potassii ferricyanidum	5 3	1 6	0 5	0 1
36	lb.	Potassii ferricyanidum coml. ..	4 6	1 4	0 5	—
18	lb.	Potassii ferrocyanidum	2 3	0 8	0 3	—
5	oz.	Potassii formas	—	—	0 9	0 2
5	oz.	Potassii glyceroph. 50% ..	—	—	0 9	0 2
12	oz.	Potassii guaiacolsulphonas ..	—	—	1 9	0 3
48	oz.	Potassii hippuras	—	—	7 0	1 0
21	oz.	Potassii hydrosquin. sulph. ..	—	—	3 1	0 10
7	oz.	Potassii hypophosphis	—	—	1 1	0 2
87	lb.	Potassii iodidum	—	3 2	0 10	0 2
13	lb.	Potassii metasulphis	1 8	0 6	0 2	—
15	lb.	Potassii nitras	2 0	0 8	0 3	—
7	lb.	Potassii nitras coml.	0 11	0 3	0 1½	—
768	cwt.	Potassii nitras coml.	7 lb.	5 10	14 lb.	10 10
20	lb.	Potassii oxalas neut. ..P.I. (8)	—	0 9	0 3	0 1
18	lb.	Potassii permanganas	2 3	0 8	0 3	—
45	lb.	Potassii persulphas	—	1 4	0 5	0 1
48	lb.	Potassii phosphas	6 0	1 9	0 6	0 1
24	lb.	Potassii phosphas coml. ..	3 0	1 0	0 3	—
48	lb.	Potassii phosph. (tribasic) ..	—	1 9	0 6	—
12	oz.	Potassii salicylas	—	—	1 9	0 3
36	lb.	Potassii silicas fus.	—	1 4	0 5	—
15	oz.	Potassii succinas	—	—	2 3	0 4
13	lb.	Potassii sulphas pulv.	—	0 7	0 2	0 1
6	lb.	Potassii sulphas coml.	0 9	0 3	0 1	—
30	lb.	Potassii sulph. c. sulph. ..	—	1 1	0 4	—
7	oz.	Potassii sulphis	—	—	1 1	0 2
5	oz.	Potassii sulphocarbolas ..	—	—	0 9	0 2
6	oz.	Potassii sulphocyanidum ..	—	—	0 11	0 2
39	lb.	Potassii tartras	4 10	1 5	0 5	0 1
16	lb.	Potassii tartras acidus	2 0	0 7	0 3	—
12	lb.	Potassii tartras acidus 92% ..	7 lb.	11 0	—	—
60	oz.	Procain. hyd. .. S.I. (4)	—	—	8 9	1 3
12	gm.	Proflavinum	per	gr.	0 2	—
85	20	Prolan pellets .. P.I. (13)		9 6	tube	
13	10	Prominal tablets ..℞ only		1 6	tube	
45	oz.	Protargol	—	—	—	1 1
22	oz.	Protargol granulate	—	—	3 3	0 6
21	lb.	Psyllii sem.	—	0 10	0 3	—
84	lb.	Pulv. acetanilidi co. P.I. (13)	—	3 0	0 10	0 2
27	lb.	Pulv. alkalinus (Maclean's) ..	—	1 0	0 4	—
26	lb.	Pulv. aloes cap c. canella ..	—	0 11	0 4	—
48	lb.	Pulv. aloes c. canella (super.) ..	—	1 9	0 6	0 1
48	lb.	Pulv. amygdalæ co.	—	1 9	0 6	0 1
48	lb.	Pulv. antimonialis S.I. (5)	—	—	0 6	0 1
264	lb.	Pulv. aromaticus co.	—	9 7	2 7	0 5
32	lb.	Pulv. bismuth. co. N.I.F. ..	—	1 2	0 4	—
54	lb.	Pulv. catechu co.	—	2 0	0 7	0 1
60	lb.	Pulv. cinnamomi co.	—	2 2	0 8	0 2
90	lb.	Pulv. conf. aromat.	—	3 3	0 11	0 2
16	lb.	Pulv. cretæ aromaticus	—	0 7	0 3	—
32	lb.	Pulv. cretæ aromat. c. op. S.I. (5)	—	1 2	0 4	0 1
48	oz.	Pulv. elaterini co.	—	—	7 0	1 3
15	lb.	Pulv. glycyrrhizæ co.	2 0	0 7	0 3	0 1
8	oz.	Pulv. ipecacuanhæ et opii S.I. (5)	—	—	1 2	0 2
36	lb.	Pulv. jalapæ co.	—	1 4	0 5	0 1

Pu—Ro

Cost d.	per	Pu—Ro	Selling Price 16 oz. s. d.	4 oz. s. d.	1 oz. s. d.	1 dr. s. d.
7	oz.	Pulv. kino co. .. S.I. (5)	—	—	1 1	0 2
27	lb.	Pulv. lobeliæ co. B.P.C. ..	—	1 0	0 4	—
10	oz.	Pulv. opii co. .. .. D.D.	—	—	1 6	0 3
8	oz.	Pulv. pepsini co.	—	—	1 2	0 2
26	lb.	Pulv. pro mist. cretæ	3 3	1 0	0 4	0 1
30	lb.	Pulv. rhei co.	—	1 2	0 4	0 1
72	lb.	Pulv. scammonii co.	—	2 7	0 10	0 2
20	lb.	Pulv. seidlitz	ea.	3d.	—	—
24	lb.	Pulv. stramon. co. B.P.C. ..	—	1 0	0 4	—
39	lb.	Pulv. tragacanthæ co.	—	1 3	0 4	0 1
12	lb.	Pulv. zinc. amylo ac. bor. ..	1 6	0 6	—	—
28	oz.	Pyramidon .. ℞ only	—	—	—	0 7
30	lb.	Pyrethri radicis pulvis	—	1 1	0 4	—
18	oz.	Pyridina pura	—	—	2 8	0 5
24	oz.	Pyrocatechin	—	—	3 6	0 6
39	oz.	Pyrogallol monoacet. sol. ..	—	—	5 9	1 0
36	oz.	Pyrogallol triacetas	—	—	5 3	1 0
		Q				
8	lb.	Quassiæ ligni rass.	1 0	0 4½	0 2	—
14	lb.	Quassiæ ligni pulvis.	—	0 7	0 3	0 1
108	dr.	Quassinum amorph.	—	—	—	15 0
48	lb.	Quebracho cortex S.I. (4)	—	1 9	0 6	—
10	lb.	Quercus cortex	1 3	0 5	0 2	—
12	lb.	Quillaiæ cortex	—	0 6	0 2	—
15	lb.	Quillaiæ cortex contusus ..	2 0	0 7	0 2	—
18	lb.	Quillaiæ corticis pulvis ..	—	0 8	0 3	—
			Gr.x.			
96	oz.	Quinidina	0 5	—	—	2 0
69	oz.	Quinidinæ sulph.	0 4	—	—	1 6
72	oz.	Quinina	0 3	—	—	1 6
92	oz.	Quinin. acetylsalicylas	0 4	—	—	2 0
68	oz.	Quinin. ethylcarbonas	0 3	—	—	1 6
80	oz.	Quinin. glycerophosphas ..	0 4	—	—	1 8
92	oz.	Quinin. hydriodidum acidum ..	0 4	—	—	2 0
55	oz.	Quinin. hydrobromidum ..	0 3	—	—	1 2
55	oz.	Quinin. hydrobromid. acidum ..	0 3	—	—	1 2
55	oz.	Quinin. hydrochlor.-bi. ..	0 3	—	—	1 2
92	oz.	Quinin. hypophosphis	0 4	—	—	2 0
72	oz.	Quinin. phosphas	0 3	—	—	1 6
68	oz.	Quinin. salicylas	0 3	—	—	1 6
38	oz.	Quinin. sulphas	0 2	—	—	0 10
42	oz.	Quinin. sulphas acidus	0 2	—	—	0 11
58	oz.	Quinin. et ureæ hydrochl. ..	0 3	—	—	1 3
66	oz.	Quinin. urethane	—	—	8 9	1 6
89	oz.	Quinin. valerianas	0 4	—	—	1 8
		R				
11	lb.	Rapii semina	1 5	0 6	0 2	—
20	lb.	Red squill compound	2 6	0 9	0 3	—
8	lb.	Resina (amber)	1 0	0 4	0 1	—
11	lb.	Resin. flav. pulv.	1 5	0 6	0 2	—
11	oz.	Resorcinol	—	—	1 8	0 3
20	25c.c.	Radiostoleum	—	—	3 6	0 6
27	oz.	Resorcini acetas	—	—	4 0	0 8
28	lb.	Rhei rhizoma Ang. pulv. ..	—	1 0	0 4	—
264	lb.	Rhei rhiz. "E. I." elect. ..	—	9 5	2 9	0 5
210	lb.	Rhei rhiz. "E. I." (trimmed) ..	—	7 8	2 4	0 4
156	lb.	Rhei rhiz. "E. I." sec. ..	—	5 7	1 7	0 3
162	lb.	Rhei rhiz. "E. I." pulv. elect...	—	5 10	1 8	0 3
120	lb.	Rhei rhiz. "E. I." pulv. sec. ..	—	4 3	1 2	0 2
84	lb.	Rhei rhiz. "E. I." pulv. ..	—	3 0	0 10	0 2
63	dr.	Rhubidii iodidum	—	—	—	9 2
20	lb.	Ringworm oint. (vet.) P.L.F ..	2 6	0 9	—	—
14	lb.	Rosmarini folia	1 8	0 6	0 2	—
36	lb.	Rouge, jewellers'	4 6	1 4	0 5	—
192	lb.	Rosæ pet. Ang.	—	6 10	2 0	—
96	lb.	Rosæ pet. exot.	—	3 0	0 10	—

Cost d.	per	Sa—Se	Selling Price 16 oz. s. d.	4 oz. s. d.	1 oz. s. d.	1 dr. s. d.
		S				
54	oz.	Saccharinum 550	per	gr.	0 1	1 2
48	oz.	Saccharinum solubile	per	gr.	0 1	1 0
6	lb.	Saccharum pur. pulv. subtil. ..	—	0 2½	0 1	—
		Saccharum lactis (tins)	½ lb.	1 6	1 lb.	2 8
14	lb.	Saccharum lactis pulv.	1 9	0 7	0 2	—
18	lb.	Saccharum ustum Ang. ..	2 3	0 9	0 3	—
10	lb.	Saccharum ustum exot. ..	1 3	0 5	0 2	—
		Sachet powder opt. (var.) P.L.F.	—	—	1 4	—
		Sachet powder sec. P.L.F. ..	—	3 4	1 0	—
54	lb.	Safrol	—	1 9	0 6	0 1
24	lb.	Sal acetos. pulv.P.L.F. P.II. (10)	—	0 11	0 3	—
18	lb.	Sal acetos. pulv. P.II. (10)	—	0 8	0 3	—
14	lb.	Sal Carlsbad artif. N.F. ..	1 9	0 7	0 2	—
36	lb.	Sal Carol. fact. eff. pulv. ..	4 6	1 4	0 5	0 1
18	lb.	Sal Cheltenham artif.	2 3	0 8	0 3	—
33	lb.	Sal Harrogate, artif.	4 2	1 3	0 5	—
—	3 oz.	Sal hepatica	—	—	0 9	0 2
12	lb.	Sal Kissingen artif.	1 6	0 6	0 2	—
54	lb.	Sal limonis P.L.F. P.II. (10)	—	2 0	0 7	—
48	lb.	Sal limon. (non-toxic) P.L.F. ..	—	1 9	0 6	—
13	lb.	Sal prunella glob.	1 9	0 7	0 2	—
19	lb.	Sal prunella glob. parv. ..	2 4	0 9	0 3	—
18	lb.	Sal Vichy artif.	2 3	0 8	0 3	—
19	oz.	Salicinum	—	—	2 10	0 5
24	lb.	Saline effervesc. P.L.F. ..	3 0	1 0	0 3	—
45	oz.	Salipyrine	—	—	—	1 1
7	oz.	Salol	—	—	—	0 2
42	oz.	Salophen	—	—	6 2	1 6
33	lb.	Sambuci flores sicc.	4 3	1 3	0 4	—
39	lb.	Sandaraca	5 0	1 5	0 5	—
24	lb.	Sanguinariæ radix	—	1 0	0 4	—
27	dr.	Sanguinarin.	—	—	—	4 0
150	lb.	Sanguis draconis pulv. opt. ..	—	5 4	1 6	0 3
108	lb.	Sanguis draconis pulv. sec. ..	13 6	3 11	1 1	0 2
30	lb.	Santal. flav. lig. pulv.	3 6	1 0	0 4	—
54	dr.	Santoninum	per	gr.	0 3	8 0
18	lb.	Sapo albus pulv.	2 3	0 8	0 3	—
24	lb.	Sap. alc. sol. indust.	—	0 10	0 3	—
13	lb.	Sapo animalis	1 7	0 6	0 2	—
18	lb.	Sapo animal. pulv.	2 3	0 8	0 3	—
36	lb.	Sapo ars. (taxid.) P.L.F .S.I. (6)	4 6	1 4	0 5	—
15	lb.	Sapo Cast. mottled	1 10	0 7	0 2	—
24	lb.	Sapo " coconut oil "	3 0	1 0	0 3	—
18	lb.	Sapo durus	2 3	0 8	0 3	—
28	lb.	Sapo durus pulv.	3 6	1 0	0 3	—
48	lb.	Sapo ethereal P.L.F.	—	1 8	0 7	—
174	lb.	Sapo Hebra rect.	—	6 2	1 8	0 3
24	lb.	Sapo kalinus	3 0	0 11	0 4	—
13	lb.	Sapo mollis viridis	1 9	0 6	0 2	—
9	lb.	Sapo mollis coml. opt.	1 2	0 4	—	—
36	lb.	Sapo Napol.	4 6	1 4	0 5	—
12	oz.	Saponinum	—	—	1 9	0 4
39	lb.	Sarsæ radix Jam.	4 10	1 5	0 5	0 1
48	lb.	Sarsæ radix Jam. incis. ..	6 0	1 10	0 6	0 1
18	lb.	Sassafras radix incis.	2 3	0 9	0 3	—
7	oz.	Scammoniæ resinæ pulv. ..	—	—	1 1	0 2
23	dr.	Scammoniæ virgin. pulv. ..	—	—	—	3 5
42	oz.	Scarlet red	—	—	6 2	1 0
60	lb.	Schlippe's salt	7 6	2 2	0 7	0 1
3	oz.	Scilla pulv.	—	—	0 6	0 1
146	100	Sedobrol tablets	doz.	2 4	—	—
242	gross	Seltzogene charges 3-pt. ..	doz.	2 3	—	—
312	gross	Seltzogene charges 5-pt. ..	doz.	4 6	—	—
36	lb.	Senegæ rad.	—	1 4	0 5	—
42	lb.	Senegæ rad. pulv.	—	1 6	0 5	—
54	lb.	Sennæ folia Alex. opt.	6 9	2 0	0 7	—

Cost d.	per	Se—So	Selling Price 16 oz. s. d.	4 oz. s. d.	1 oz. s. d.	1 dr. s. d.
24	lb.	Sennæ fol. Alex. pulv.	3 0	0 11	0 4	—
30	lb.	Sennæ fol. Tinnev.	3 9	1 1	0 4	—
18	lb.	Sennæ fol. Tinnev. pulv. ..	2 3	0 8	0 3	—
96	lb.	Sennæ fructus Alex. (picked) ..	12 0	3 5	1 0	—
18	lb.	Sennæ fructus Tinnev. ..	2 3	0 8	0 3	—
54	lb.	Serpentariæ rhizoma	—	2 0	0 7	0 1
40	lb.	Sevum benzoatum	—	1 6	0 5	—
36	lb.	Sevum præparatum	—	1 5	0 5	—
11	oz.	Sevum phosphoratum P.I. (9)	—	—	1 8	0 4
28	lb.	Shampoo pdr. (borax soap) ..	—	1 0	0 4	—
21	lb.	Shampoo pdr. (coconut soap) ..	2 8	0 10	0 3	—
36	lb.	Shellac alb.	4 6	1 4	0 5	—
24	lb.	Shellac aurant.	3 0	0 11	0 3	—
17	lb.	Shellac aurant. sec.	2 2	0 8	0 3	—
19	lb.	Sherbet P.L.F.	2 5	0 9	0 3	—
4	oz.	Silica pur. præcip.	—	—	0 8	—
6	lb.	Silica coml.	0 10	0 3	0 1	—
10	lb.	Sinapis albæ semina	1 3	0 5	0 2	—
		Sodium				
30	lb.	Soda caustic.(sticks)pur.P.II. (15)	3 9	1 2	0 4	—
11	lb.	Soda caustic.(gran.or fl.)P.II. (15)	1 5	0 6	0 2	—
15	lb.	Soda lime	2 0	0 7	0 2	—
15	lb.	Sodii acetas pur. cryst. ..	1 10	0 7	0 2	—
18	oz.	Sodii acetylsalicylas	—	—	2 8	0 6
27	lb.	Sodii ammon. phos.	—	1 0	0 4	—
6	oz.	Sodii arsenas anhyd. S.I.,P.II. (4)	—	—	0 11	0 2
30	oz.	Sodii benzoas nat.	—	—	4 5	0 8
36	lb.	Sodii benzoas artif.	—	1 4	0 5	—
6	lb.	Sodii bicarb. (Howards) ..	0 9	0 3	0 2	—
5	lb.	Sodii bicarb. opt. pulv. ..	0 8	0 3	0 1	—
		Sodii bicarb. opt. pkd.	—	0 4½	0 1½	—
4	lb.	Sodii bicarb. coml. pulv. ..	0 6	0 2	0 1	—
264	cwt.	Sodii bicarb. coml. pulv. ..	7 lb.	1 8	14 lb.	3 0
11	lb.	Sodii bichromas	1 6	0 6	0 2	—
15	lb.	Sodii bisulphas pur.	1 11	0 7	0 2	—
54	lb.	Sodii bitartras	6 9	2 0	0 7	0 1
35	lb.	Sodii bromidum	4 6	1 4	0 5	—
36	oz.	Sodii cacodylas .. S.I. (4)	—	—	5 3	0 9
5	lb.	Sodii carbonas cryst.	0 8	0 3	0 1	—
8	lb.	Sodii carbonas exsic.	1 0	0 4	0 1	—
3	lb.	Sodii carbonas coml.	0 5	0 2	0 1	—
54	oz.	Sodii chaulmoogras	—	—	—	1 2
21	lb.	Sodii chlorate	2 8	0 9	0 3	—
10	lb.	Sodii chloridum pur.	1 3	0 6	0 2	—
14	oz.	Sodii cinnamas	—	—	2 0	0 4
35	lb.	Sodii citras	4 5	1 4	0 5	0 1
42	lb.	Sodii citro-tartras eff.	5 3	1 6	0 6	—
30	lb.	Sodii cyanid. .. S.I. (4)	3 9	1 1	0 4	—
2	oz.	Sodii formas	—	—	0 4	0 1
9	oz.	Sodii glycerophos. pulv. ..	—	—	1 4	0 3
26	oz.	Sodii guaiacas	—	—	3 9	0 8
42	oz.	Sodii hippuras	—	—	6 2	1 0
54	oz.	Sodii hydnocarpas	—	—	8 0	1 4
26	lb.	Sodii hydroxid. sticks P.II. (15)	—	1 0	0 4	—
6	oz.	Sodii hypophosphis	—	—	0 11	0 2
4.5	lb.	Sodii hyposulphis opt.	0 8	0 3	0 1	—
3	lb.	Sodii hyposulphis (photog.) ..	0 5	—	—	—
11	oz.	Sodii iodidum	—	—	1 8	0 3
6	lb.	Sodii lactas (syrupy)	—	—	1 3	0 3
7.5	oz.	Sodii lith. cit. co.	—	—	1 2	0 2
28	oz.	Sodii Mandelas	—	—	4 1	0 7
21	lb.	Sodii manganas coml.	2 9	0 9	0 3	—
18	lb.	Sodii metasulphis	2 3	0 8	0 3	—
54	oz.	Sodii morrhuas	—	—	8 0	1 4
18	lb.	Sodii nitras pur.	—	0 8	0 3	—
4.5	lb.	Sodii nitras coml.	0 7	0 3	0 1	—
21	lb.	Sodii nitris pur. cryst.	—	0 10	0 3	0 1

So—Sp

Cost d.	per	Sodium—(cont.)	Selling Price 16 oz. s. d.	4 oz. s. d.	1 oz. s. d.	1 dr. s. d.
24	oz.	Sodii nitroprussidum	—	—	3 6	0 7
60	oz.	Sodii nucleinas	—	—	8 9	1 3
42	lb.	Sodii oleas	—	1 6	0 5	—
26	lb.	Sodii oxalas .. P.I. (8)	—	1 0	0 4	—
24	lb.	Sodii perboras	3 0	0 11	0 4	0 1
39	lb.	Sodii peroxidum	—	1 5	0 5	0 1
66	lb.	Sodii persulphas	—	2 4	0 8	0 2
3	lb.	Sodii phenas .. P.I. (8)	—	—	0 6	0 1
13	lb.	Sodii phosphas "pea" ..	1 9	0 6	0 2	—
14	lb.	Sodii phosphas "feathery" ..	2 0	0 8	0 2	—
16	lb.	Sodii phosph. pulv.	2 3	0 8	0 3	—
24	lb.	Sodii phosph. pulv. exsic. ..	—	0 11	0 3	—
24	lb.	Sodii phosph. acidus	—	0 11	0 4	—
36	lb.	Sodii phosph. eff.	4 6	1 4	0 5	—
24	lb.	Sodii phosph. (tribasic) ..	—	1 0	0 4	—
18	lb.	Sodii et potas. tart. pulv. ..	2 3	0 8	0 3	—
18	lb.	Sodii pyrophosph.	2 3	0 9	0 3	—
32	lb.	Sodii salicylas cryst.	—	1 2	0 4	0 1
30	oz.	Sodii salicylas nat.	—	—	4 5	0 8
4.5	lb.	Sodii silicatis solut. (wgt.) ..	0 8	0 3	—	—
36	lb.	Sodii stearas	—	1 4	0 5	—
18	oz.	Sodii succinas	—	—	2 8	0 6
5	lb.	Sodii sulphas "pea"	0 8	0 3	0 2	—
5	lb.	Sodii sulphas "feathery" ..	0 9	0 3	0 2	—
6	lb.	Sodii sulph. pulv.	0 10	0 4	0 2	—
7	lb.	Sodii sulph. pulv. exsic. ..	1 0	0 5	0 2	—
216	cwt.	Sodii sulph. coml. cryst. ..	0 4	—	7 lb.	1 8
294	cwt.	Sodii sulph. coml. pulv. ..	0 5	—	7 lb.	2 4
27	lb.	Sodii sulph. eff.	3 6	1 0	0 4	—
176	cwt.	Sodii sulph. vet.	7 lb.	1 5	14 lb.	2 8
21	lb.	Sodii sulphidum cryst.	—	0 9	0 3	—
5	lb.	Sodii sulphis	0 9	0 3	0 1	—
32	lb.	Sodii sulphocarbolatis pulv. ..	—	1 2	0 4	0 1
6	oz.	Sodii sulphocyanid.	—	—	0 9	0 2
36	lb.	Sodii tartras (neutral)	—	1 4	0 5	0 1
18	oz.	Sodii tauroglycocholas B.P.C. ..	—	—	2 8	0 5
66	lb.	Sodii tungstas pur.	—	—	0 8	0 2
20	oz.	Sodii valerianas	—	—	2 11	0 5
108	lb.	Sol. ætheris nitrosi (1-7) ..	—	3 6	1 0	—
129	oz.	Sozoiodol, hydrarg.	—	—	—	2 2
54	oz.	Sozoiodol, zinc.	—	—	—	1 4
14	dr.	Sparteinæ sulphas	—	—	—	2 0
72	lb.	Spigelia	—	2 7	0 9	0 2
		Spiritus				
72	lb.	Spiritus ætheris	—	2 4	0 8	0 2
96	lb.	Spt. ætheris comp.	—	3 2	0 10	0 2
67	lb.	Spt. ætheris nitrosi	7 6	2 2	0 7	0 1
24	lb.	Spt. ætheris nit. substit. P.L.F.	3 0	—	—	—
52	lb.	Spt. ammoniæ aromaticus ..	5 9	1 7	0 6	0 1
		Spt. ammon. ar. pkd. (std. bot.)	—	2 6	℥ij.	1 6
96	lb.	Spt. ammoniæ fetidus	—	3 2	0 10	0 2
24	oz.	Spt. anisi	—	—	3 4	0 6
66	lb.	Spt. armoraciæ co.	—	2 2	0 8	0 2
96	lb.	Spt. cajuputi	—	3 2	0 11	0 2
78	lb.	Spt. camphoræ	—	2 7	0 9	0 2
68	lb.	Spt. chloroformi	—	2 2	0 8	0 2
33	oz.	Spt. cinnamomi	—	—	4 4	0 8
102	lb.	Spt. juniperi	—	3 5	1 0	0 2
18	oz.	Spt. juniperi co. P.L.	—	—	2 6	0 5
630	lb.	Spt. lavandulæ Ang.	—	—	4 9	0 9
426	lb.	Spt. lavandulæ exot.	—	15 0	4 2	0 7
32	oz.	Spt. menthæ pip. Ang. ..	—	—	4 3	0 8
312	lb.	Spt. menthæ pip. exot.	—	10 6	2 9	0 5
26	oz.	Spt. myristicæ	—	—	3 9	0 7
126	lb.	Spt. nucis juglandis	—	4 0	1 1	0 2
300	lb.	Spt. rosmarini exot.	—	10 0	2 8	0 5
62	lb.	Spt. saponatus	6 9	2 0	0 7	—

Sp—Sy

Cost d.	per	Spiritus—(cont.)	Selling Price 16 oz. s. d.	4 oz. s. d.	1 oz. s. d.	1 dr. s. d.
24	lb.	Spt. saponis kalini meth. ..	3 0	0 11	0 3	—
72	gal.	Spt. sick-room (Surgical) ..	pint	1 2	—	—
54	gal.	Spt. vini meth. 64 o.p. (min'l) ..	0 10	0 3	0 1	—
41	gal.	Spt. vini meth. 64o.p.(10gal.lots)	pint	0 6	—	—
29	gal.	Spt. vini meth. 64 o.p. (indust.) (10 gall. lots)	pint	0 7	gal.	4 0
40	gal.	Spt. vini meth. (indust.) 64 o.p.	pint	0 8	—	—
28	80	Stannoxyl tablets, unstd. ..	doz.	0 6	—	—
57	lb.	Stanni oxid. pulv. coml. opt. ..	7 2	2 1	0 8	—
78	lb.	Stannum gran. pur.	9 9	2 9	0 8	0 2
48	lb.	Staphisagria sem. ..S.I. (4)	—	1 9	0 6	—
57	lb.	Staphisagria sem. pulv. S.I. (4)	—	2 1	0 8	—
13	gm.	Stovaine .. .. S.I. (4)	—	—	—	—
18	lb.	Stramonii folia .. S.I. (4)	2 3	0 8	0 3	—
18	lb.	Stramonii fol. pulv. S.I. (4)	2 3	0 8	0 3	—
6	oz.	Strontii bromidum cryst. ..	—	—	0 11	0 2
8	oz.	Strontii bromid. exsic.	—	—	1 2	0 2
20	oz.	Strontii iodidum	—	—	3 0	0 6
18	oz.	Strontii lactas	—	—	2 8	0 6
17	lb.	Strontii nitras coml. pulv. ..	2 3	0 8	0 3	—
18	oz.	Strontii salicylas	—	—	2 8	0 6
9	gr.	Strophanthinum S.I. (4)	per	gr.	1 4	—
53	oz.	Strychnina cryst. S.I. (4)	—	—	7 9	1 2
53	oz.	Strych. pulv. .. S.I. (4)	—	—	7 9	1 2
50	oz.	Strych. hydrochlor. S.I. (4)	—	—	7 4	1 1
50	oz.	Strych. nitras .. S.I. (4)	—	—	7 4	1 1
50	oz.	Strych. sulphas S.I. (4)	—	—	7 4	1 1
27	20	Stypticin tablets S.I. (4)	doz.	1 10	—	—
29	20	Styptol tablets .. S.I. (4)	doz.	2 1	—	—
61	oz.	Styracol	—	—	—	1 6
84	lb.	Styrax præparatus	—	3 1	0 11	0 2
48	lb.	Succus allii	—	1 9	0 6	—
39	lb.	Succus belladonnæ P.I. (10)	—	1 5	0 5	—
38	lb.	Succus conii .. P.I. (9)	—	1 5	0 5	—
48	lb.	Succus digitalis .. S.I. (4)	—	1 10	0 7	—
42	lb.	Succus glycyrrhizæ (Solazzi) ..	—	1 6	0 5	—
16	lb.	Succus glycyrrhizæ (block) ..	2 0	0 7	0 3	0 1
36	lb.	Succus hyoscyami P.I. (9)	—	1 4	0 5	—
108	gal.	Succus limettæ	1 6	0 6	0 2	—
108	gal.	Succus limonis	1 6	0 6	0 2	—
32	lb.	Succus scoparii	—	1 3	0 5	—
34	lb.	Succus taraxaci	—	1 3	0 5	—
28	oz.	Sulphonal .. ℞ only	—	—	4 1	0 7
9	lb.	Sulphur lotum	1 2	0 4	0 1½	—
12	lb.	Sulphur præcipitatum	—	0 6	0 2	—
5	lb.	Sulphur rotundum	0 9	0 3	0 1	—
6	lb.	Sulphur sublimatum	0 9	0 3	0 1	—
264	cwt.	Sulphur sublimatum sec. ..	7 lb.	2 1	14 lb.	3 10
5	lb.	Sulphur vivum	0 9	0 3	—	—
312	cwt.	Sulphur vivum	7 lb.	2 4	—	—
18	lb.	Sulphur hair wash P.L.F. ..	—	8 oz.	1 4	—
6	lb.	Sulphur wash P.L.F.	1 0	—	—	—
26	lb.	Sulphuris chloridum (liq.) ..	—	1 8	0 6	—
20	oz.	Sulphuris iodidum	—	—	3 0	0 6
		Suppositoria (*see* Pricing Prescriptions)				
		Syrupi				
8	lb.	Syrupus	1 6	0 6	0 2	—
21	lb.	Syr. ac. hydriodici	—	1 0	0 4	—
28	lb.	Syr. allii	—	1 6	0 5	—
16	lb.	Syr. althææ	—	0 10	0 4	—
24	lb.	Syr. anisi	—	1 3	0 5	—
39	lb.	Syr. apomorphinæ B.P.C. P.I. (9)	—	2 0	0 7	0 1
42	lb.	Syr. aromaticus	—	2 0	0 7	0 1
33	lb.	Syr. aurantii	—	1 7	0 5	—
24	lb.	Syr. aurantii floris	—	1 2	0 4	—

Sy

Cost d.	per	Syrupi—(cont.)	Selling Price 16 oz. s. d.	4 oz. s. d.	1 oz. s. d.	1 dr. s. d.
54	lb.	Syr. bromoformi (Martind.) ..	—	2 3	0 8	—
27	lb.	Syr. butyl-chloral hydratis P.I. (10)	—	1 4	0 7	0 1
28	lb.	Syr. calcii chlor. B.P.C. ..	—	1 6	0 6	—
18	lb.	Syr. calcii hypophosphitis ..	—	1 0	0 4	—
16	lb.	Syr. calcii lactophosphatis ..	—	0 10	0 4	0 1
22	lb.	Syr. calcii lactophosphatis c. ferro	—	1 2	0 4	—
18	lb.	Syr. camphoræ co. ..P.I. (9)	—	0 10	0 4	—
54	lb.	Syr. cascaræ aromaticus ..	—	2 10	0 10	0 2
24	lb.	Syr. chloral .. ..P.I. (9)	—	1 1	0 4	0 1
48	lb.	Syr. cocillanæ co. P.I. (10)	—	2 2	0 7	0 1
87	16 oz.	Syr. cocillanæ co. (P.D.) P.I. (10)	—	3 3	0 11	0 2
33	lb.	Syr. codeinæ phosph. P.I. (9)	—	1 6	0 5	0 1
27	lb.	Syr. croci B.P.C.	—	1 4	0 5	0 1
42	lb.	Syr. cydoniæ	—	2 0	0 7	—
48	lb.	Syr. eucalypti gummi	—	2 2	0 7	0 1
24	lb.	Syr. ferri bromidi	—	1 3	0 5	0 1
51	lb.	Syr. ferri bromidi c. quin. ..	—	2 4	0 8	0 2
48	lb.	Syr. ferri bromidi c. quin. et strych. .. ..P.I. (9)	—	2 2	0 8	0 2
19	lb.	Syr. ferri dial.	—	1 0	0 4	—
20	lb.	Syr. ferri hypophosphitis ..	—	1 0	0 4	—
18	lb.	Syr. ferri iodidi	—	0 10	0 3	—
24	lb.	Syr. ferri lactophosphatis ..	—	1 3	0 5	—
15	lb.	Syr. ferri phosphatis	2 9	0 10	0 4	—
12	lb.	Syr. ferri phosphatis co. ..	2 3	0 9	0 3	—
		Syr. ferri phosphatis co. pkd. ..	—	1 0	℥ viij	1 9
38	lb.	Syr. ferri phosphatis c. mang. ..	—	1 6	0 5	—
32	lb.	Syr. ferri phosphatis c. quin. ..	—	1 7	0 5	—
18	lb.	Syr. fer. phos. c. quin. et str. P.I. (9)	—	0 10	0 4	—
21	lb.	Syr. fici	3 4	1 0	0 4	—
30	lb.	Syr. format. co... P.I. (13)	—	1 6	0 5	—
12	lb.	Syr. glucosi	—	0 8	0 3	—
30	lb.	Syr. glycerophosph. flav. ..	5 0	1 5	0 5	0 1
24	lb.	Syr. glyceroph. c. form. P.I. (9)	4 0	1 3	0 4	—
17	lb.	Syr. glycerophos. co. ..P.I. (9)	2 10	0 11	0 4	—
48	lb.	Syr. glycerophosph. co. c. medulla rub. .. ..P.I. (9)	8 0	2 4	0 8	0 2
24	lb.	Syr. glycerophos. co. (Robin) P.I. (9)	—	1 3	0 4	—
24	lb.	Syr. hemidesmi	—	1 3	0 4	—
72	lb.	Syr. hydrobrom. co. (Hewlett) ..	—	3 5	0 11	0 2
13	lb.	Syr. hypophos. co. B.P.C. P.I. (9)	2 2	0 8	0 3	—
		Syr. hypophos. co. pkd. P.I. (9)	—	1 0	℥ ij.	0 8
42	lb.	Syr. iodotannicus	—	2 0	0 7	0 1
30	lb.	Syr. ipecacuanhæ	—	1 6	0 5	—
22	lb.	Syr. limonis	3 6	1 0	0 4	—
18	lb.	Syr. marrubii	3 3	1 0	0 4	—
33	lb.	Syr. mori	5 6	1 9	0 6	—
22	lb.	Syr. papaveris albæ ..P.I. (9)	—	1 0	0 4	—
18	lb.	Syr. picis liquidæ	—	1 0	0 4	—
30	lb.	Syr. pini B.P.C.	—	1 5	0 5	—
36	lb.	Syr. pruni cerasi	—	1 9	0 6	—
12	lb.	Syr. pruni serot.	—	0 8	0 3	—
39	lb.	Syr. quininæ hypophositis ..	—	2 0	0 7	—
39	lb.	Syr. quininæ iodidi	—	2 0	0 7	—
39	lb.	Syr. quininæphosph.	—	2 0	0 7	—
17	lb.	Syr. rhamni	—	0 10	0 4	—
30	lb.	Syr. rhamni frang.	—	1 6	0 5	—
14	lb.	Syr. rhei	—	0 10	0 3	—
16	lb.	Syr. rhœados	2 8	0 10	0 4	—
21	lb.	Syr. ribis nig.	—	1 0	0 4	0 1
51	lb.	Syr. ribis rub.	—	2 6	0 8	0 2
63	lb.	Syr. robor. (Roberts), unstd. fl.	—	2 3	0 7	0 2
36	lb.	Syr. rosæ	—	1 6	0 5	—
35	lb.	Syr. rubi fructicosi	—	1 6	0 5	—
27	lb.	Syr. rubi idæi	—	1 3	0 4	—
27	lb.	Syr. rutæ	—	1 3	0 4	—
12	lb.	Syr. scillæ	—	0 8	0 3	—

Sy—Ti

Cost d.	per	Syrupi—(cont.)	Selling Price 16 oz. s. d.	4 oz. s. d.	1 oz. s. d.	1 dr. s. d.
38	lb.	Syr. senegæ	—	1 10	0 7	—
30	lb.	Syr. sennæ Alex.	—	1 5	0 5	—
18	lb.	Syr. sennæ	—	0 11	0 4	—
30	lb.	Syr. sennæ fruct. Alex. ..	—	1 5	0 5	0 1
22	lb.	Syr. tamarindi	—	1 1	0 4	—
11	lb.	Syr. tolutanus	—	0 8	0 3	—
21	lb.	Syr. triplex B.P.C. P.I. (10)	—	1 1	0 4	—
24	lb.	Syr. tussilaginis	—	1 4	0 5	—
16	lb.	Syr. violæ	—	0 10	0 4	—
15	lb.	Syr. zingiberis	—	0 10	0 3	—
		T				
104	oz.	Taka diastase (P.D.)	—	—	13 0	2 0
36	4 oz.	Taka diastase elixir	—	4 6	1 2	0 2
32	4 oz.	Taka diastase liq.	—	4 0	1 0	0 2
77	100	Taka diastase tablets gr. 2½ ..	doz.	1 3	—	—
22	ea.	Takazyma	2 9	each	—	—
18	lb.	Talcum opt.	2 3	0 8	0 2½	—
5.5	lb.	Talcum coml.	0 8	0 2½	0 1	—
10	lb.	Tallow	1 3	0 5	0 1½	—
38	lb.	Tamarindi pulpa	4 9	1 5	0 5	—
17	lb.	Tamarindus W.I.	2 3	0 8	0 3	—
24	oz.	Tannalbin	—	—	3 6	0 6
20	20	Tannalbin tablets gr. 7½ ..	doz.	1 6	—	—
30	25 gm	Tannoform	—	—	—	0 8
26	lb.	Taraxaci radix Ang. incis. ..	3 3	1 0	0 4	—
36	lb.	Terebenum	—	1 3	0 5	—
72	lb.	Terebinth. Canad.	—	2 7	0 9	—
14	oz.	Terebinth. chia.	—	—	2 0	0 4
15	lb.	Terebinth. Venet. fact. ..	2 0	0 8	0 3	—
36	lb.	Terebinth. Venet. ver.	4 6	1 4	0 5	—
6	oz.	Terpini hydras	—	—	0 11	0 2
6	oz.	Terpineol	—	—	1 0	0 2
5	oz.	Terpinol	—	—	0 9	0 2
30	lb.	Terra rosæ	3 9	1 2	0 4	—
108	oz.	Tetronal .. .. ..℞ only	—	—	—	2 10
72	oz.	Thallii acetas .. ..S.I. (4)	—	—	—	1 8
189	oz.	Thallii sulph. .. ..S.I. (4)	—	—	—	5 8
90	6	Theelin ampoules 1.0	10 0	per	box	—
90	6	Theelin amps. in oil	10 0	per 6	amps.	—
103.5	20	Theelol capsules	11 6	—	—	—
15	oz.	Theobromina	—	—	2 3	0 4
28	oz.	Theobrominæ acetylsal. ..	—	—	4 1	0 7
14	oz.	Theobrominæ-sod. acet. ..	—	—	2 0	0 4
13	oz.	Theobrominæ-sod. sal. ..	—	—	1 11	0 4
22	oz.	Theobromin. et sodii benz. ..	—	—	3 3	0 7
39	oz.	Theobromin. et sodii iod. ..	—	—	5 9	0 10
24	oz.	Theobromin. salicyl	—	—	3 6	0 6
144	oz.	Theocinæ-sod. acet.	—	—	—	3 5
58	50	Theominal tablets ..℞ only	doz.	2 2	—	—
96	oz.	Theophyllin.-sod. acet. ..	—	—	—	2 0
6	lb.	Theriaca	—	—	0 3	0 1
33.6	50c.c.	Thilocologne	3 6	per	tube	—
37.6	100cc	Thilocologne	4 9	per	tube	—
65	oz.	Thiocol	—	—	—	1 7
43	6 oz.	Thiocol syrup	—	—	0 11	0 2
27	25	Thiocol tablets	doz.	1 8	—	—
28	oz.	Thioform	—	—	3 6	0 8
60	oz.	Thiol	—	—	7 6	1 8
30	gm.	Thiol. amino. methyl. glyox. hyd.	0 4	per	grain	—
36	oz.	Thiosinamina	—	—	5 3	0 9
12	oz.	Thio-urea	—	—	1 9	0 3
24	oz.	Thorii nitras pur.	—	—	3 6	0 6
18	lb.	Thus	2 3	0 8	0 3	—
13	oz.	Thymol	—	—	1 11	0 4
84	oz.	Thymol carbonas	—	—	12 4	1 0
36	oz.	Thymol iodidum	—	—	5 3	0 9
42	oz.	Thyroideum	—	—	6 4	1 0
24	lb.	Tiliæ flores	3 0	0 11	0 3	—

Cost d.	Cost per	Th—Ti	Selling Price 16 oz. s. d.	4 oz. s. d.	1 oz. s. d.	1 dr. s. d.
84	lb.	Thymotussin	—	3 3	0 10	—
		Tincturæ				
68	lb.	Tr. aconiti .. S.I. (5)	—	2 5	0 9	0 2
93	lb.	Tr. aconiti Fleming S.I. (5)	—	3 3	0 11	0 2
87	lb.	Tr. adonis vernalis	—	3 0	0 10	0 2
9	oz.	Tr. alii	—	—	1 4	0 3
45	lb.	Tr. aloes	—	1 7	0 5	0 1
96	lb.	Tr. aloes co. B.P.C.	—	3 4	0 11	0 2
57	lb.	Tr. ammoniæ co. B.P.C. ..	7 0	2 0	0 7	—
75	lb.	Tr. anthemidis	—	2 8	0 9	0 2
84	lb.	Tr. antiperiodica B.P.C. P.I. (9)	—	3 0	0 10	0 2
80	lb.	Tr. apocyni	—	2 10	0 10	0 2
48	lb.	Tr. arnicæ florum	5 10	1 8	0 6	0 1
72	lb.	Tr. arnicæ radicis	9 0	2 7	0 9	0 2
72	lb.	Tr. asafetidæ	—	2 5	0 8	0 2
210	lb.	Tr. aurantii	—	7 0	2 0	0 4
282	lb.	Tr. aurantii dulcis	—	9 6	2 5	0 4
75	lb.	Tr. baptisiæ	—	—	0 9	0 2
63	lb.	Tr. belladonnæ P.I. (9)	—	2 3	0 8	0 2
64	lb.	Tr. benzoini comp.	7 4	2 2	0 7	0 1
78	lb.	Tr. benzoini simp.	—	2 7	0 8	0 2
98	lb.	Tr. berberidis	—	3 2	0 11	0 2
75	lb.	Tr. boldo	—	2 9	0 9	0 2
68	lb.	Tr. bryoniæ	—	2 5	0 8	0 2
70	lb.	Tr. buchu	—	2 5	0 8	0 2
96	lb.	Tr. calendulæ	—	3 4	0 11	0 2
57	lb.	Tr. calumbæ	—	2 0	0 7	0 1
48	lb.	Tr. camphoræ co. P.I. (9)	—	1 6	0 5	0 1
32	oz.	Tr. cannabis ind. .. D.D.	—	—	4 8	0 8
84	lb.	Tr. cantharidini S.I. (5)	—	3 0	0 10	0 2
92	lb.	Tr canthar. B.P. '98 S.I. (6)	—	3 3	0 11	0 2
102	lb.	Tr. cantharidis acet. S.I. (6)	—	3 7	1 0	0 2
52	lb.	Tr. capsici	—	1 9	0 7	0 1
96	lb.	Tr. capsici fortior B.P.C. ..	—	3 4	1 0	0 2
80	lb.	Tr. cardamomi	—	2 10	0 9	0 2
48	lb.	Tr. cardamomi co.	—	1 9	0 6	0 1
108	lb.	Tr. carminativa	—	4 0	1 1	0 2
86	lb.	Tr. cascaræ	—	3 0	0 11	0 2
90	lb.	Tr. cascarillæ	—	3 2	0 11	0 2
16	oz.	Tr. castorei	—	—	2 4	0 4
42	lb.	Tr. catechu	—	1 6	0 6	0 1
80	lb.	Tr. caulophylli	—	2 10	0 9	0 2
11	oz.	Tr. cerei B.P.C.	—	—	1 8	0 3
60	lb.	Tr. chiratæ	—	2 2	0 7	0 1
68	lb.	Tr. chloroformi comp.	—	2 6	0 9	0 2
38	lb.	Tr. chlor.et morph. B.P.C. S.I.(5)	—	1 6	0 6	0 1
144	lb.	Tr. chlorof. et morph. co. D.D.	—	—	1 8	0 3
57	lb.	Tr. cimicifugæ	—	2 0	0 7	0 1
69	lb.	Tr. cinchonæ	—	2 5	0 8	0 2
69	lb.	Tr. cinchonæ co.	—	2 5	0 8	0 2
23	oz.	Tr. cinnamomi	—	—	3 5	0 6
69	lb.	Tr. cinnamomi co.	—	2 5	0 9	0 2
84	lb.	Tr. cocæ .. .. D.D.	—	3 0	0 10	0 2
15	oz.	Tr. cocci	—	—	2 3	0 4
60	lb.	Tr. colchici .. ..P.I. (9)	—	2 0	0 7	0 1
68	lb.	Tr. colch. sem. B.P. '98 P.I. (10)	—	2 2	0 7	0 1
84	lb.	Tr. colchici cormi P.I. (10)	—	3 0	0 10	0 2
84	lb.	Tr. collinsoniæ canad.	—	3 0	0 10	0 2
10	oz.	Tr. colocynthidis	—	—	1 6	0 3
90	lb.	Tr. condurango	—	3 1	0 11	0 2
8	oz.	Tr. conii .. S.I. (6)	—	—	1 2	0 2
7	oz.	Tr. convallariæ	—	—	1 1	0 2
120	lb.	Tr. coto	—	4 3	1 2	0 2
13	oz.	Tr. croci	—	—	1 10	0 4
9	oz.	Tr. cubebæ	—	—	1 4	0 3
26	oz.	Tr. curcumæ	—	—	3 9	0 7
86	lb.	Tr. cusparisæ	—	3 0	0 10	0 2
81	lb.	Tr. damianæ	—	2 10	0 11	0 2

Cost d.	Cost per	Ti Tincturæ—(cont.)	Selling Price 16 oz. s. d.	4 oz. s. d.	1 oz. s. d.	1 dr. s. d.
10	oz.	Tr. daturæ sem. P.I. (10)	—	—	1 6	0 3
66	lb.	Tr. digitalis .. S.I. (5)	—	2 5	0 9	0 2
9	oz.	Tr. droseræ rot.	—	—	1 4	0 3
114	lb.	Tr. ergotæ B.P. '85 S.I. (6)	—	4 1	1 2	0 2
102	lb.	Tr. ergotæ ammoniata S.I. (5)	—	3 8	1 0	0 2
7	oz.	Tr. eucalypti fol.	—	—	1 1	0 2
9	oz.	Tr. eucalypti gum.	—	—	1 4	0 3
7	oz.	Tr. euonymi	—	—	1 1	0 2
10	oz.	Tr. euonymin. virid.	—	—	1 5	0 3
72	lb.	Tr. euphorbiæ	—	2 7	0 9	0 2
54	lb.	Tr. ferri acetatis	—	2 0	0 7	0 1
21	lb.	Tr. ferri perchloridi	2 9	0 11	0 4	0 1
51	lb.	Tr. ferri pomati	—	1 10	0 6	0 1
84	lb.	Tr. gallæ	—	3 0	0 10	0 2
54	lb.	Tr. gelsemii .. ..P.I. (9)	—	2 0	0 7	0 1
42	lb.	Tr. gentianæ co.	5 2	1 5	0 5	0 1
7	oz.	Tr. gossypii	—	—	1 1	0 2
7	oz.	Tr. grindeliæ	—	—	1 1	0 2
81	lb.	Tr. guaiaci	—	2 10	0 10	0 2
81	lb.	Tr. guaiaci ammoniata	—	3 0	0 10	0 2
12	oz.	Tr. guaranæ	—	—	1 9	0 3
50	lb.	Tr. hamamelidis	—	1 9	0 7	0 1
99	lb.	Tr. hellebori nigri	—	3 7	1 0	0 2
15	oz.	Tr. hibisci	—	—	2 3	0 4
102	lb.	Tr. hydrastis	—	3 7	1 0	0 2
66	lb.	Tr. hyoscyami .. ..P.I. (9)	—	2 4	0 8	0 2
9	oz.	Tr. ignatiæ amaræ ..P.I. (9)	—	—	1 4	0 3
200	lb.	Tr. iodi ætherea	—	7 0	1 10	0 4
75	lb.	Tr. iodi decolorata	—	2 8	0 9	0 2
96	lb.	Tr. iodi decolorat. fort. B.P.C.	—	3 5	0 11	0 2
32	lb.	Tr. ipecacuanhæ ..P.I. (9)	—	1 2	0 4	—
8	oz.	Tr. ipecacuanhæ et opii D.D.	—	—	1 2	0 2
25	oz.	Tr. iridis	—	—	3 8	0 7
54	lb.	Tr. jaborandi .. ..P.I. (9)	—	2 0	0 7	0 1
78	lb.	Tr. jalapæ	—	2 7	0 9	0 2
78	lb.	Tr. jalapæ co.	—	2 7	0 9	0 2
66	lb.	Tr. kino	—	2 4	0 8	0 2
66	lb.	Tr. kolæ	—	2 4	0 8	0 2
60	lb.	Tr. krameriæ	—	2 2	0 8	0 2
10	oz.	Tr. laricis	—	—	1 6	0 3
87	lb.	Tr. lavandulæ co.	—	3 2	0 11	0 2
204	lb.	Tr. limonis	—	7 3	2 2	0 4
62	lb.	Tr. lobeliæ	—	2 2	0 7	0 1
84	lb.	Tr. lobeliæ ætherea	—	3 0	0 10	0 2
66	lb.	Tr. lupuli	—	2 4	0 9	0 2
14	oz.	Tr. lycopodii	—	—	2 0	0 4
7	oz.	Tr. maticæ	—	—	1 1	0 2
87	lb.	Tr. myrrhæ	—	3 1	0 11	0 2
69	lb.	Tr. myrrhæ co. vet.	8 6	2 5	0 9	—
90	lb.	Tr. myrrhæ et boracis P.L.F. ..	11 3	3 0	0 11	0 2
104	lb.	Tr. myrrhæ et boracis B.P.C. ..	—	3 9	1 0	0 2
262	lb.	Tr. myrrhæ et boracis c. eau de Cologne P.L.F.	—	8 6	2 3	—
45	lb.	Tr. nuc. vomicæ ..P.I. (9)	—	1 8	0 6	0 1
183	lb.	Tr. odontalg. P.L.F. P.I. (13)	—	—	1 8	0 4
72	lb.	Tr. opii .. .. .. D.D.	—	2 7	0 9	0 2
69	lb.	Tr. opii B.P. '98 .. D.D.	—	2 5	0 8	0 2
72	lb.	Tr. opii ammoniata ..P.I. (9)	—	2 7	0 9	0 2
54	lb.	Tr. opii aq. (1% morph.) D.D.	—	2 0	0 7	0 1
180	lb.	Tr. opii crocata B.P.C. D.D.	—	6 5	1 10	0 4
90	lb.	Tr. opii deod. U.S.P. .. D.D.	—	3 2	0 10	0 2
36	lb.	Tr. persionis B.P.C.	—	1 4	0 5	0 1
13	oz.	Tr. phosphori co. ..P.I. (9)	—	—	2 0	0 4
96	lb.	Tr. podophylli	—	3 4	0 11	0 2
84	lb.	Tr. podophylli ammoniata ..	—	3 0	0 10	0 2
57	lb.	Tr. pruni virginianæ	—	2 0	0 7	0 1
78	lb.	Tr. pulsatillæ	—	2 9	0 10	0 2
84	lb.	Tr. pyrethri	—	2 10	0 11	0 2

Ti—Un

Cost d.	per	Tincturæ—(cont).	Selling Price 16 oz. s. d.	4 oz. s. d.	1 oz. s. d.	1 dr. s. d.
86	lb.	Tr. pyrethri florum	—	3 0	0 10	0 2
45	lb.	Tr. quassiæ	—	1 8	0 6	0 1
45	lb.	Tr. quillaiæ	—	1 8	0 6	0 1
264	lb.	Tr. quininæ	—	9 5	2 9	0 5
54	lb.	Tr. quininæ ammoniata	6 9	2 0	0 7	0 1
		Tr. quin. am. pkd. (std. bot.)	—	2 4	1 6	℥ij.
78	lb.	Tr. quin. ammon. c. cinnam.	—	2 9	0 10	0 2
45	lb.	Tr. rhei co.	5 6	1 7	0 6	0 1
92	lb.	Tr. rhei '85	11 0	3 2	0 11	0 2
7	oz.	Tr. rhus toxicod.	—	—	1 1	0 2
51	lb.	Tr. scillæ	—	1 11	0 7	0 1
68	lb.	Tr. senegæ	—	2 5	0 8	0 2
54	lb.	Tr. sennæ co. Alex.	—	2 0	0 7	0 1
45	lb.	Tr. sennæ co. Tinnev.	—	1 7	0 6	0 1
78	lb.	Tr. serpentariæ	—	2 9	0 9	0 2
45	lb.	Tr. stramonii ..P.I. (9)	—	1 7	0 6	0 1
64	lb.	Tr. stramonii sem. ..P.I. (9)	—	2 3	0 8	0 2
96	lb.	Tr. strophanthi ..S.1. (5)	—	3 5	1 0	0 2
7	oz.	Tr. sumbul	—	—	1 1	0 2
84	lb.	Tr. tolutana	—	3 0	0 10	0 2
60	lb.	Tr. valerianæ	—	2 2	0 8	0 2
92	lb	Tr. valerianæ ætherea	—	3 0	0 10	0 2
57	lb.	Tr. valerianæ ammoniata	—	2 1	0 8	0 2
87	lb.	Tr. veratri ..P.I. (9)	—	3 0	0 10	0 2
7	oz.	Tr. viburni prunifol.	—	—	1 1	0 2
84	lb.	Tr. zingiberis	—	3 0	0 10	0 2
96	lb.	Tr. zingiberis fort.	—	3 4	0 11	0 2
		Tr. zingiberis fort., pkd.	℥ij.	1 9	℥j.	1 0
179	lb.	Toilet vinegar P.L.F.	—	6 9	1 10	0 4
84	lb.	Toncæ fabæ Para frosted	—	3 0	0 10	0 2
198	lb.	Tonca fabæ Angostura	—	7 0	2 1	0 4
36	oz.	Totaquina	—	—	5 3	0 9
90	lb.	Tragacantha	—	3 3	0 10	—
168	lb.	Tragacanthæ pulv. opt.	—	6 10	1 11	0 4
108	lb.	Tragacanthæ pulv. sec.	—	4 0	1 1	0 2
42	oz.	Triferrin	—	—	—	1 0
24	30	Triferrin tablets gr. 5	doz.	1 3	—	—
8	oz.	Trinitrophenol ..P.I. (8)	—	—	1 2	0 2
10	lb.	Trinitrophenol 1% sol...P.I. (8)	1 3	0 5	0 2	—
21	lb.	Trinitrophenol alc. sol.	2 6	0 10	0 3	—
21	lb.	Tripoli photographic	2 8	0 9	0 3	—
10	lb.	Tripoli polishing	1 3	0 5	0 2	—
15	dr.	Trypsin	—	—	—	2 3
18	oz.	Tumenol ammon.	—	—	—	0 8
		U				
33	lb.	Ulmi fulvæ cortex	—	1 3	0 4	—
24	lb.	Ulmi fulvæ corticis pulv.	3 0	0 11	0 4	—
30	lb.	Ultramarine	3 9	1 2	0 4	—
58	15	Unden pellets	—	6 6	tube	—
		Unguenta				
39	lb.	Unguentum acidi benzoici co.	4 6	1 4	0 5	—
15	lb.	Ung. acidi borici	1 10	0 7	0 3	—
13	lb.	Ung. acidi borici flavum	1 8	0 7	0 2	—
60	lb.	Ung. acidi carbolici co. P.I. (10)	7 6	2 2	0 8	—
21	lb.	Ung. acidi salicylici	2 8	0 10	0 3	—
54	lb.	Ung. ac. tannic	—	2 0	0 7	—
78	oz.	Ung. aconitinæ ..S.1. (9)	—	—	—	1 9
22	lb.	Ung. adipis lanæ hydros.	2 9	0 10	0 3	—
15	oz.	Ung. adrenalini ..P.I. (9)	—	—	2 3	0 4
27	lb.	Ung. althææ	3 6	1 0	0 4	—
33	lb.	Ung. anilin. vir. (1 : 1,000)	—	1 3	0 5	—
48	lb.	Ung. anilin. coccin. 5%	—	1 9	0 6	0 1
84	lb.	Ung. anilin. coccin. 8%	—	3 0	0 10	0 2
63	lb.	Ung. antim. tart. ..S.1. (6)	7 10	2 3	0 8	—
78	lb.	Ung. aquæ rosæ	—	2 10	0 9	—

Un

Cost d.	per	Unguenta—(cont.)	Selling Price 16 oz. s. d.	4 oz. s. d.	1 oz. s. d.	1 dr. s. d.
30	lb.	Ung. aquos	3 9	1 2	0 4	—
18	oz.	Ung. atropinæ ..S.1. (5)	—	—	2 8	0 5
7	oz.	Ung. belladonnæ ..S.1. (5)	—	—	1 1	0 2
48	lb.	Ung. bismuthi oleat. B.P.C	6 0	1 9	0 6	0 1
28	lb.	Ung. boracis	3 6	1 0	0 4	—
11	oz.	Ung. cadmii iodidi	—	—	1 8	0 3
18	lb.	Ung. calamin. N.H.I.	2 3	0 8	0 3	—
18	lb.	Ung. calaminæ	2 3	0 8	0 3	0 1
33	lb.	Ung. camphoræ B.P.C.	4 2	1 3	0 5	—
63	lb.	Ung. cantharidini ..S.1. (5)	—	2 4	0 8	—
57	lb.	Ung. cantharidis ..S.1. (5)	—	2 1	0 7	0 1
24	lb.	Ung. capsici	3 0	0 11	0 4	0 1
8	oz.	Ung. capsici Co.	—	—	1 2	0 2
28	lb.	Ung. cetacei	3 6	1 0	0 4	—
38	lb.	Ung. chaulmoogræ	—	1 5	0 6	—
20	lb.	Ung. chrom. (factory)	2 6	0 9	0 3	—
26	lb.	Ung. chrysarobini	3 3	1 0	0 4	0 1
42	oz.	Ung. cocainæ .. D.D.	—	—	6 4	1 0
54	lb.	Ung. creosoti	—	2 0	0 7	—
42	lb.	Ung. cupri oleatis	5 3	1 6	0 6	—
72	lb.	Ung. elemi	—	2 7	0 9	0 2
22	lb.	Ung. eucalypti	2 9	0 10	0 3	—
16	lb.	Ung. flav. dil. 1-4	—	0 7	0 2	—
30	lb.	Ung. gallæ	—	1 2	0 4	—
60	lb.	Ung. gallæ c. opio S.1. (5)	—	2 2	0 7	0 1
48	lb.	Ung. glycer. et ichthamol "jelly"	6 0	1 9	0 6	—
41	lb.	Ung. glycer. et zinc. " jelly "	5 2	1 6	0 5	—
26	lb.	Ung. glyc. plumb. subac. '98 P.I.(9)	—	1 0	0 4	—
69	lb.	Ung. hæmamol (D.F.)	—	2 2	0 7	0 1
27	lb.	Ung. hamamelidis	3 6	1 0	0 4	—
28	Tube	Ung. histamine	3 6	per	tube	—
46	lb.	Ung. hydrargyri	5 9	1 8	0 6	—
24	lb.	Ung. hyd. ammoniati ..P.I. (9)	3 0	0 11	0 4	—
22	lb.	Ung. hyd. ammoniati dil. P.I. (9)	2 9	0 10	0 3	—
42	lb.	Ung. hyd. co.	5 3	1 6	0 5	—
51	lb.	Ung. hyd. iodidi rubri ..S.1. (5)	6 5	1 10	0 7	—
39	lb.	Ung. hyd. nitratis ..S.1. (5)	—	1 5	0 5	—
21	lb.	Ung. hyd. nitratis dil.	2 8	0 10	0 3	—
36	lb.	Ung. hyd. oleatis ..S.1. (5)	4 6	1 4	0 5	—
16	lb.	Ung. hyd. oxidi flavi ..P.I. (9)	2 0	0 7	0 2	—
33	lb.	Ung. hyd. oxidi rubri ..P.I. (9)	4 2	1 3	0 5	—
48	lb.	Ung. hyd. subchloridi	—	1 9	0 6	0 1
20	lb.	Ung. ichthamol	—	0 9	0 3	—
48	lb.	Ung. ichthamol. co. B.P.C.	—	1 9	0 6	0 1
33	lb.	Ung. iodi	—	1 3	0 5	0 1
24	lb.	Ung. iodi denigrescens	—	1 0	0 4	—
24	lb.	Ung. iodi denigresc. N.H.I.	—	1 0	0 4	—
51	lb.	Ung. iodoformi	—	2 0	0 7	0 1
30	lb.	Ung. lanæ co.	3 9	1 1	0 4	0 1
48	lb.	Ung. mentho. 5%	—	1 9	0 6	0 1
32	lb.	Ung. mercuriale (" Trooper ")	4 0	1 2	0 4	—
24	lb.	Ung. metallorum B.P.C.	3 0	0 11	0 4	—
36	lb.	Ung. methyl salicyl.	—	1 4	0 5	0 1
21	lb.	Ung. methyl salicyl. dil.	—	0 10	0 3	—
66	lb.	Ung. methyl salicyl. co.	—	2 6	0 9	0 2
32	lb.	Ung. methyl salicyl. co. dil.	—	1 2	0 4	0 1
8	oz.	Ung. oleoresinæ capsici	—	—	1 2	0 2
9	oz.	Ung. oleoresinæ capsici co.	—	—	1 4	0 3
15	oz.	Ung. opii .. D.D.	—	—	2 3	0 4
15	lb.	Ung. paraf. alb.	1 10	0 7	0 2	—
13	lb.	Ung. paraf. flav.	1 9	0 7	0 3	—
19	lb.	Ung. phenol. .. P.II. (9)	—	0 9	0 3	—
21	lb.	Ung. picis carb.	2 8	0 10	0 3	—
24	lb.	Ung. picis carb. co.	3 0	0 11	0 4	—
22	lb.	Ung. picis liq.	2 9	0 10	0 3	—
42	lb.	Ung. pini sedat. (D.F.)	—	1 6	0 5	0 1
26	lb.	Ung. plumbi acetatis ..P.I. (9)	3 3	0 11	0 4	—

Cost d.	Cost per	Un—Ve Unguenta—(cont.)	Selling Price 16 oz. s. d.	4 oz. s. d.	1 oz. s. d.	1 dr. s. d.
38	lb.	Ung. plumbi carb.	—	1 6	0 5	—
60	lb.	Ung. plumbi iodidi	—	2 2	0 8	0 2
54	lb.	Ung. plumbi oleatis ..S.1. (5)	6 0	1 9	0 6	0 1
24	lb.	Ung. plumbi subacetatis ..	3 0	0 11	0 3	—
42	lb.	Ung. potass. polysulph. ..	—	1 6	0 6	—
36	lb.	Ung. potassæ sulphuratæ ..	4 6	1 4	0 5	—
66	lb.	Ung. potassii iodidi	—	2 5	0 9	0 2
20	lb.	Ung. resinæ	2 6	0 9	0 3	—
33	lb.	Ung. resinæ co. B.P.C. ..	—	1 3	0 4	—
38	lb.	Ung. resorcini B.P.C.	—	1 5	0 5	0 1
30	lb.	Ung. resorcini co. B.P.C. ..	—	1 1	0 4	0 1
63	lb.	Ung. resorcini et bismuthi co. B.P.C.	—	2 4	0 8	0 2
72	lb.	Ung. rosæ album B.P.C. ..	—	2 7	0 9	—
24	lb.	Ung. rusci co.	—	0 11	0 4	—
51	lb.	Ung. sabinæ .. S.1. (6)	—	2 0	0 7	0 1
42	lb.	Ung. sambuci flor.	5 3	1 6	0 5	0 1
30	lb.	Ung. sambuci viride	3 9	1 1	0 4	0 1
17	lb.	Ung. simplex alb.	2 1	0 8	0 3	—
14	lb.	Ung. simpl. flav.	—	0 7	0 2	—
54	lb.	Ung. staphisagriæ	—	2 0	0 7	0 1
13	lb.	Ung. sulphuris	1 8	0 6	0 2	—
24	lb.	Ung. sulphuris co.	3 0	0 11	0 4	—
28	lb.	Ung. sulphuris et resorcini ..	—	1 2	0 4	—
10	oz.	Ung. sulphuris hypochloritis ..	—	—	1 6	0 3
60	lb.	Ung. sulphuris iodidi	—	2 2	0 8	0 2
36	lb.	Ung. terebinthinæ	4 6	1 4	0 5	—
90	lb.	Ung. thymol 5%	—	3 3	0 11	0 2
93	lb.	Ung. thymol co. B.P.C. ..	—	3 4	1 0	—
51	lb.	Ung. thymol comp. dilut. B.P.C.	—	2 0	0 7	—
10	oz.	Ung. veratrinæ S.1. (5)	—	—	1 6	0 3
16	lb.	Ung. zinci oxid.	2 0	0 7	0 2	—
26	lb.	Ung. zinci c. ol. ricini	3 3	1 0	0 4	—
20	lb.	Ung. zinci c. ac. borici ..	2 6	0 9	0 3	—
36	lb.	Ung. zinci oleatis	4 6	1 4	0 5	0 1
45	lb.	Ung. zinci stearat. B.P.C. ..	—	1 9	0 6	—
20	lb.	University cream P.L.F. ..	2 6	0 9	—	—
102	oz.	Uradal B.P.C.	—	—	14 10	2 2
26	oz.	Uranii acetas	—	—	3 9	0 7
20	oz.	Uranii nitras	—	—	3 0	0 5
24	lb.	Urea	—	0 11	0 4	0 1
24	oz.	Ureæ hydrochlor.	—	—	3 6	0 6
13	oz.	Urethanum .. ..℞ only	—	—	2 3	0 4
36	oz.	Urotropin	—	—	5 3	0 11
12	lb.	Uvæ ursi folia	—	0 6	0 2	—
		V				
84	lb.	Valerianæ rhizoma Ang. ..	—	3 0	0 10	0 2
14	lb.	Valerianæ rhizoma Belg. ..	—	0 7	0 3	—
103	oz.	Validol	—	—	—	3 6
103	100	Validol perles	doz.	1 6	—	—
27	25	Valyl perles gr. 2	doz.	1 6	—	—
26	oz.	Vanillæ fabæ	—	—	3 9	0 7
26	oz.	Vanillinum	—	—	3 9	0 7
42	lb.	Vap. menthol N.I.F.	—	1 6	0 6	—
189	12 v.	Ventriculin, P., D. & Co. ..	12	vials	21 0	—
122	100 gr	Ventriculin with iron, P., D.&Co.	100	grs.	12 6	—
98	oz.	Veramon .. ..℞ only	—	—	—	2 3
126	100	Veramon tablets gr. 6 ..℞ only	doz.	2 0	—	—
19	lb.	Veratri alb. rhiz. pulv. S.1. (4)	—	0 9	0 3	—
60	lb.	Veratri virid. rhiz. pulv. S.1. (4)	—	2 3	0 8	0 2
20	dr.	Veratrina S.1. (4)	—	—	—	3 0
36	oz.	Veronal .. .. ..℞ only	—	—	—	0 9
22	25	Veronal tablets, gr. 5 ..℞ only	doz.	1 6	—	—
36	oz.	Veronal, sodium ..℞ only	—	—	—	0 9
22	25	Veronal sodium tabs ..℞ only	doz.	1 6	—	—

Cost d.	Cost per	Vi—Zi	Selling Price 16 oz. s. d.	4 oz. s. d.	1 oz. s. d.	1 dr. s. d.
		Vina				
42	lb.	Vinum aloes	—	1 6	0 6	—
24	lb.	Vin. antimoniale ..P.I. (9)	—	0 11	0 4	—
126	gal.	Vin. aurantii	pint	2 0	—	—
198	gal.	Vin. aurantii detan.	pint	3 3	0 4	—
54	lb.	Vin. cinchonæ	—	2 0	0 7	0 1
66	lb.	Vin. cocæ .. .. D.D.	—	2 5	0 9	0 2
27	lb.	Vin. colchici .. ..P.I. (9)	—	1 0	0 4	0 1
36	lb.	Vin. colchici sem. ..P.I. (9)	—	1 4	0 5	0 1
30	lb.	Vin. ferri	3 9	1 1	0 4	—
24	lb.	Vin. ferri citratis	3 0	1 0	0 4	—
38	lb.	Vin. ipecacuanhæ '14	—	1 5	0 5	—
84	lb.	Vin. opii .. .. .. D.D.	—	3 0	0 10	0 2
42	lb.	Vin. pepsini	6 4	1 10	0 7	—
18	lb.	Vin. quininæ	2 3	0 8	0 3	—
66	lb.	Vin. rhei	—	2 4	0 8	—
30	oz.	Virid Nitens	per	gr.	0 2	0 9
		W				
4.5	lb.	Waterglass, pkd.	2 lb.	0 10	4 lb.	1 4
8	lb.	Water softener P.L.F.	1 4	—	—	—
31	lb.	White oils P.L.F.	4 0	1 1	0 4	—
		X				
57	oz.	Xeroform	—	—	—	1 5
24	lb.	Xylol rectif.	—	1 0	0 4	—
		Y				
4	oz.	Yeast (dried)	—	—	0 7	0 1
5	gr.	Yohimbinæ hydrochlor. S.1. (4)	per	gr.	0 10	—
11	10	Yohimbine tablets . S.1. (4)	per	tube	1 6	—
		Z				
26	lb.	Zinci acetas	—	1 0	0 4	0 1
15	oz.	Zinci benzoas ver.	—	—	2 3	0 4
11	oz.	Zinci bromidum	—	—	1 8	0 3
24	lb.	Zinci carbonas	—	1 0	0 4	0 1
32	lb.	Zinci chloridum (fused) ..	4 0	1 2	0 4	0 1
11	oz.	Zinci chloridum (sticks) ..	—	—	1 8	0 3
14	lb.	Zinci chloridum coml.	1 9	0 7	0 2	—
33	oz.	Zinci et hydrarg. cyan. S.1. (4)	—	—	4 10	0 9
24	oz.	Zinci iodidum	—	—	3 6	0 6
12	oz.	Zinci lactas	—	—	1 9	0 3
48	lb.	Zinci oleas præcip.	—	1 9	0 6	0 1
51	lb.	Zinci oleostearas	—	1 10	0 7	0 1
16	lb.	Zinci oxidum	2 0	0 7	0 2	—
66	lb.	Zinci oxidum (Howards) ..	—	2 5	0 9	—
19	lb.	Zinci oxidum (Hubbuck) ..	2 5	0 9	0 3	—
12	lb.	Zinci oxid. c. amylo	1 6	0 6	0 2	—
12	lb.	Zinci oxid. c. amylo et ac. bor.	1 6	0 6	0 2	—
14	oz.	Zinci permanganas	—	—	2 3	0 4
15	oz.	Zinci peroxidum 20%	—	—	2 3	0 5
42	lb.	Zinci phosphas	—	1 6	0 5	0 1
15	oz.	Zinci phosphidum	—	—	2 3	0 4
45	lb.	Zinci stearas	—	1 8	0 7	0 1
12	oz.	Zinci sulphanilas	—	—	1 9	0 3
9	lb.	Zinci sulphas	1 2	0 5	0 2	—
6	lb.	Zinci sulphas coml.	0 9	0 3	0 1	—
8	oz.	Zinci sulphidum pur.	—	—	1 1	0 2
34	lb.	Zinci sulphocarb. pulv. ..	—	1 3	0 5	0 1
16	oz.	Zinci tannas	—	—	2 4	0 4
16	oz.	Zinci valerianas pulv.	—	—	2 4	0 4
38	lb.	Zincum granulatum pur. ..	—	1 4	0 5	—
13	lb.	Zincum granulatum coml. ..	1 8	0 7	0 2	—
16	lb.	Zingiberis rhizoma Afric. ..	2 0	0 7	0 2	—
18	lb.	Zingib. rhiz. Afric. pulv. ..	2 3	0 7	0 2	—
17	lb.	Zingib. rhiz. Afric. pulv. crs. ..	2 1	0 7	0 2	—
42	lb.	Zingib. rhiz. Jam. opt.	5 3	1 6	0 6	—
36	lb.	Zingib. rhiz. Jam. pulv. opt. ..	4 6	1 4	0 5	0 1
32	oz.	Zircon nit.	—	—	4 8	0 8

Ampullæ		Cost per ½ doz. d.	Sell per ½ doz. s. d.	Cost per doz. d.	Sell per doz. s. d.
Acetyl choline 0.05		40	5 0	—	—
Acetyl choline 0.1		48	6 0	—	—
Adrenalin	P.I. (8)	18	2 3	34	4 3
Apomorphinæ hydroch. gr. $\frac{1}{20}$	S.I. (6)	18	2 3	34	4 3
Atropinæ sulph. gr. $\frac{1}{100}$	P.I. (13)	18	2 3	34	4 3
Benzamin. hyd. gr. $\frac{1}{8}$, adrenalin. gr. $\frac{1}{1000}$		18	2 3	34	4 3
Bismuth. 0.2 gm.		30	3 9	52	6 6
Bismuth. salicyl. 1.2 c.c.		26	3 3	46	5 9
Caffein. sod.-sal. gr. 3		18	2 3	34	4 3
Caffein. sodii benz. 3.75		18	2 3	34	4 3
Camph. in ol. olivæ gr. 1½, gr. 3		18	2 3	34	4 3
Camphor. æther, ol. oliv.		26	3 3	48	6 0
Choline hyd. 0.1 c.c.		46	5 9	—	—
Cocain. hydroch. gr. $\frac{1}{6}$, gr. $\frac{1}{3}$, gr. $\frac{1}{2}$	D.D.	18	2 3	34	4 3
Cocain. hydroch. gr. $\frac{1}{8}$ adrenalin. gr. $\frac{1}{1000}$	D.D.	18	2 3	34	4 3
Cocain. hydroch. gr. $\frac{1}{3}$ adrenalin. gr. $\frac{1}{200}$	D.D.	18	2 3	34	4 3
Digitalin. gr. $\frac{1}{10}$	S.I. (6)	22	2 9	30	5 0
Emetinæ hydroch. gr. ½	S.I. (6)	30	3 9	52	6 6
Emetin. hydroch. gr. 1	S.I. (6)	42	5 3	78	9 6
Ephedrine sulph. gr. ¾	P.I. (13)	22	2 9	40	5 0
Ergometrine	S.I. (6)	32	4 0	64	8 0
Ergotoxin. ethanesulph. 0.5 mg.	S.I. (6)	30	3 9	52	6 6
Ergotoxin. phosphate 0.5 mg.	S.I. (6)	30	3 9	52	6 6
Ethyl chaulmoogratis 2 c.c.		27	3 9	56	7 0
Ethyl morrhuatis		24	3 0	23	5 8
Ethyl hydnocarpate with creosote, camph., olive oil E.C.C.O.		22	2 9	40	5 0
Extract. ergotæ gr. 1½	S.I. (6)	18	2 3	34	4 3
Extract. ergotæ gr. 3½	S.I. (6)	26	3 3	48	6 0
Extract. ergotæ gr. 7	S.I. (6)	40	5 3	78	9 6
Ext. pituitary liq. 0.5	P.I. (13)	30	3 9	56	7 0
Ext. pituitary liq. 1.0	P.I. (13)	48	6 0	88	11 0
Ferri et ammon. cit. vir. gr. ½		18	2 3	34	4 3
Glucosi 2 fl. oz. for 1 pt.		16	2 0	—	—
Gum saline conc. 50 c.c.		20	2 6	each	—
Hyoscin. hydrobr. gr. $\frac{1}{100}$	P.I. (13)	18	2 0	34	4 3
Indigo carmine 0.4 per cent.		32	4 0	60	7 6
Iodi, boxes of 6		10	1 6	—	—
Manganese butyrate 1.5 c.c.		32	4 0	60	7 6
Mercurial cream ♏ 10		20	2 6	36	4 6
Morph. hydroch. gr. $\frac{1}{6}$, gr. ¼, gr. $\frac{1}{3}$, gr. ½	D.D.	20	2 6	38	4 9
Morph. hydroch. gr. ½ atropin. sulph. gr. $\frac{1}{200}$	D.D.	20	2 6	38	4 9
Ol. cinerei (grey oil) ½ c.c.		18	2 3	34	4 3
Peptoni 7½% 1.5 c.c.		30	3 9	56	7 0
Pilocarpin. nit. gr. ¼	S.I. (6)	22	2 9	40	5 0
Pituitrin ½ c.c.	P.I. (13)	—	4 6	—	8 0
Pituitrin 1 c.c.	P.I. (13)	—	7 6	—	14 0
Quinine urethane 2 c.c.		22	2 9	40	5 0
Scopolamin. hydrobr. gr. $\frac{1}{100}$ morph. acet. gr. ¼	D.D.	18	2 3	34	4 3
Sodii cacodyl. gr. ½, gr. $\frac{2}{3}$	S.I. (6)	18	2 3	34	4 3
Sodii cacodyl. gr. $\frac{1}{3}$, ferri cac. gr. $\frac{1}{3}$	S.I. (6)	22	2 9	40	5 0
Strophanthin. gr. $\frac{1}{500}$	S.I. (6)	18	2 3	34	4 3
Strychnin. sulph. gr. $\frac{1}{60}$, gr. $\frac{1}{30}$	S.I. (6)	18	2 3	34	4 3
Symmetrical ureas S.U.M. 36 (0.01 gm.)		30	4 6	64	8 0
Symmetrical ureas S.U.P. 36 (0.01 gm.)		30	4 6	64	8 0
Symmetrical ureas S.U.P. 468 (0.001 gm.)		60	7 6	—	—
Tetraiodophthalein T.I.P. 3.5 gm. 28 c.c.		22	2 9	each	—
Thiosinamin.-sod. sal. 2.3 c.c.		42	5 3	76	9 6

Cost d.	Cost per	Capsulæ vel Perles	Selling Price	s. d.		s. d.
270	1,000	Caps. apiol. ♏ 3	36	2 0	24	1 4
381	1,000	Caps. apiol. ♏ 5	36	2 6	24	1 9
468	1,000	Caps. apiol (3) et ext. ergot. (2) S.I. (6)	36	3 0	24	2 0
326	1,000	Caps. apiol steel pulegii ♏ 5	36	2 1	24	1 6
180	1,000	Caps. benzyl benz. ♏ 3	36	1 6	24	1 1
141	1,000	Caps. Blaudii gr. 10	36	1 3	24	1 0
174	1,000	Caps. Blaudii gr. 15	36	1 5	24	1 1
129	1,000	Caps. Blaudii pil. gr. 5	36	1 1	24	0 11
153	1,000	Caps. Blaudii pil. (5) et hæmoglob. (3)	36	1 3	24	1 0
153	1,000	Caps. Blaudii pil. (5) et ac. arsenios ($\frac{1}{50}$) S.I. (6)	36	1 3	24	1 0
153	1,000	Caps. Blaudii pil. (5) et ac. arsenios. et strych. S.I (6)	36	1 3	24	1 0
186	1,000	Caps. Blaudii pil. (10) et ext. casc. sag. (1)	36	1 6	24	1 1
276	1,000	Caps. carbon tetrachlor. 1 c.c.	36	2 0	24	1 6
402	1,000	Caps. carbon tetrachlor. 2 c.c.	36	2 9	24	1 11
192	1,000	Caps. casc. sag. ext. liq. ♏ 20	36	1 6	24	1 1
222	1,000	Caps. casc. sag. ext. liq. ♏ 30	36	1 8	24	1 2
357	1,000	Caps. casc. sag. ext. liq. ♏ 60	36	2 5	24	1 8
252	1,000	Caps. cinnam. et quin.	36	1 10	24	1 3
252	1,000	Caps. colch. sal. gr. $\frac{1}{250}$ S.I. (6)	36	2 1	24	1 6
390	1,000	Caps. colch. sal. gr. $\frac{1}{50}$ S.I. (6)	36	3 0	24	2 0
132	1,000	Caps. copaibæ (Maran.) ♏ 5	36	1 2	24	0 11
222	1,000	Caps. copaibæ (Maran.) ♏ 10	36	1 9	24	1 2
305	1,000	Caps. copaibæ (Maran.) ♏ 15	36	2 1	24	1 6
372	1,000	Caps. copaibæ et cubebæ et buchu ♏ 10	36	2 6	24	1 9
396	1,000	Caps. copaibæ et cubebæ et ol. santali ♏ 10	36	2 8	24	1 9
129	1,000	Caps. creos. in oleo ♏ 1 P.I. (13)	36	1 2	24	0 11
141	1,000	Caps. creos. in oleo ♏ 2 P.I. (13)	36	1 3	24	0 11
174	1,000	Caps. creos in oleo ♏ 3 P.I. (13)	36	1 6	24	1 1
384	1,000	Caps. ergotæ ext. gr. 3 S.I. (6)	36	2 6	24	1 9
207	1,000	Caps. filicis maris ♏ 5	36	1 8	24	1 2
306	1,000	Caps. filicis maris ♏ 10	36	2 3	24	1 6
414	1,000	Caps. filicis maris ♏ 15	36	3 2	24	1 9
483	1,000	Caps. filicis maris ♏ 20	36	3 1	24	2 3
666	1,000	Caps. filicis maris ♏ 30	36	4 1	24	2 10
156	1,000	Caps. guaiacol. in oleo ♏ 1	36	1 3	24	1 0
204	1,000	Caps. guaiacol. in oleo ♏ 2	36	1 8	24	1 2
309	1,000	Caps. guaiacol. in oleo ♏ 5	36	2 1	24	1 6
168	1,000	Caps. hæmoglobin. gr. 3	36	1 4	24	1 0
192	1,000	Caps. hæmoglobin. gr. 5	36	1 7	24	1 2
60	100	Caps. Halibut Oil ♏ 3	—	—	25	2 8
336	1,000	Caps. lecithin. gr. 2½	36	2 4	24	1 7
450	1,000	Caps. lecithin. (1½) et. paraf. liq. (30)	36	2 11	24	2 0
486	500	Caps. menthol valer. ♏ 5	36	5 7	24	3 8
132	1,000	Caps. ol. cajuputi ♏ 1	36	1 2	24	0 11
162	1,000	Caps. ol. caryophylli ♏ 2	36	1 4	24	1 1
174	1,000	Caps. ol chaulmoogra ♏ 5	36	1 6	24	1 1
246	1,000	Caps. ol. chaulmoogra ♏ 10	36	1 6	24	1 1
540	1,000	Caps. ol. chenopodii ♏ 5	36	3 4	24	2 4
228	1,000	Caps. ol. cinnamomi ♏ 1	36	1 8	24	1 3
348	1,000	Caps. ol. cinnamomi ♏ 2	36	2 4	24	1 8
270	1,000	Caps. ol. methylene Blue gr. 2	36	2 0	24	1 6
162	1,000	Caps. ol. morrhuæ ♏ 10	36	1 4	24	1 1
258	1,000	Caps. ol. morrhuæ ♏ 15	36	2 0	24	1 5
274	1,000	Caps. ol. morrhuæ ♏ 20	36	2 4	24	1 8
321	1,000	Caps. ol. morrhuæ ♏ 30	36	2 4	24	1 8
276	1,000	Caps. ol. morrhuæ (20) et creosot. (1)	36	2 0	24	1 4
360	1,000	Caps. ol. morrh. (30) et creos. (2)	36	2 4	24	1 8
246	1,000	Caps. ol. olivæ ♏ 15	36	1 9	24	1 3
348	1,000	Caps. ol. olivæ ♏ 30	36	2 4	24	1 8
222	1,000	Caps. ol. ricini ♏ 15	36	1 7	24	1 2
300	1,000	Caps. ol. ricini ♏ 30	36	1 10	24	1 5

Cost d.	per	Capsulæ vel Perles (cont.)	Selling Price	s. d.		s. d.
396	1,000	Caps. ol. ricini ♏ 60	36	2 8	24	1 10
264	500	Caps. ol. santali ♏ 5	36	3 3	24	2 3
345	500	Caps. ol. santali ♏ 7½	36	4 1	24	2 10
492	500	Caps. ol. santali ♏ 10	36	5 9	24	3 8
456	1,000	Caps. ol. santali (5) c. copaiba (5)	36	2 11	24	2 0
129	1,000	Caps. ol. terebinthinæ rect. ♏ 5	36	1 2	24	0 11
168	1,000	Caps. ol. terebinthinæ rect. ♏ 10	36	1 5	24	1 1
150	1,000	Caps. perichthol. ♏ 3	36	1 3	24	1 0
180	1,000	Caps. perichthol. ♏ 5	36	1 6	24	1 1
143	1,000	Caps. picis ♏ 5	36	1 6	24	0 11
228	1,000	Caps. syr. East. ♏ 30 S.I. (6)	36	1 9	24	1 2
321	1,000	Caps. syr. East. ʒj. S.I. (6)	36	2 3	24	1 6
228	1,000	Caps. syr. glyce. co. ♏ 30 P.I. (13)	36	1 9	24	1 2
324	1,000	Caps. syr. glyc. co. ʒj. P.I. (13)	36	2 3	24	1 7
228	1,000	Caps. syrup. hypophosphitum co. ♏ 30 .. P.I. (13)	36	1 9	24	1 2
324	1,000	Caps. syrup. hypophosphitum co. ʒj. .. P.I. (13)	36	2 3	24	1 7
147	1,000	Caps. terebeni	36	1 6	24	1 4
222	1,000	Caps. tinct. quininæ am. ♏ 30	36	1 9	24	1 2
321	1,000	Caps. tinct. quininæ am. ʒj. ..	36	2 3	24	1 8

Cost d.	per	Tabellæ	Selling Price (in containers) 100 s. d.	50 s. d.	25 s. d.
63	1,000	Acidi arseniosi gr. $\frac{1}{100}$ .. S.I. (6)	1 6	1 1	0 9
63	1,000	Acidi arseniosi gr. $\frac{1}{60}$ .. S.I. (6)	1 6	1 1	0 9
51	1,000	Acetanilidi gr. 3 .. P.I. (13)	1 3	0 10	0 7
63	1,000	Acetanilidi gr. 5 .. P.I. (13)	1 5	1 1	0 9
63	1,000	Acetanilidi co. .. .. P.I. (13)	1 5	0 11	0 7
72	1,000	Acetanilidi (3) caffein. (½) ammon. carb. (1) .. .. P.I. (13)	1 6	1 1	0 9
78	1,000	Acetanilidi (3) caffein. (½) sod. bic. (1) P.I. (13)	1 6	1 1	0 9
75	1,000	Aloes et ferri gr. 4	1 9	1 1	0 9
87	1,000	Aloes et myrrhæ	1 11	1 2	0 9
75	1,000	Aloini gr. ½	1 9	1 1	0 9
75	1,000	Aloini gr. ¼	1 9	1 1	0 9
69	1,000	Aloini co.	1 9	1 1	0 9
246	1,000	Amidopyrinæ gr. 5 .. .. ℞ only	4 1	2 3	1 3
63	1,000	Ammonii bromidi gr. 5	1 5	1 0	0 7
63	1,000	Antacid (Roberts)	1 6	1 1	0 9
38	1,000	Aspirin gr. 5	1 2	0 9	0 6
105	1,000	Aspirin gr. 10	2 0	1 4	0 11
108	1,000	Aspirin (4) et caffein. (1)	2 0	1 3	0 10
87	1,000	Aspirin (2½) et phenac. (2½)	1 9	1 1	0 9
120	1,000	Aspirin (2½) et phenac. (2½) et caffein. (1)	2 4	1 6	0 11
111	1,000	Aspirin compound N.I.F. P.I. (13)	2 2	1 3	0 10
108	1,000	Aspirin (3) et pulv. ipec. co. (2) P.I. (13)	2 0	1 3	0 9
171	1,000	Aspirin (4) et quininæ sulphatis (1) ..	3 0	1 9	1 1
252	1,000	Barbitoni gr. 5 .. .. .. ℞ only	4 1	2 4	1 4
273	1,000	Barbitoni solubile gr. 5 .. ℞ only	4 5	2 6	1 6
186	1,000	Benzonaphthol gr. 5	3 3	1 10	1 2
87	1,000	Beta-naphthol gr. 3	1 11	1 2	0 9
11	1,000	Beta-naphthol. gr. 5	2 3	1 4	0 11
87	1,000	Beta-naphthol co.	1 11	1 2	0 9
69	1,000	Bismuthated magnesia	—	1 1	—
62	1,000	Bismuthi carbonatis gr. 5	2 0	1 8	1 1
99	1,000	Bismuthi carb. (2½) et sod. bic. (2½) ..	2 0	1 2	0 9
99	1,000	Bism. carb. (2) sod. bic. (2) p. zingib. (1)	2 0	1 2	0 9
99	1,000	Bismuthi carb. (2) sod. bic. (1½) p. zingib. (½) p. rhei (1)	2 0	1 2	0 9
111	1,000	Bismuthi carb. (2) pepsin (1) carb. lig. (2)	2 3	1 4	0 10
150	1,000	Bismuthi salicylatis gr. 5	2 10	1 7	1 0
35	1,000	Bismuthi subnitratis gr. 5	2 6	1 6	0 11
51	1,000	Blaud pil. gr. 5	1 4	0 11	0 8

Cost d.	per	Tabellæ (cont.)	Selling Price (in containers) 100 s. d.	50 s. d.	25 s. d.
51	1,000	Blaud pil. (5) et ac. arsen. ($\frac{1}{100}$) S.I. (6)	1 6	1 1	0 9
63	1,000	Blaud pil. (5) ac. arsenios. ($\frac{1}{100}$) strychninæ ($\frac{1}{100}$) .. .. ..S.I. (6)	1 6	1 1	0 9
51	1,000	Blaud pil. (5) aloin. ($\frac{1}{10}$)	1 6	1 1	0 9
51	1,000	Blaud pil. (5) et casc. sag. (½)	1 4	0 11	0 8
84	1,000	Blaud pil. mang. diox. (1) ac. arsen. ($\frac{1}{64}$) ..	1 7	1 1	0 9
99	1,000	Caffeinæ citratis gr. 2	2 0	1 3	0 11
102	500	Calcii acetylsalicylatis	3 6	2 0	1 2
45	1,000	Calcii lactatis gr. 5	1 2	0 10	0 7
51	1,000	Calcii sulphid. ad gr. 1	1 3	0 11	0 7
38	1,000	Carbonis lig. (salicis) gr. 5	1 2	0 10	0 7
39	1,000	Cascaræ sag. ext. gr. 2	1 2	0 9	0 6
75	1,000	Cascaræ sag. ext. gr. 3	1 8	1 1	0 7
111	1,000	Cascaræ sag. ext. gr. 5	2 3	1 4	0 11
39	1,000	Cerevisiæ ferm. gr. 2	1 0	0 10	0 6
51	1,000	Cerevisiæ ferm. gr. 5	1 2	0 11	0 7
273	1,000	Cinchophenum gr. 5 .. ..℞ only	4 5	2 4	1 4
120	1,000	Cinnam. et quin. .. ..℞ only	2 3	1 8	1 1
264	1,000	Codeinæ gr. ¼ .. .. ..S.I. (6)	4 5	2 5	1 4
222	500	Codeinæ gr. ½ .. .. ..S.I. (6)	7 0	3 9	2 0
200	250	Codeinæ gr. 1 .. .. ..S.I. (6)	12 3	6 4	3 4
210	1,000	Codeinæ phosphatis gr. ¼ ..S.I. (6)	3 7	2 0	1 2
173	500	Codeinæ phosphatis gr. ½ ..S.I. (6)	5 7	3 1	1 9
151	250	Codeinæ phosphatis gr. 1 ..S.I. (6)	9 4	5 0	2 8
225	500	Cotamin. hydrochl. gr. ¾ ..S.I. (6)	—	4 0	2 6
225	500	Cotamin. pthal. gr. ¾ .. ..S.I. (6)	—	4 0	2 6
69	1,000	Cretæ arom. pulv. gr. 5	1 8	1 1	0 9
75	1,000	Cretæ arom. c. op. gr. 5	1 9	1 1	0 9
216	1,000	Diamorph. hyd. gr. $\frac{1}{12}$ .. .. D.D.	3 8	2 0	1 2
162	1,000	Diamorph. hyd. gr. $\frac{1}{24}$ .. .. D.D.	2 11	1 9	1 1
180	1,000	Digitalin. amorph. $\frac{1}{100}$ .. ..S.I. (6)	3 3	2 0	1 2
126	1,000	Digitalis fol. gr. 1 .. ..S.I. (6)	2 8	—	—
96	1,000	Doveri pulv. gr. 5 .. S.I. (6)	2 0	1 2	0 9
60	25	Emetin. bism. iod. gr. 1 ..S.I. (6)	—	—	6 9
75	1,000	Ephedrinæ hydrochloridi gr. ¼ P.I. (13)	2 9	—	1 0
117	1,000	Ephedrinæ hydrochloridi gr. ½ P.I. (13)	4 9	—	1 6
312	1,000	Ergotæ ext. gr. 2 .. ..S.I. (6)	4 8	2 8	1 6
432	1,000	Ergotæ ext. gr. 3 .. ..S.I. (6)	6 2	3 4	1 10
270	1,000	Ferri alginatis gr. 5	3 6	1 11	1 2
69	1,000	Ferri redact. gr. 3	1 9	1 1	0 9
72	1,000	Ferri carb. sacch. gr. 5	1 6	1 0	0 8
57	1,000	Formaldeh. B.P.C. gr. 15	—	1 1	—
57	1,000	Formald. et cinnam. gr. 12	—	1 1	—
96	1,000	Fuci ext. gr. 4	1 11	1 2	0 9
108	1,000	Fuci ext. gr. 5	2 0	1 3	0 9
126	1,000	Galvani pil. co. gr. 4	2 8	1 9	1 1
75	1,000	Glycyrrh. pulv. co. gr. 30	—	(40) 10	—
96	1,000	Guaiaci resinæ gr. 5	1 11	1 2	0 9
75	1,000	Guaiaci resinæ (3) sulph. (3)	1 8	1 1	0 9
194	1,000	Guaiacol. carbonatis gr. 5	3 1	1 9	1 1
90	1,000	Hæmoglobin. co.	1 11	1 2	0 9
57	1,000	Hexaminæ gr. 5	1 4	0 11	0 8
33	1,000	Hydrargyri c. creta gr. ½	1 0	0 9	0 7
33	1,000	Hydrargyri c. creta gr. 1	1 0	0 9	0 7
48	1,000	Hydrargyri c. creta gr. 2	1 2	0 10	0 8
126	1,000	Hydrargyri c. creta (1) et p. ipec. co. (1)	2 0	1 2	0 11
36	1,000	Hydrargyri c. creta (½) sod. bic. (½) ..	1 1	0 9	0 7
45	1,000	Hydrargyri c. creta (1) sod. bic. (3) ..	1 3	0 10	0 7
60	1,000	Hydrargyri iodidi rub. gr. $\frac{1}{16}$ ..S.I. (6)	1 6	1 1	0 9
60	1,000	Hydrargyri iodidi rub. gr. $\frac{1}{20}$ ..S.I. (6)	1 6	1 1	0 9
60	1,000	Hydrargyri iodidi vir. gr. ⅛	1 6	1 1	0 9
60	1,000	Hydrargyri iodidi vir. gr. ¼	1 6	1 1	0 9
39	1,000	Hydrargyri subchloridi gr. ½	1 1	0 10	0 7
51	1,000	Hydrargyri subchloridi gr. 1	1 2	0 10	0 7
93	1,000	Hydrargyri subchloridi gr. 3	1 5	1 0	0 8
138	1,000	Hydrargyri subchloridi gr. 5	2 6	1 6	1 0

Tabellæ (cont.)

Cost d.	Cost per	Tabellæ (cont.)		Selling Price (in containers) 100 s. d.	50 s. d.	25 s. d.
180	1,000	Hyoscinæ hydrobr. gr. $\frac{1}{100}$	S.I. (6)	3 3	1 9	1 1
144	1,000	Hyoscinæ hydrobr. gr. $\frac{1}{200}$	S.I. (6)	2 8	1 7	0 11
57	1,000	Iodised throat		—	1 1	—
300	1,000	Lactic. bacilli		4 10	2 10	1 8
147	1,000	Lithii carbonatis gr. 5		2 10	1 8	1 1
147	1,000	Lithii citratis gr. 5		2 10	1 8	1 1
252	1,000	Lithii citratis eff. gr. 5 in gr. 15 ..		4 1	2 10	1 4
173	500	Methylsulphonal gr. 5 ..	℞ only	5 7	3 1	1 9
63	1,000	Nitroglyc. gr. $\frac{1}{100}$, $\frac{1}{150}$, $\frac{1}{200}$	P.I. (13)	1 6	1 1	0 9
240	1,000	Ox bile (purif.) gr. 5		4 1	2 3	1 3
132	1,000	Pepsini gr. 2½ (coated)		2 6	1 6	0 11
81	1,000	Phenacetini gr. 5		1 8	1 1	0 9
159	1,000	Phenacetini, quin., caffein.		2 10	1 8	1 1
87	1,000	Phenacetini (4) et caff. cit. (1) ..		1 8	1 2	0 9
180	1,000	Phenazoni gr. 5		3 1	1 9	1 1
156	1,000	Phenazoni (4) et caff. cit. (1)		2 9	1 7	1 0
54	1,000	Phenolphthaleini gr. 1		1 4	0 11	0 7
60	1,000	Phenolphthaleini gr. 2		1 4	1 0	0 8
87	1,000	Phenolphthaleini gr. 5		1 6	1 2	0 9
51	1,000	Potassii bicarbonatis gr. 5		1 3	1 0	0 7
57	1,000	Potassii bromidi gr. 5		1 3	1 0	0 8
16	1,000	Potassii chloratis gr. 5		0 9	0 7	0 6
22	1,000	Potassii chloratis et boracis gr. 5 ..		0 11	0 8	0 6
105	1,000	Potassii chlor. et bor. et cocain. (gr. [illegible])	D.D.	2 0	1 3	0 10
87	1,000	Quininæ ammon. ♏ 30		1 10	1 1	0 9
136	1,000	Quininæ ammon. ʒj.		2 6	1 6	1 0
168	1,000	Quininæ ammon. et cinnam. ʒj. ..		2 11	1 8	1 1
102	1,000	Quininæ bisul. gr. 1		2 3	1 4	0 11
210	1,000	Quininæ bisul. gr. 2		3 8	2 1	1 3
147	500	Quininæ bisul. gr. 3		5 0	2 9	1 7
231	500	Quininæ bisul. gr. 5		7 4	4 0	2 3
300	500	Quininæ ethyl carb. gr. 5		9 6	5 3	2 10
120	1,000	Quininæ hydrobrom. gr. 1		2 6	1 6	1 0
246	1,000	Quininæ hydrobrom. gr. 2		4 3	2 4	1 5
246	1,000	Quininæ hydroch. gr. 2		4 3	2 4	1 5
174	500	Quininæ hydroch. gr. 3		5 9	3 1	1 9
278	500	Quininæ hydroch. gr. 5		8 9	4 7	2 6
264	1,000	Quininæ salicyl. gr. 2		4 7	2 6	1 6
286	500	Quininæ salicyl. gr. 5		8 2	4 3	2 6
87	1,000	Rhei (3) et sod. bic. (2)		1 11	1 2	0 9
87	1,000	Rhei (3) zingib. (½) sod. bic. (1½) ..		1 9	1 2	0 10
78	1,000	Rhei pil. co. gr. 4		1 9	1 1	0 9
57	1,000	Rhei pulv. co. gr. 5		1 6	0 11	0 7
48	1,000	Saccharini 550 gr. 0.3 (500—200—100)		3 3	1 7	1 0
270	1,000	Salicini gr. 5		4 5	2 6	1 5
123	1,000	Salol. gr. 5		2 4	1 4	0 11
84	100	Santonini gr. 1		—	—	3 6
84	100	Santonini co. B.P.C.		—	—	3 6
111	250	Santonini (½) et hyd. subchl. (½) ..		—	—	2 0
13	1,000	Soda-mint gr. 5		0 9	0 7	0 5
22	1,000	Sodii bicarbonatis gr. 5		0 9	0 7	0 6
32	1,000	Sodii citratis gr. 2		1 1	0 9	0 7
63	1,000	Sodii citratis gr. 5		1 6	1 1	0 9
108	1,000	Sodii phosph. ac. (5) hexamin. (5) ..		2 0	1 3	0 10
159	500	Sulphonal gr. 5	℞ only	5 0	2 8	1 6
51	1,000	Sulph. præcip. (5) et pot. bitart. (1) ..		1 5	1 0	0 8
69	1,000	Syr. Eastoni ♏ 30 ..	S.I. (6)	1 6	1 0	0 8
111	1,000	Syr. Eastoni ʒj. ..	S.I. (6)	2 3	1 4	0 10
162	1,000	Syr. glyceroph. co. ♏ 30	P.I. (13)	2 11	1 9	1 1
111	1,000	Syr. hypoph. co. ʒj. ..	P.I. (13)	2 3	1 4	0 11
192	1,000	Theobrom. et sod. sal. gr. 5		3 5	1 11	1 2
108	100	Theophyllin-sod. acet. gr. 4		—	8 4	4 3
111	500	"Three bromides"		2 3	1 4	0 10
143	1,000	"Three syrups" ..	P.I. (13)	2 8	1 7	1 0
309	1,000	"Three valerianates"		5 0	2 8	1 6
73	100	Trypsogen		per	doz.	1 4

Tabellæ, Hypodermic

(Tubes of ten tablets)

Cost d.	Cost per	Tabellæ, Hypodermic		Sell per	s. d.
63	doz.	Adrenalini gr. $\frac{1}{200}$	P.I. (13)	tube	0 10
99	doz.	Apomorphinæ hydrochloridi gr. $\frac{1}{10}$	S.I. (6)	tube	1 6
54	doz.	Atropinæ sulphatis gr. $\frac{1}{100}$ ..	S.I. (6)	tube	0 9
75	doz.	Caffeinæ sodio-salic. gr. ½		tube	1 0
111	doz.	Cocainæ hydrochloridi gr. ¼	D.D.	tube	1 8
150	doz.	Cocainæ hydrochloridi gr. ½	D.D.	tube	2 3
63	doz.	Diamorphinæ hydrochloridi gr. $\frac{1}{12}$ ..	D.D.	tube	1 0
69	doz.	Diamorphinæ hydrochloridi gr. ⅙ ..	D.D.	tube	1 1
57	doz.	Digitalini gr. $\frac{1}{100}$	S.I. (6)	tube	1 0
63	doz.	Hyoscinæ hydrobromidi gr. $\frac{1}{200}$	S.I. (6)	tube	1 0
75	doz.	Morphinæ sulphatis gr. ⅛	D.D.	tube	1 2
75	doz.	Morphinæ sulphatis gr. ⅙	D.D.	tube	1 2
75	doz.	Morphinæ sulphatis gr. ¼	D.D.	tube	1 2
105	doz.	Morphinæ sulphatis gr. ½	D.D.	tube	1 7
75	doz.	Morph. sulph. (⅛) et atrop. sulph. ($\frac{1}{200}$)	D.D.	tube	1 2
75	doz.	Morph. sulph. (⅙) et atrop. sulph. ($\frac{1}{180}$)	D.D.	tube	1 2
75	doz.	Morph. sulph. (¼) et atrop. sulph. ($\frac{1}{150}$)	D.D.	tube	1 2
75	doz.	Morph. sulph. (¼) et atrop. sulph. ($\frac{1}{100}$)	D.D.	tube	1 2
87	doz.	Morph. sulph. (⅓) et atrop. sulph. ($\frac{1}{120}$)	D.D.	tube	1 4
81	doz.	Morphinæ tartratis gr. ⅛	D.D.	tube	1 2
93	doz.	Morphinæ tartratis gr. ¼	D.D.	tube	1 4
57	doz.	Physostigminæ salicylatis gr. $\frac{1}{100}$	S.I. (6)	tube	0 11
75	doz.	Pilocarpinæ nitratis gr. $\frac{1}{10}$ ..	S.I. (6)	tube	1 2
81	doz.	Pilocarpinæ nitratis gr. ¼ ..	S.I. (6)	tube	1 2
81	doz.	Pilocarpinæ nitratis gr. ⅓ ..	S.I. (6)	tube	1 2
75	doz.	Quininæ hydrobrom. gr. ½		tube	1 1
57	doz.	Strophanthin $\frac{1}{100}$–$\frac{1}{500}$	S.I. (6)	tube	0 11
57	doz.	Strychninæ hydrochloridi gr. $\frac{1}{60}$	S.I. (6)	tube	0 11
57	doz.	Strychninæ hydrochloridi gr. $\frac{1}{30}$	S.I. (6)	tube	0 11
57	doz.	Strychninæ sulphatis gr. $\frac{1}{100}$ ..	S.I. (6)	tube	0 11
57	doz.	Strychninæ sulphatis gr. $\frac{1}{30}$ ..	S.I. (6)	tube	0 11

Organotherapeutic Tablets

The term gland is used as a synonym for the desiccated material, and the figures in brackets indicate the approximate equivalence of desiccated and fresh material.

Cost d.	Cost per	Organotherapeutic Tablets		Selling Price (in containers) 100 s. d.	50 s. d.	25 s. d.
168	1,000	Cerebrinin (1-7) gr. ¾		2 10	1 8	1 1
240	1,000	Corpus luteum (1-5) gr. ½		4 0	2 3	1 3
480	1,000	Corpus luteum (1-5) gr. 1		7 5	4 0	2 2
168	1,000	Didymin (1-7) gr. ¾		2 10	1 8	1 1
270	1,000	Duodenin (1-7) gr. ¾		4 5	2 5	1 4
210	1,000	Lymphatic (1-7) gr. ¾		3 6	2 0	1 1
168	1,000	Mammary (1-8) gr. ¾		2 10	1 9	1 1
228	1,000	Ovarian (1-6) gr. ½		3 9	2 0	1 2
392	1,000	Parathyroid (1-10) gr. $\frac{1}{20}$		5 10	3 2	1 9
555	1,000	Parathyroid (1-10) gr. $\frac{1}{10}$		8 9	4 7	2 5
246	1,000	Parathyroid gr. $\frac{1}{40}$, calc. lact. gr. 5 ..		4 1	2 3	1 4
444	1,000	Pituitary (whole) (1-5) gr. ½ ..	P.I.	7 0	3 8	2 0
840	1,000	Pituitary (whole) (1-5) gr. 1 ..	P.I.	12 6	6 9	3 5
690	1,000	Pituitary ant. (1-5) gr. 1 ..	P.I.	10 6	5 5	2 10
600	1,000	Pituitary post. (1-6) gr. $\frac{1}{12}$ ..	P.I.	9 3	4 10	2 6
240	1,000	Placenta (1-6) gr. 1		4 0	2 3	1 2
228	1,000	Prostate (1-6) gr. 1		3 9	2 0	1 2
240	1,000	Spleen (1-5) gr. 1		4 0	2 3	1 2
270	1,000	Suprarenal (1-5) gr. 1		4 7	2 6	1 4
261	1,000	Thymus (1-6) gr. 1		4 3	2 4	1 4
45	1,000	Thyroid gr. $\frac{1}{10}$	P.I.	1 2	0 10	0 7
45	1,000	Thyroid gr. ¼	P.I.	1 2	0 10	0 7
57	1,000	Thyroid gr. ½	P.I.	1 4	0 11	0 7
75	1,000	Thyroid gr. 1	P.I.	1 8	1 1	0 8
123	1,000	Thyroid gr. 2	P.I.	2 3	1 4	0 11
162	1,000	Thyroid gr. 3	P.I.	2 10	1 9	1 0
246	1,000	Thyroid gr. 5	P.I.	4 1	2 4	1 4

Solvellæ

Cost d.	Cost per	Solvellæ		Selling Price (in containers) 100 s. d.	50 s. d.	25 s. d.
50	1,000	Alum. et zinci sulph. aa. gr. 15 ..		3 2	1 9	1 1
180	1,000	Alum. et zinci s'carb. aa. gr. 30 ..		3 3	1 11	1 2
96	1,000	Boracis co. B.P.C.		2 0	1 3	0 10
174	1,000	Hyd. perchlor. gr. 8.75	S.I. (6)	3 3	1 11	1 2
309	1,000	Hyd. et pot. iod. gr. 8.75		5 3	2 10	1 8
108	1,000	"Mouth-wash. eff."		2 0	1 3	0 10
57	1,000	Nasal., alk. N.H.I. ..	P.II. (10)	1 6	1 1	0 9
66	1,000	Nasal., alk. co. gr. 10		1 8	1 1	0 9
99	1,000	Nasai., eucal. co. gr. 18		2 0	1 3	0 10
111	1,000	Nasal., phenol. co. gr. 15	P.II. (10)	2 3	1 4	0 11
160	1,000	Nasal-pharyng. co. N.I.F. ..	D.D.	3 0	1 9	1 1
87	1,000	Sodii chloridi gr. 60		1 10	1 2	0 10

Surgical Dressings and Appliances

Bandages

(Completely wrapped)

Cost d.	Cost per	Bandages (Completely wrapped)	Sell	s. d.
		Calico, bleached : M.O.H.		
16	doz.	2 in. × 4 yd.	each	0 3
19·5	doz.	2½ in. × 4 yd.	each	0 4
22·5	doz.	3 in. × 4 yd.	each	0 5
		Calico, unbleached : M.O.H.		
14·5	doz.	2 in. × 4 yd.	each	0 2
17·5	doz.	2½ in. × 4 yd.	each	0 3
21	doz.	3 in. × 4 yd.	each	0 4
		Crepe, cream or flesh : M.O.H.		
68	doz.	2 in.	each	0 11
86	doz.	2½ in.	each	1 1
102	doz.	3 in.	each	1 4
120	doz.	3½ in.	each	1 6
138	doz.	4 in.	each	1 9
		Domette : M.O.H.		
58	doz.	2 in. × 6 yd.	each	0 9
72	doz.	2½ in. × 6 yd.	each	0 10
84	doz.	3 in. × 6 yd.	each	1 0
		Elastic web : M.O.H.		
54	doz. yds.	2 in.	per yd.	0 9
63	doz. yds.	2½ in.	per yd.	0 10
75	doz. yds.	3 in.	per yd.	1 0
		Flannel (wool) : M.O.H.		
72	doz.	2½ in. × 4 yd.	each	0 10
132	doz.	3 in. × 6 yd.	each	1 5
		Indiarubber : M.O.H.		
204	doz.	3 ft. × 2½ in., plain	each	2 3
252	doz.	3 ft. × 2½ in., perforated	each	2 8
252	doz.	3 ft. × 3 in., plain	each	2 8
299	doz.	3 ft. × 3 in., perforated	each	3 2
264	doz.	5 ft. × 2½ in., plain	each	3 5
300	doz.	5 ft. × 2½ in., perforated	each	4 0
300	doz.	5 ft. × 3 in., plain	each	3 9
396	doz.	5 ft. × 3 in., perforated	each	4 5
396	doz.	7½ ft. × 2½ in., plain	each	4 9
432	doz.	7½ ft. × 2½ in., perforated	each	5 6
492	doz.	7½ ft. × 3 in., plain	each	6 0
576	doz.	7½ ft. × 3 in., perforated	each	6 8
		Muslin, bleached : M.O.H.		
16	doz.	2½ in. × 6 yd.	each	0 3
20	doz.	3 in. × 6 yd.	each	0 4
27	doz.	4 in. × 6 yd.	each	0 5
		Open wove, white (water dressing) : M.O.H.		
51	gross	1 in. × 3 yd.	each	0 1
84	gross	1½ in. × 4 yd.	each	0 2
108	gross	2 in. × 4 yd.	each	0 3
135	gross	2½ in. × 4 yd.	each	0 3
108	gross	3 in. × 4 yd.	each	0 3
		Open wove, white (water dressing) : M.O.H. —cont.		
312	gross	4 in. × 6 yd.	each	0 4
456	gross	6 in. × 6 yd.	each	0 6
		Plaster of Paris : M.O.H.		
105	doz.	3 in. × 4 yd.	each	1 4
128	doz.	4 in. × 4 yd.	each	1 10
		Ambulance, fast edge :		
54	doz.	2 in. × 6 yd.	each	0 8
66	doz.	2½ in. × 6 yd.	each	0 9
78	doz.	3 in. × 6 yd.	each	0 10
		Ambulance, loose edge :		
150	gross	2 in. × 6 yd.	each	0 2
188	gross	2½ in. × 6 yd.	each	0 3
224	gross	3 in. × 6 yd.	each	0 4
		Binders, twill :		
36	each	12 in. × 54 in.	each	5 3
40	each	18 in. × 54 in.	each	7 0
8	each	Suspensory, cotton, best	each	1 2
30	doz.	Triangular, plain	each	0 6

Cost d.	Cost per		Selling Price 16 oz. s. d.	4 oz. s. d.	1 oz. s. d.	1 dr. s. d.
7	lb.	Tow	1 2	—	—	—
9	lb.	Tow, carbolised	1 4	—	—	—
		First-Aid Cases (refills)				
5	doz.	Finger dressings	doz.	0 10	—	—
9	doz.	Hand dressings	doz.	1 4	—	—
13	doz.	Body dressings	doz.	2 0	—	—
7	doz.	Burn dressings, finger ..	doz.	1 2	—	—
9	doz.	Burn dressings, small ..	doz.	1 6	—	—
16	doz.	Burn dressings, large ..	doz.	2 4	—	—
10	doz.	Cotton wool (¼ oz.)	doz.	1 6	—	—
12	doz.	Cotton wool (½ oz.) ..	doz.	1 9	—	—
13	doz.	Eye pad	doz.	3 6	—	—
6.5	lb.	Cellulose wadding	per lb.	1 0	—	—
12	lb.	Cellulose tissue	per lb.	1 9	—	—
24	ea.	Elastic adhesive bandage 2½ in.	ea.	2 10	—	—
30	ea.	Elastic adhesive bandage 3 in.	ea.	3 6	—	—
22	ea.	Elastic adhesive bandage N.H.I. 2½ in.	ea.	2 6	—	—
26	ea.	Elastic adhesive bandage N.H.I. 3 in.	ea.	3 0	—	—
14	ea.	Zinc Paste bandage, 3½ in. × 6 yds.	ea.	1 9	—	—
		Emp. adhesiv., spools :				
16	doz.	½ inch × 1 yd.	ea.	0 3	—	—
90	doz.	½ inch × 5 yd.	ea.	1 2	—	—
138	doz.	½ inch × 10 yd.	ea.	1 9	—	—
24	doz.	1 inch × 1 yd.	ea.	0 4	—	—
129	doz.	1 inch × 5 yd.	ea.	1 8	—	—
228	doz.	1 inch × 10 yd.	ea.	2 10	—	—
210	doz.	2 inch × 5 yd. ..	ea.	2 8	—	—
		Cotton-wool (net weight pkts.)				
14	doz.	Medium (M.O.H.) oz. ..	—	—	0 2	—
42	doz.	Med. (M.O.H.) 4 oz. ..	—	0 7	—	—
150	doz.	Med. (M.O.H.) 16 oz. ..	1 7	—	—	—
24	doz.	Superfine, oz. cartons ..	—	—	0 3	—
66	doz.	Superfine, 4 oz. packets ..	—	0 8	—	—
240	doz.	Superfine, 16 oz.	2 9	—	—	—
21	doz.	Boric, oz.	—	—	0 3	—
70	doz.	Boric, 4 oz.	—	0 9	—	—
240	doz.	Boric, 16 oz.	2 9	—	—	—

Catheters, gum-elast. : cost 6d. each, sell **1s. 0d.** Catheters, soft rubber Jaques (to size 12) : cost 5½d. ea., sell **10d.**; over size 12, **1s. 0d.**

Gauzes (M.O.H. sealed packets	3 yd. Cost doz. d.	3 yd. Sell each s. d.	1 yd. Cost doz. d.	1 yd. Sell each s. d.	½ yd. Cost doz. d.	½ yd. Sell each s. d.
Absorbent sterilised	42	0 6	18	0 3	10	0 2
Absorbent plain	41	0 6	16	0 3	9	0 2
Boric	48	0 8	19	0 3	12	0 2
Carbolic	48	0 8	20	0 3	12	0 2
Double cyanide P.I. (9)	51	0 9	21	0 4	13	0 2
Iodoform	64	0 10	28	0 5	16	0 3
Picric	64	0 10	28	0 5	16	0 3
Salalembroth .. P.I. (9)	51	0 9	21	0 4	12	0 2
Sublimate .. P.I. (9)	51	0 9	21	0 4	12	0 2

	Size	Cost doz. d.	Sell each s. d.	Size	Cost doz. d.	Sell each s. d.
Gauze tissue, M.O.H. ..	4 oz.	54	0 9	16 oz.	183	2 0
Lint, plain, M.O.H. (sealed pkts.)	1 oz.	18	0 3	2 oz.	33	0 5
	4 oz.	62	0 9	8 oz.	120	1 5
	16 oz.	228	2 8			
Lint, Boric, M.O.H. (sealed pkts.)	1 oz.	15	0 3	2 oz.	26	0 4
	4 oz.	46	0 7	8 oz.	94	1 1
	16 oz.	174	2 0			
Ice Bags, Check circ. ..	9 in.	264	2 9			
Rubber black ..	9 in.	278	3 0			

Protectives (M.O.H.)	12in. × 12in. Cost doz. d.	12in. × 12in. Sell each s. d.	12in. × 18in Cost doz. d.	12in. × 18in Sell each s. d.	36in. × 36in. Cost doz. d.	36in. × 36in. Sell each s. d.
Gutta percha	42	0 6	—	—	252	3 0
Jaconet	36	0 6	—	—	180	3 6
Oiled silk	—	—	70	1 6	396	5 6
Oiled cambric	39	0 6	—	—	288	3 6

Serological Products—
Abridged List

	Selling Price A. & H. s. d.	B. W. s. d.	P. D. s. d.	Evans s. d.
acillus coli .. .. 10 c.c.	—	3 6	—	—
ick Test Products test and control 1 c.c.	—	1 6	—	1 6
iphtheria (conc.) .. .. 500 units	1 6	1 6	1 3	1 3
iphtheria conc. .. .. 1,000 units	2 0	2 0	—	1 9
iphtheria conc. .. .. 2,000 units	3 3	3 3	3 6	3 3
iphtheria conc. .. .. 3,000 units	—	4 9	5 0	5 0
iphtheria, conc. .. .. 4,000 units	6 0	6 0	6 0	6 0
iphtheria, conc. .. .. 6,000 units	8 9	8 9	8 9	8 9
iphtheria, conc. .. .. 8,000 units	9 6	9 6	9 6	9 6
iphtheria, prophyl. A.P.T. .. 0·5 c.c.	—	2 6	—	—
iphtheria, prophyl. A.P.T. .. .. 1 c.c.	—	4 0	—	3 6
iphtheria, prophyl. A.P.T. .. .. 5 c.c.	—	16 0	—	—
iphtheria, prophyl. A.P.T. .. .. 10 c.c.	—	—	—	21 0
iphtheria, prophyl. F.T. .. .. 1 c.c.	—	2 6	—	2 0
iphtheria, prophyl. T.A.F. .. .. 1 c.c.	—	3 0	—	3 0
iphtheria, prophyl. T.A.M. .. .. 1 c.c.	—	2 6	—	2 6
ysentery .. .. 20 or 25 c.c.	—	8 6	8 6	—
ysentery conc. .. .. 10,000 units	8 6	—	—	—
rysipelas streptococcus ant. .. 10 c.c.	—	—	—	15 0
as gangrene (perfringens) .. 4,000 units	6 6	6 6	6 6	—
as gangrene (perfringens) .. 10,000 units	15 0	15 0	15 0	—
æmostatic .. .. 2 c.c.	—	—	—	5 0
emoplastin .. .. 2 c.c.	—	—	6 0	—
emoplastin, oral .. .. .. 5 c.c.	—	—	9 6	—
mmunogens, various .. .. .. 10 c.c.	—	—	12 6	—
fluenza (equine) .. .. .. 30 c.c.	—	—	8 0	—
eningococcus antitox. 10,000 units 30 c.c.	—	—	30 0	—
eningococcus .. 3 c.c. conc. = 10 c.c.	3 6	3 6	—	—

Serological Products—
Abridged List—*cont.*

	Selling Price A. & H. s. d.	B. W. s. d.	P. D. s. d.	Evans s. d.
Meningococcus .. 5 c.c. conc. = 15 c.c.	5 0	—	—	—
Meningococcus .. .. .. 20 c.c.	—	—	—	—
Meningococcus .. .. .. 25 c.c.	—	8 6	—	—
Meningococcus 10 c.c. conc. = 30 c.c.	10 0	—	—	—
Normal (horse) .. .. .. 10 c.c.	1 6	1 6	—	1 6
Normal (horse) .. .. .. 25 c.c.	3 0	3 0	—	3 0
Phylacogens (boxes of 5) .. .. 1 c.c.	—	—	9 0	—
Phylacogens .. .. 10 c.c.	—	—	11 8	—
Pneumococcus conc. Type 1 .. 4,000 units	4 0	—	—	—
Pneumococcus Type 1 .. 20,000 units	—	30 0	—	—
Pneumococcus Type 1 high potency (unconc.) 25,000 units	—	20 0	—	—
Pneumococcus anti (Felton) Types 1 & 2 10,000 units	—	30 0	33 9	—
Pneumococcus anti (Felton) Types 1 & 2 20,000 units	—	—	65 0	—
Pneumococcus Type 2 .. 25,000 units	—	20 0	—	—
Pneumococcus Type 2 conc. .. 20,000 units	—	30 0	—	—
Poliomyelitis serum, anti .. .. 5 c.c.	7 6	—	—	—
Puerperal streptococcus, ant. conc. 10 c.c.	—	—	20 0	15 0
Scarlet fev. strept. ant. .. .. 10 c.c.	—	—	12 6	12 6
Scarlet fev. strept. ant. .. .. 30 c.c.	—	—	32 0	32 0
Schick Test Products .. .. 1 c.c. per set	—	2 6	—	2 6
Schick Test Products .. .. 5 c.c. per set	—	8 6	18 0	8 6
Staphylococcus, antitoxin conc. 2,000 units	10 6	—	—	—
Staphylococcus conc .. .. .. 10 c.c.	—	10 6	—	—
Streptococcus, erysipelas .. .. 25 c.c.	—	8 6	—	—
Streptococcus, erysipelas ant. .. 10 c.c.	—	—	—	15 0
Streptococcus, polyval. (3 c.c. conc. = 10 ord.) .. 10 c.c.	3 6	3 6	4 7	3 6
Streptococcus, polyval. conc. (10 c.c. conc. = 30 ord.) .. 10 c.c.	10 6	—	20 0	—
Streptococcus, polyval. conc. .. 20 c.c.	—	—	—	6 6
Streptococcus, polyval. (8 c.c. conc. = 25 ord.) .. 25 c.c.	8 6	8 6	8 6	—
Streptococcus, puerp. fever (conc. P.D.) 10 c.c.	3 6	3 6	20 0	—
Streptococcus, puerp. fever .. .. 25 c.c.	8 6	8 6	—	—
Streptococcus, puerperal ant. .. 10 c.c.	—	—	—	15 0
Streptococcus (scarlatina) 10 c.c. 3,000 U.S.A. units	—	12 6	—	—
Tetanus :—				
1,000 international units	1 6	1 9	2 0	1 9
3,000 international units	4 0	4 0	4 7	4 0
10,000 international units	12 0	—	—	12 0
16,000 international units	17 6	—	—	—
20,000 units	20 0	—	25 0	—
Thromboplastin .. .. .. 20 c.c.	—	—	5 3	—
Typhoid conc. .. .. 10 c.c.	10 0	—	—	—
Typhoid ,, ... 25 c.c.	21 0	—	—	—

Veterinary Sera

	Selling Price A. & H. s. d.	B. W. s. d.	P. D. s. d.	Evans s. d.
Anti-leptospira (canine) .. .. 10 c.c.	—	3 6	—	—
Lamb dysentery .. .. 100 c.c.	—	18 0	—	18 0
Streptococcus (equine) .. .. 30 c.c.	—	—	8 0	—
Swine erysipelas .. .. .. 10 c.c.	—	1 0	—	1 0
Swine erysipelas .. .. 100 c.c.	—	6 0	—	6 0
Tetanus .. .. .. 1,000 units	—	—	—	1 6
Tetanus .. .. .. 2,000 units	—	2 6	—	—
Tetanus .. .. .. 3,000 units	—	—	—	3 3
Tetanus .. .. .. 6,000 units	—	5 0	—	5 0
Tetanus (vet.) American .. 3,000 units	—	5 0	6 0	—
Tetanus (vet.) ,, .. 5,000 units	—	—	9 6	8 0
Tetanus (vet.) ,, .. 10,000 units	—	—	—	15 0
White scour (bovine) .. .. 10 c.c.	—	—	4 0	—
White scour (bovine) .. .. 30 c.c.	—	—	8 0	—

Printed in the USA
CPSIA information can be obtained
at www.ICGtesting.com
LVHW051534110923
757835LV00003B/101